Bacteria for Breakfast
Probiotics for Good Health

Kelly Dowhower Karpa, PhD, RPh

Trafford Publishing
Victoria, BC, Canada

Note for Librarians: a cataloguing record for this book that includes Dewey Classification and US Library of Congress numbers is available from the National Library of Canada. The complete cataloguing record can be obtained from the National Library's online database at:
www.nlc-bnc.ca/amicus/index-e.html
ISBN 1-4120-0925-0

Information in this book is based upon experience and research conducted by the author. Every effort has been made to ensure that the information contained in this book is accurate and complete. However, neither the publisher nor the author is engaged in rendering professional services to the individual reader. This book is intended for informational purposes and is not meant to diagnose, prescribe, or substitute for appropriate medical care. You must seek advice of a health care professional before using any product or procedure described in this book. The ideas, procedures, and recommendations contained in this book are not intended to substitute for a consultation with your physician. All matters regarding your health require medical supervision.

Neither the author nor publisher shall be liable or responsible for any loss, injury, or damage allegedly arising from any information contained in this book. Mention of any product, company, physician, scientist, or research organization should in no way be misconstrued as endorsement of a particular product or technique, nor should it be misinterpreted as an endorsement of these individuals or organizations for this book.

Neither the author nor publisher condones or condemns any health treatment described in this book, but believes the information presented herewithin should be available to the public for educational purposes. Opinions expressed in this book represent the personal views of the author and not the publisher.

Cover Photography: Barry Dowhower
Editorial Assistants: Linda Lee Karpa, Patricia Dowhower, Lisa Bonfanti
Artwork: Karl Karpa
Publication Design: Ann Messner, Messner Publications, Inc.

TRAFFORD

This book was published *on-demand* in cooperation with Trafford Publishing.
On-demand publishing is a unique process and service of making a book available for retail sale to the public taking advantage of on-demand manufacturing and Internet marketing.
On-demand publishing includes promotions, retail sales, manufacturing, order fulfilment, accounting and collecting royalties on behalf of the author.

Suite 6E, 2333 Government St., Victoria, B.C. V8T 4P4, CANADA
Phone 250-383-6864 Toll-free 1-888-232-4444 (Canada & US)
Fax 250-383-6804 E-mail sales@trafford.com
Web site www.trafford.com TRAFFORD PUBLISHING IS A DIVISION OF TRAFFORD HOLDINGS LTD.
Trafford Catalogue #03-1294 www.trafford.com/robots/03-1294.html

10 9 8 7 6 5 4 3 2

Dedication

This book is dedicated to all those who have experienced chronic, persistent *Clostridium difficile* diarrhea or watched a loved one suffer from it. May this book help you find a cure.

Acknowledgements

I would like to acknowledge first and foremost my husband and children, whose love and patience have made this book possible. I would be remiss if I didn't also acknowledge my father, Barry Dowhower, and Dr. Mike McCann. Both of these men encouraged me to sit down and put the knowledge I gained from countless hours of literature searches on paper for the benefit of others. A special thanks to all who have shared their time, talents, and stories to help this book become a reality.

Contents

Introduction

Kix®, Cheerios®, or bacteria? These breakfast selections are a standard joke around our house ever since my son became seriously ill. Every morning before we eat our Wheaties®, we begin the day with a healthy dose of bacteria.

If you are reading this book, it is probably because you or a loved one has also been diagnosed with a medical condition. The ailment may be a problem within the gastrointestinal tract, perhaps recurrent urogenital infections, or maybe an allergic condition. For many reading this book, it is likely that traditional therapies have failed. Alternatively, perhaps you are hoping to try a more "natural" approach in place of conventional medicines.

Regardless of why you have picked up this book, it is important for you to understand that this book is not intended to substitute for appropriate medical intervention. Please don't use information in this book for self-diagnosis or self-medication. Instead, please take any knowledge you gain from reading this book to your physician so that together you can make an informed decision about the best way to approach your care.

As a health care professional, I did not fully appreciate the merits of probiotics until I was faced with a life threatening illness in my two-year old son. Medical training teaches health care professionals to prescribe and dispense only pharmaceuticals that have been extensively studied and reviewed by the FDA. Getting over the idea that probiotics are not "FDA-approved medications" is often the first hurdle that physicians and patients must overcome.

So what are probiotics? Probiotics are live microorganisms that have potential to benefit the host. The word probiotic literally means "for life." Think about that for a minute..."for life". Now contrast "probiotic" with "antibiotic". We all know what antibiotics do — they kill bacteria. Probiotics, then, are the opposite of antibiotics. In other words, this book describes the merits of using bacteria and other microorganisms to treat illnesses. Of course, this notion runs counter-intuitive to what we have been taught for nearly a century. Ever since the advent of antibiotics like penicillins and sulfas, we have relied, perhaps, too much, on antibiotics. Now, I'm about to describe for you why we need bacteria in our bodies. It is often difficult to overcome this mental hurdle.

When you consider that probiotics have been used successfully for thousands of years, the idea of using them becomes less daunting. Fermented milk products, which contain probiotics, have been used for centuries. According to Persian tradition, Abraham of the Old Testament owed his longevity to ingestion of fermented milk. King Francis I of France was reportedly cured of an illness after eating yogurt in the early 1500s. More recently, in the early 1900s, Metchnikoff, a Russian Nobel laureate, believed high numbers of lactobacilli in the gastrointestinal tract held the keys to a long and healthy life. To prove this, he reportedly experimented on himself. Metchnikoff experienced improved health and well-being with regular ingestion of sour milk. He supposedly said,

"When people have learnt how to cultivate a suitable flora in the intestines of children as soon as they are weaned from the breast, the normal life may extend to twice my 70 years" (Van de Water et al., 1999). From his experience, Metchnikoff believed lactic acid-producing bacteria were antagonistic to disease-causing microorganisms and would prevent illness and disease. So you see, this "probiotic stuff" isn't new. Probiotics have been around for more than 5000 years.

Where do we find probiotics? The most common place to find probiotics is yogurt. In fact, you may have eaten some already today. Remember the statement found on the carton of yogurt that you ate for lunch (or sent to school in your children's lunches), "This product contains live and active cultures." Have you ever thought about what that means? It means you are ingesting bacteria, live microscopic organisms, with each delicious spoonful. Yogurt is not a probiotic per se. However, when yogurt contains microorganisms that bring about health benefits, it then becomes a probiotic-containing food. The notion that yogurt is a health food has been established for centuries. In fact, some of you may have already used yogurt in the past to treat diarrhea, prevent urinary tract infections, or treat recurrent yeast infections. Although yogurt contains probiotics, it probably doesn't contain enough microorganisms to bring about major changes in our digestive systems. That's why probiotic supplements (capsules and powders) are necessary.

When traditional medicine failed to eradicate my son's illness, we were left with little in the way of alternatives. As a result, I began reading the medical literature and was astounded at the huge body of knowledge supporting the use of probiotics for treating a variety of different diseases — ranging from food allergies to eczema; from Crohn's disease to antibiotic-associated diarrhea. Interestingly, as I continued reading and learning more about probiotics, I saw how not only the current life-threatening gastrointestinal infection that my son was battling, but also other common medical conditions that my son had been previously diagnosed with, all pointed unanimously to a single underlying problem — that of an imbalance in gut bacteria, probably dating back to his birth.

It was then, that I began to see the need to have all the data on probiotics compiled into one neat handbook or guide that could be read by both the lay public and practitioners, alike. Some physicians claim that there isn't enough data showing the benefits of probiotics. Clearly, they have never looked. If all of the data was compiled and put it together in one easy-to-read format, physicians would come to realize the merits of probiotics, and patients would be better off because of it. So that is exactly what I have set out to do. I have compiled the data on probiotics, and have written this book using language that even the medical novice can understand.

Frankly, I have written this book in hopes of reaching out to two entirely different audiences. First, I want to introduce probiotics and their uses to the general public. Second, at the same time, I want to provide physicians with clinical documentation on the uses of probiotics. I want physicians to see that probiotics aren't "voodoo medicine". Quite the contrary, we already know and understand many of the immunologic reasons why probiotics are effective. Because of the dual audience that I am trying to reach, lay readers may find parts of the text too detailed or complicated for their needs. However, let me encourage you, don't simply stop reading! Keep going! Skim over parts that aren't of interest to you. You will find that if you keep going, you will understand the "bottom line", through "down-to-earth" explanations. In this book you will read about medical procedures that you've never even heard of and will meet fascinating people, who were formerly ill —even close to death — as I relay their true-to-life experiences and tell you how probiotics made them well and gave them their lives back again. Additionally, for the medical novice, there is a glossary in the back of the book that defines terms that are unclear.

It is also important for me to let you know that, unlike some other authors who have written books touting the merits of probiotics, I am not promoting any product or any brand of probiotics in particular. At times, I may share with you, based upon my experience, the name of a specific product that worked/failed to work for my family, but please understand I don't have a hidden agenda. I stand to gain nothing financially from any particular probiotic that is sold. It doesn't matter to me which specific product you use to improve your health, as long as you find one that works. In this book, I don't spend a great deal of time discussing specific probiotic manufacturers, specific products by trade name, or individual dosages. So please, don't interpret this book as promoting any particular product. My job, as I see it, is to simply compile the data for you and relay the facts in a relatively easy to understand format. It is up to you and your physician to decide what to do with the information from there.

A mentor once told me, "A single study in the medical/scientific literature should never be accepted as fact. Rather, a study should be repeated a minimum of three times by independent investigators (researchers who don't stand to profit in any way from the outcome) before it is accepted." This is why, as you will see, I have included numerous references at the end of each chapter for clinicians who wish to look up the details about various studies. The data supporting use of probiotics for health benefits is enormous; with all of this knowledge, the merits of probiotics can finally be accepted as fact, rather than just hearsay.

My goal in writing this book is to arm you with more knowledge than I had when I was faced with a situation similar to the one you find yourself in right now. This book is not intended to diagnose or treat any disease nor is it intended to substitute for medical advice given by your physician. Instead, this book is designed purely for educational purposes. I want to educate you, so you and your physician can decide, together, if probiotics may be right for you. I hope you will sit back and learn some information that will be useful to you, your loved ones, or your patients, as you continue your quest for good health.

Reference

Van de Water J, Keen CL, and Gershwin ME. The influence of chronic yogurt consumption on immunity. J Nutr. 1999;129:S1492-S1495.

Chapter 1

Bacteria 101: Bacteria Within

Most folks know that there are "bad" bacteria — bacteria that cause disease. But did you know that there are also "good" bacteria — bacteria that actually prevent disease? That's right. Some bacteria prevent disease. It surprises some people when they learn that both good and bad bacteria co-exist within our bodies. The good bacteria play a part in keeping us healthy. The bad bacteria, if not kept in check, can make us ill. But, how many bacteria are there? What are they called? Where do they come from? What is their effect on our bodies? In the first chapter of this book, we will explore the answers to these questions and more.

Normal Flora

It is estimated that the human body is comprised of 100 trillion cells. But guess what? At least 90% of these cells are **not** of human origin. Instead, the vast majority of the cells are bacteria! (Dai and Walker, 1999; Savage, 1977). The bacteria that reside inside or on the human body are known collectively as "**normal flora**". Various "normal" bacterial species are found on the skin, in the lungs, and within the urogenital tract, but the vast majority of normal flora live inside the gastrointestinal tract. The gastrointestinal tract, with a surface area of 300-400 m^2 — the approximate size of one or two tennis courts — is the largest body surface that connects the inside of the body with the outside world. As a result of such a large surface area, quite a lot of bacteria can potentially reside here (See figure 1-1).

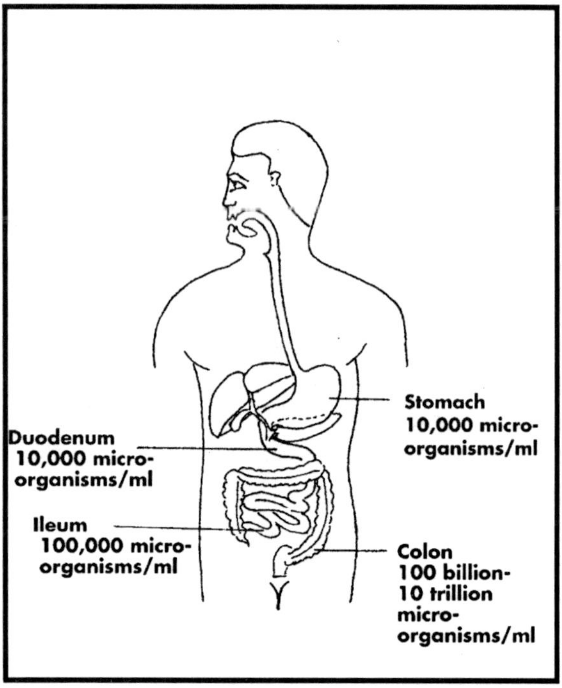

Figure 1-1. Number of bacteria found in various segments of the digestive tract. Modified from Human Physiology and Mechanisms of Disease, 4th edition, Guyton AC., Movement of Food through the Alimentary Tract, page 487, 1992, with permission from Elsevier.

It is the large intestines that are home to the majority of bacteria that live in our gastrointestinal tracts. In fact, estimates suggest that there are 1 trillion bacterial microorganisms in every gram of fecal matter or, another way to look at it, bacteria account for approximately 30% of the entire weight of dry fecal matter.

Although the medical community refers to the bacteria that live in the gut as "normal," these microorganisms are essentially a collection of parasites that have become well adapted to living inside the intestinal tract. Normal flora is found inside everyone, especially healthy humans. At the present time, science and medicine are only just beginning to define the roles of normal gut flora, but our current understanding suggests that there is a **symbiotic** relationship between humans and the bacteria living in our intestines. Bacteria benefit from this relationship because they obtain nutrients from us — through undigested dietary components and intestinal secretions. Likewise, we receive numerous benefits from the bacteria, too. We now know that gut bacteria are involved with: producing essential vitamins for us, providing us with energy in the form of short chain fatty acids, stimulating our immune systems, and protecting us from disease. Yes, contrary to what is commonly believed about bacteria, the microorganisms residing in our guts do not cause disease under normal circumstances. Instead, we now understand that normal flora actually protects us from disease. Interestingly, just like fingerprints, the normal flora carried by each individual is unique. As a result, we are either uniquely protected from certain health ailments or at risk for disease — based upon the types of "normal" bacteria that we accumulate in our guts.

Where Does Normal Flora Come From?

Role of environment

Prior to birth, as you can imagine, the womb — or the environment in which babies grow — is remarkably sterile. In fact, it has to be that way. In rare instances when the uterus is colonized by bacteria or viruses, these disease-causing invaders are responsible for extensive damage to the developing child — triggering premature labor, causing birth defects, and even leading to fetal death.

At birth, infants leave the sterile environment of the womb and quickly become colonized by bacteria. Bacteria that are established first in the gastrointestinal tracts of infants originate from the mother's birth canal, for babies born vaginally. Infants are exposed to these bacteria for the first time during the birthing process. It makes sense, then, that the normal gut flora of vaginally-delivered infants closely resembles the gut flora of their mothers. But other external environments, such as hospital personnel or neonatal incubators, can also supply microbes that colonize an infant's digestive tract early in life. Of course, babies delivered by cesarean section also acquire normal flora, but there are differences both in (a) how rapidly bacterial colonization occurs and (b) the type of bacteria that take up residence in these infants — when compared to vaginally-delivered infants.

Numerous studies have followed the patterns by which gut flora are acquired in infants early in life when exposed to various environments. It is clear that the method of delivery — vaginal or cesarean section — plays an important role in determining which microbes colonize the gut after birth. Consider the following examples:

> Fecal flora from 34 vaginally-delivered infants was compared to flora of 30 infants born by a cesarean delivery. Stool samples were collected and analyzed periodically during the first 6 months of life. It was determined that normal fecal colonization was delayed in infants born by cesarean delivery (Gronlund et al., 1999). These infants had fewer lactobacilli in their guts until 10 days of age, less bifidobacteria until 30 days of age, and these infants were still less likely to be colonized by *Bacteroides fragilis* even at six months of age. These results are in agreement with reports by others that found decreases in bifidobacteria and bacteroides counts in infants delivered by cesarean section. (Long and Swenson, 1977; Bennet and Nord,1987; Neut et al., 1987). Furthermore, the number of a potentially harmful bacteria, *Clostridium perfringes,* was elevated in infants born via cesarean delivery. This bacterial species has been associated with gastrointestinal discomfort, diarrhea, and bloody stools (Gronlund et al.,1999).

Taken all together, these studies clearly indicate that the immediate environmental conditions imposed by the method of delivery during the birthing process can have a profound impact upon the species of bacteria in the gastrointestinal tract of newborns. Furthermore, these differences persist for more than 6 months. The different normal bacterial colonization patterns in infants delivered by cesarean section versus those delivered vaginally are probably related to two factors: (a) lack of contact with flora inside the birth canal and (b) maternal administration of **antibiotics** prior to cesarean surgery.

Yes, that's right, I said antibiotics. But, aren't antibiotics good things? Where would we be without penicillin and the rest of them? This is a good time to introduce a key concept — a point that will be revisited many times throughout this book. Antibiotics kill normal flora. Antibiotics do not discriminate between "good" bacteria and "bad" bacteria. Any time antibiotics are used, the drugs kill not only bacteria causing an infection, they also kill "healthy" bacteria. It is especially of concern when antibiotics kill bacteria that are part of the normal gastrointestinal flora. Altered gut normal flora is the reason diarrhea occurs as a side effect in at least 25% of people taking antibiotic drugs. As we will see in subsequent chapters, alterations in gut normal flora not only cause diarrhea, but also contribute to allergies and other medical ailments.

In addition to the *method of delivery during the birthing process,* other environmental factors play a significant role in the establishment of intestinal flora. While healthy, full-term breast-fed infants acquire a complex bacterial normal flora within days of birth, infants requiring intensive care tend to be colonized much more slowly than healthy babies. Furthermore, infants in intensive care units (ICU) tend to acquire atypical or abnormal organisms as part of their "normal flora". This is unfortunate, but it is easily understood. In an intensive care environment, organisms are easily spread from person to person, so it is not surprising that atypical organisms spread easily from infant to infant and overtly cause disease (Bennet et al., 1986; Bell et al., 1984) or create subtle imbalances that aren't detected until much later. Additionally, antibiotics contribute to the establishment of atypical microorganisms in infants who receive intensive care. In neonatal intensive care units, antibiotics are widely used. It is well known that antibiotics like ampicillin, cefuroxime, and cloxacillin contribute to colonization of potentially harmful bacteria like *Clostridium* and *Klebsiella* species. Overgrowth of some of these harmful microorganisms can lead to potentially fatal diarrhea if not dealt with immediately.

Role of diet

"We are what we eat" applies to infants, too. We now understand that the process of acquiring normal gut flora also depends heavily upon dietary intake. Great differences exist in the bowel flora of infants depending upon whether they are breast-fed or formula-fed.

> Although the earliest bacteria to colonize the gut in infants are enterobacteria, at six days of age, bifidobacteria outnumber enterobacteria by 1000 to 1 in breast-fed infants. In contrast, at this same time point enterobacteria exceed bifidobacteria by a rate of 10 to 1 in formula-fed babies (Yoshioka H et al., 1983).
>
> It is clear that breast feeding encourages the growth of bifidobacteria. In fact, human breast milk is said to contain a "Bifidus factor", a substance not found in any other milk that specifically promotes the growth of bifidobacteria (Levy, 1998).

It is well established that at one month of age, bifidobacteria are the predominant bacterial species in both breast-fed and formula-fed babies. However, the number of these "healthy bacteria" in formula-fed infants' stools is only a fraction — a mere 10% — of that found in stools of breast-fed babies. Furthermore, formula-fed babies have a more complex variety of microorganisms in their bowels including enterococci, coliforms, and clostridial species.

Bifidobacteria continue to be the dominant bacterial species in infants until solid foods are introduced. As solids are added to their diets, the normal gut flora of breast-fed infants undergoes dramatic changes, as bacteroides, clostridia, and streptococci numbers increase sharply. The changes in formula-fed infants are more moderate since they are likely to have been colonized by these types of bacteria already. By one year of age, the bacterial populations in both breast-fed and formula-fed infants begin to resemble that of adults — both in numbers and composition (Stark and Lee, 1982).

The reasons for early differences in gut flora between breast-fed infants and formula-fed babies are not entirely clear; however, some theories have been suggested. For example, the type of proteins that are passed to infants via breast milk differs in composition from that found in infant formulas. In breast milk, whey is the most common protein found. In contrast, casein is typically the predominant protein in formula. (Balmer SE et al., 1989c; Balmer et al., 1989a). It appears that whey-based formulas stimulate growth of flora that more closely resembles the flora found in breast-fed infants (Balmer et al., 1989a).

Another factor that may play a role in the different flora between formula-fed and breast-fed babies involves the availability of iron. Obviously, the amount of iron that reaches the gut of formula-fed infants is dictated by the amount of iron present in the formula. In contrast, for breast-fed infants, the amount of iron received is determined by the presence of lactoferrin in breast milk. Lactoferrin is a protein that binds very tightly to iron and is thought to aid in iron delivery. Lactoferrin also stimulates growth of some "good" bacterial species.

> Several studies have investigated the role of lactoferrin in altering gut flora. In laboratory experiments, lactoferrin is a potent stimulator of gut bacteria like *Bifidobacteria infantis* and *Bifidobacteria breve* (Petschow et al., 1991).
>
> Iron is a necessary component for some harmful bacterial species to grow. If lactoferrin binds all available iron, the harmful bacteria are essentially iron-depleted and cannot overgrow (Levy, 1998).

Lactoferrin is not added to infant formulas. Thus, either the very presence of lactoferrin or the enhanced iron delivery by lactoferrin, alters the viability of specific bacterial species in the gut and may account for some differences in gut flora between breast-fed and formula-fed infants (Balmer et al., 1989b; Roberts et al., 1992).

There are also other components of breast milk that account for different bowel microorganisms in breast-fed infants. For example, breast milk contains complex sugars such as N-acetylglucosamine.

> Certain complex sugars are believed to act as "growth factors" for some bifidobacterial species including *Bifidobacterium bifidum* (Petshow, 1991; Gyorgy et al., 1974).

Additionally, human breast milk does not neutralize the acidic environment of the stomach the way that cow's milk-based formulas do. Stomach acids inhibit growth of many species of bacteria, but cow's milk tends to neutralize the acidic environment of the stomach. As a result, breast-fed infants pass more acidic feces than formula-fed infants, and the acids suppress growth of harmful bacteria.

> It is not entirely clear why breast milk does not neutralize acids like cow's milk does, but there are several theories. Some of those theories involve specific components of breast milk, like high levels of lactose and low concentrations of protein and phosphate. (Bullen and Tearle, 1976).

Breast feeding is clearly nature's way of promoting healthy gut flora in infants, ensuring colonization by "healthy" bifidobacteria and maintaining an acidic environment to suppress the growth of harmful bacterial invaders. For some women, however, breast feeding is just not an option. Yet, as we are finding out, it may still be possible for formula-fed infants to obtain a healthy repertoire of gut flora. Experiments are showing us that adding probiotics to infant formulas may make up for the factors found in breast milk that are missing in formula.

> Supplementing infant formulas with the "good bacteria," *Bifidobacterium bifidum*, results in a gut flora that more closely resembles that of breast-fed infants rather than that of formula-fed infants in terms of the number of bifidobacteria present in feces and the acid content of stools (Pahwa and Mathur, 1987).

In fact, it has become commonplace in some European countries to manufacture infant formulas that contain probiotics. In this way, food manufacturers and health care industries have united to promote good intestinal health, beginning at an early age.

Once initially colonized by bacteria in infancy, an individual's gut flora remains remarkably constant throughout the rest of life. This is because the gut's immune system quickly learns to recognize and tolerate the bacteria acquired during infancy. As such, you can imagine that it is extremely important to acquire a *healthy* repertoire of bacteria early in life. With aging, it becomes increasingly difficult to permanently alter the composition of one's gastrointestinal tract normal flora; it is hard to "reprogram" the body to recognize and tolerate healthy bacteria, once it has become home to unhealthy ones. However, there are probiotic supplements available to help compensate when the flora isn't quite as "normal" as we'd like. We will learn more about these in subsequent chapters.

Additionally, it is interesting to note that numerous studies have now discovered that "normal" intestinal flora varies with geographical location. For example, in western Europe — in industrialized countries with a market economy — the intestinal flora of adults contains different strains of bacteria and yeasts than the flora found in Uganda, Japan, and southern India. Perhaps dietary differences like the high consumption of meat and fats in Europe as opposed to the more vegetarian diets eaten in many other parts of the world account for these discrepancies (Sepp et al., 1997). Indeed, studies have shown major dietary changes — like eating an uncooked vegetarian diet only and then converting to a conventional Western diet — can cause major changes in fecal flora (Sepp et al., 1997).

Likewise, there are distinct differences in fecal normal bacterial flora in infants depending upon their location. Different species of bacteria are found in the intestines of Pakistani infants than are present in Swedish babies' intestines. Similarly, there are differences between Estonian and Finnish infants' fecal flora, as well as distinct changes when comparing fecal flora of one year olds residing in Estonia versus Switzerland (Sepp et al., 1997). Certainly, there have been major improvements in general standards of living in western societies during the past few decades (Sepp et al., 1997). And for the most part, these changes have been good. But as we will see in subsequent chapters, it appears that highly effective sterilization techniques and cleansing procedures, as well as increased use of antibiotics, in industrialized countries, has altered normal flora towards an "unhealthy" type of "normal".

Normal Flora: What Keeps it "Normal"?

Throughout life, the digestive tract is exposed to numerous microorganisms. Most of these microbes have only a brief existence in our bodies — they just pass right through the gastrointestinal system. However, others take up a more permanent residence. What keeps gut bacterial growth in check? Why don't they multiply out-of-control and cause widespread infection? What permits some bacteria to grow and proliferate, while other bacterial species are rapidly eliminated and destroyed? Various control mechanisms exist throughout the entire length of the digestive tract. Some of the players involved in this regulation include (a) the structure and functions of the gastrointestinal tract, (b) the actions of the immune system, and (c) the metabolic activities of bacteria. All of these components function together to prevent bacterial overgrowth within the digestive system, to keep the system running smoothly. Under ideal conditions, these controls serve as a system of "checks and balances" to regulate the numbers and types of bacteria that survive in the gut. To fully comprehend what can go wrong within the gastrointestinal tract that leads to an imbalance in gut flora and causes illness or disease, it is first necessary to understand how the digestive tract is supposed to work. So let's take a moment to consider the anatomy and physiology of the gastrointestinal system (See figure 1-2).

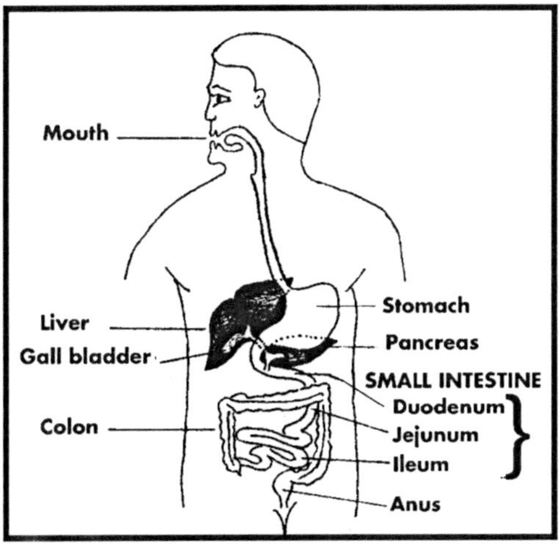

Figure 1-2. Components of the human digestive tract.
Modified from Human Physiology and Mechanisms of Disease, 4th edition, Guyton AC., Movement of Food through the Alimentary Tract, page 487, 1992, with permission from Elsevier.

The gastrointestinal tract can be thought of as a long tube that begins with the mouth and ends with the anus. Of course, there are some other important organs lying in between — such as the stomach, as well as the small intestines and the large intestines. Additionally, the liver, pancreas, and gall bladder — while located outside the "tube" — each contribute to normal digestive tract function and regulation of bacterial activities in their own special ways.

Mouth and throat

Let's begin our journey through the gastrointestinal tract by starting in the mouth. The first line of defense for eliminating bacteria that threaten to invade the gastrointestinal tract is the saliva. Saliva is secreted by salivary glands in the oral cavity. Although we rarely think about it, saliva is secreted almost constantly, even when food is not present.

There are several different ways saliva suppresses bacterial overgrowth. First, the constant flow of saliva and the very action of swallowing helps remove bacteria from the mouth, sending them into the acidic environment of the stomach. Saliva also tends to wash food particles away from the teeth and gums — preventing nutrition for bacterial growth in the mouth. Additionally, saliva contains several components — **enzymes** and **antibodies** — that directly destroy bacteria. Thus, the properties of saliva eliminate many bacterial species before they have the opportunity to establish a permanent residence and cause disease.

Stomach

Moving down the digestive tract we come to the stomach. What effect does its environment have on the bacteria that pass into it? Early studies suggested that the stomach was sterile due to its highly acidic environment. However, more recent studies indicate that streptococci, staphylococci, lactobacilli and fungi — up to 10,000 microorganisms per milliliter — live in the stomach. Not surprisingly, immediately after eating, this number of organisms increases. Estimates suggest that approximately 100,000 microbes are found within each milliliter of gastric juices in the stomach immediately following each meal. These organisms originate from bacteria that reside in the mouth, as well as from microorganisms found in many types of foods.

> Examples of individual species found in the stomach just after eating include streptococci, prevotella, lactobacilli, bifidobacteria, and enterobacteriaceae.

Soon after eating, however, the stomach environment becomes very acidic due to the production of hydrochloric acid. As a result of increased acidity, bacterial counts fall to almost undetectable levels in the stomach after each meal. Interestingly, in the first week of life, babies' stomachs do not produce much stomach acid. This probably assists their gastrointestinal tracts in the initial acquisition of normal flora. At the opposite end of the aging spectrum, elderly folks also tend to produce low levels of stomach acid; this may put those over the age of 60 years at an increased risk of gastrointestinal infections caused by *Salmonella* (Sarker and Gyr, 1992) and other harmful species. In addition to protecting against invading microorganisms, hydrochloric acid has another function. It aids in digestion, by breaking down complex sugars and indirectly contributes to protein degradation.

Ultimately, the stomach is a hostile environment for bacteria because the acidity of the stomach protects against most invading microorganisms. However, because food (1) enters as a **bolus** (mass), (2) is mixed with saliva which buffers the acids somewhat, and (3) is subjected to rapid emptying into the intestines, some disease-causing microorganisms survive and can potentially disrupt **homeostasis** in lower portions of the digestive tract. Additionally, some individuals have risk factors that make them susceptible to colonization by potentially harmful bacteria. For example, some diseases or medications decrease the stomach's capability to manufacture sufficient quantities of stomach acids. Over long periods of time, these circumstances increase the likelihood of becoming colonized by disease-causing bacteria.

Glands that secrete mucus also help to keep things "normal" in the stomach. Mucus forms a thin gel layer of lubrication inside the stomach — as well as the rest of the gastrointestinal tract — to protect against harsh gastric acids and digestive enzymes. Additionally, mucus protects the gastrointestinal tract from abrasion as food passes through. Mucus also acts as a barrier, preventing harmful bacteria from attaching to the intestinal wall. Differences in mucus composition — healthy mucus versus mucus found in inflammatory bowel disease or colon cancer — have been noted (Quigley and Kelly, 1995).

Understandably, there is a delicate balance between **synthesis**, **secretion**, and **erosion** of the mucosal lining. When the mucus layer is broken down — as occurs during prolonged starvation or malnutrition — several deleterious effects may occur: increased gut inflammation, absorption of toxic and carcinogenic compounds, or overgrowth and attachment of harmful bacteria to the intestinal wall. In addition, some disease-causing bacteria disrupt the protective mucus layer by degrading it, penetrating through the layer, and causing ulcers and inflammation. *Helicobacter pylori*, the bacterium that causes gastric ulcers, has several mechanisms by which it disrupts and penetrates mucus (Quigley and Kelly, 1995). Other "harmful" species of bacteria use mucus molecules as energy sources, thereby reducing the protective effects of the mucus in the gut, while simultaneously permitting growth of harmful bacteria.

> The addition of mucus components to some bacterial cultures has been shown experimentally to stimulate the growth and metabolic activities of potentially harmful bacteria (Quigley and Kelly, 1995). Together, materials left over after digestion by gastric juices, mucus, and sloughed off cells from the lining of the digestive tract all contribute to the total pool of products that can be used as energy for bacteria living in the lower portions of the gastrointestinal tract (Collins and Gibson, 1999). The nature of these substances contributes to the composition (type and number) of bacteria that reside in the intestines.

Diets that are high in fruits, vegetables, and fiber offer some protection against the break down of the gastrointestinal tract's mucus layer. The mucus layer lining the gastrointestinal tract is very important, since a breach in this layer allows gut bacteria to cause various gastrointestinal diseases.

Small intestines, pancreas, and liver

Passing on down the gastrointestinal tract, bacteria that survive in the stomach begin their journey through the small intestines. The small intestines are divided into three different sections. The part of the small intestines closest to the stomach is the **duodenum**. The duodenum receives digestive juices and enzymes from the **pancreas** and the **liver**, organs that are required for appropriate food digestion — despite their location outside the gastrointestinal tract. The mid portion of the small intestines is referred to as the **jejunum**, and the end of the small intestines lying closest to the large intestines is called the **ileum**. The small intestines represent an area of transition between the relatively low bacterial count of the stomach and the high number of bacteria that live in the large intestines.

> The total number of organisms in the early segments of the small bowel ranges from nearly undetectable to 10,000 per milliliter of intestinal juices. Predominant organisms in the small intestine are largely gram-positive aerobes such as lactobacilli, streptococci, staphylococci, and yeasts; although, some coliforms and anaerobes are present in low concentrations. One key feature of the organisms in the duodenum is the absence of gram-negative species such as *Bacteroides* and *Escherichia coli,* despite their high numbers in the ileum and large intestine (Gorbach, 1967a; Gorbach et al., 1967b; Gorbach et al., 1967c). Bifidobacteria, fusobacteria, and clostridia are also present in the ileum, where the total bacterial count rises to 100,000 organisms per milliliter and gram-negative organisms begin to out-number gram-positives (Linskins et al., 2001).

The pancreas, a digestive organ located outside the "tube" of the gastrointestinal tract, is a small gland located in the middle of the abdomen, below the stomach. Many people are aware that the pancreas plays an important role in secreting insulin; however, most don't realize that it is also a big player in the game of digestion. Products secreted by the pancreas play a significant role in helping to keep the bacterial flora "normal" within the gut. The pancreas produces enzymes that break down proteins, carbohydrates, and fats. Laboratory experiments have found that pancreatic enzymes can degrade bacteria as well. Pancreatic juices protect us from illness by degrading harmful bacterial products like cholera toxins and destroying the outer layers of bacterial species like *Escherichia coli, Klebsiella pneumoniae,* and *Shigella* (Rubenstein et al., 1985; Sarker and Gyr, 1992). Pancreatic enzymes are secreted directly into the duodenum and keep the number of bacteria in the small intestine in check, to prevent "small bowel bacterial overgrowth".

Although there are numerous enzymes secreted by the pancreas, three major players are of interest to our discussion: **trypsin**, **amylase**, and **lipase**. Trypsin is, by far, the most abundant enzyme synthesized in the pancreas; its job is to digest proteins. When food has been consumed in reasonable quantities, properly chewed, and the pancreas and liver are functioning at maximum capacity, 98% of proteins are broken down into individual **amino acids**. These amino acids serve as energy sources for some species of bacteria residing in the gut.

Pancreatic amylase is the enzyme responsible for digesting most sugars, and pancreatic lipase breaks down 95-99% of all fats. The pancreas also produces bicarbonate. Bicarbonate neutralizes stomach acids that are dumped into the small intestine, making the small intestine considerably less acidic than the stomach. Thus, since the environment of the small intestines is less harsh than the stomach, more microorganisms begin to take up permanent residence there, and bacterial overgrowth can occur if all components of the system are not functioning at top notch.

The role of the liver in food digestion is primarily related to the synthesis of **bile**. Bile consists of water, bile salts, bilirubin, cholesterol, fatty acids, lecithin, and electrolytes. Bile is produced by the liver, stored in the **gall bladder** and released directly into the duodenum whenever it's needed. Bile salts are responsible for breaking up food particles, for **emulsifying** fat globules into small sizes, and for absorption of fatty acids and cholesterol from the intestinal tract. Bile acids transport fat to the wall of the intestine, where the fat dissolves and diffuses into the cells that line the digestive tract, called **epithelial cells**. The acidic nature of bile suppresses bacterial growth within the small intestines.

Why is all of this information about digestive enzymes important? It is important for several reasons. First, not only do these enzymes break down food products, but digestive enzymes also prevent bacterial overgrowth. Secondly, the combination of (1) a relative lack of digestive enzymes and (2) the presence of abnormal gut flora — which causes gut inflammation — is now recognized as a major factor in underlying allergic diseases such as food allergies, asthma, and eczema (see chapter 7 for details).

So, what we've learned so far is: stomach acids reduce the number of live bacteria that make it to the duodenum, and pancreatic digestive enzymes as well as hepatic bile acids provide other lines of defense against bacterial overgrowth in the small intestines (Kirjavainen, 1999).

> In fact, so potent are bile acids as antimicrobial agents, numerous bile acid derivatives are currently being evaluated for use as antibiotics (Li et al., 1999; Guan et al., 2000). It has previously been demonstrated that altered bile acid composition within the duodenum can lead to overgrowth of some bacterial species (Kocoshis et al., 1987).

> Another substance called lysozyme is also produced by cells that line the digestive tract. Lysozyme is a potent enzyme that attacks bacterial cell walls and is believed to be another primary control measure for preventing bacterial overgrowth within this region of the gut (Kirjavainen, 1999).

Therefore, gastric acid and digestive enzymes are important chemical barriers that help control the population of normal flora in the gut.

With all these bacteria inhabiting our intestines, what's to keep them from invading the rest of our body? I'm so glad you asked. There are four gastrointestinal factors necessary to keep gut normal flora from leaving the gut: epithelial cells, mucus, antibodies, and peristalsis.

The entire gastrointestinal tract is lined with epithelial cells that separate the contents of the intestine from the rest of the body. I like to think of epithelial cells as a picket fence. Just like the boards of a picket fence are tightly arranged, with minimal spaces to prevent invaders from entering the yard, so the epithelial cells of the gut are aligned closely together to prevent invading microorganisms from entering the rest of the body. Epithelial cells are normally packed together very tightly, with minimal amounts of space — referred to as **tight junctions** — between each cell (See figure 1-3). Lining the epithelial cells is a superficial layer of mucus that further separates the body from the complex microbial population that resides in the intestines. Together, intestinal epithelial cells, tight junctions, and the mucus layer comprise the "**mucosal barrier**" that keeps normal gut flora in the digestive tract, excluded from the rest of the body.

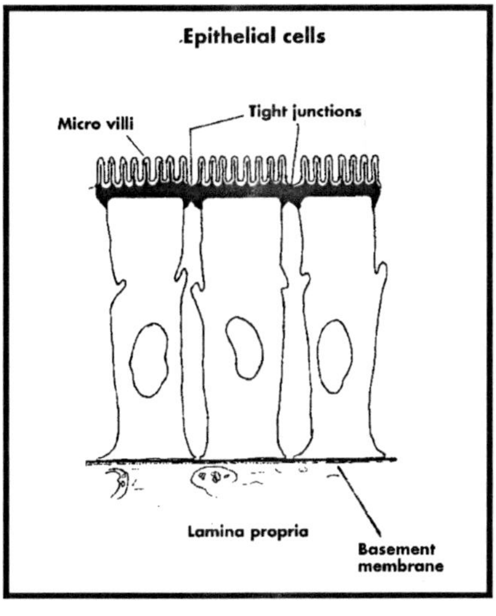

Figure 1-3. Epithelial cells line the inside of the digestive tract. These cells rest upon a basement membrane, which holds them in place. Note the tight junctions between cells — these minute pores only allow passage of substances that are smaller than 10 nanometers. Modified from Ganong WF: Review of Medical Physiology, 16th edition, 1993, Appleton and Lange, with permission of The McGraw-Hill Companies.

Although I introduced the topic of mucus when we talked about the stomach, mucus secretions are not only important in the stomach, but they are necessary in the small intestines and the large intestines, as well. As discussed earlier, mucus prevents some bacterial species from attaching to the intestinal wall. Mucus also provides a physical barrier to keep gut bacteria from leaving the digestive system and translocating to other parts of the body (Boedekar, 1994). Of course, the "mucosal barrier" is not an absolute barrier. Its design permits selective uptake of nutrients, water, and electrolytes. But, under normal circumstances, the mucosal barrier prevents disease-causing bacteria and their toxins from binding to and invading epithelial cells. On the other hand, inflammation, irritation, and infections disturb the epithelial cells that line the gastrointestinal tract. Under these circumstances, epithelial cells die faster than they can be replaced. When this occurs, large gaps are left in the mucosal barrier. There is a tendency for intestinal bacteria to leave the gastrointestinal tract through these "holes" and invade other organs of the body. In addition to causing serious infections, such disruptions may also contribute to food allergies, which will be discussed at length in chapter 7.

In the intestines, the mucosal barrier also serves as the home to a specific subset of protective antibodies (also called **immunoglobulins** or **Ig**). Immunoglobulin A (IgA) is abundant on mucosal surfaces of the intestines. It is another line of defense against bacterial disease in the gut and is secreted throughout the entire length of the gastrointestinal tract. The role of IgA is to neutralize and inactivate harmful bacterial toxins and invading viruses.

> The importance of IgA in controlling bacterial infections within the gut was demonstrated by recent studies describing a higher rate of gut-derived **sepsis** in transplant patients with IgA-deficiencies compared to those with other antibody deficits (like IgM or IgG deficiencies) (Van Thiel et al., 1992).

So far, we've discussed physical and chemical barriers that keep normal gut flora in the intestines, but there's a mechanical factor, too. It is called **peristalsis**. Sometimes — as our bellies rumble — we are painfully aware of the muscular movements in our intestines. From a mechanistic stand point, peristalsis — the constant muscular movement of the intestines — is necessary to repeatedly mix the contents (food, enzymes, bile, etc.) of the intestines. However, the constant movements of peristalsis also prevent bacteria from adhering to epithelial cells of the small intestines (Kirjavainen, 1999) (See figure 1-4). Since rapid peristaltic movements normally prevent colonization by harmful bacteria, it comes as no surprise that in situations where gastrointestinal **motility** is inhibited — due to microbial toxins or constipating drugs — there is an increased tendency for the gut to become colonized by harmful bacterial species.

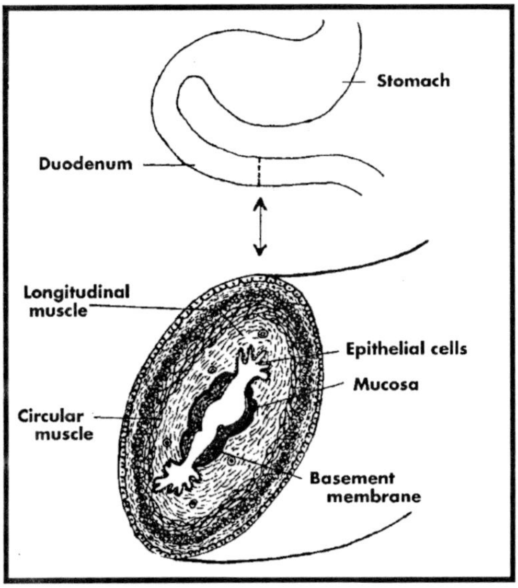

Figure 1-4. A cross section of the intestines depicts the muscle layers that are responsible for peristalsis. Modified from Human Physiology and Mechanisms of Disease, 4th edition, Guyton AC., Movement of Food through the Alimentary Tract, page 487, 1992, with permission from Elsevier.

The small intestines always propel their contents forward. If bacteria are going to survive there, they must be able to attach to the intestinal wall. To adhere, bacteria must possess adhering proteins, have their own means of locomotion, and be able to multiply rapidly enough to overcome the forward peristaltic muscular movements. Bacteria that fail to meet the criteria for attachment, motility, and propagation are passed along with fecal matter into the large intestines.

> Although the duodenum contains only a small number of bacteria, the number of bacteria increases dramatically in the ileum — the lowest portion of the small intestines. Perhaps the most striking difference between the early and late regions of the small intestines is the marked change in bacterial species. Unlike those in the duodenum, organisms found

> in the ileum are predominately gram-negative species such as enterobacteriaceae or *Bacteroides* (although, some gram positive species such as enterococci or clostridia may also be found). (Bentley et al., 1972; Gorbach et al., 1967b; Gorbach, et al., 1967c). The ileum — with its larger number of bacteria and obvious changes in resident species — serves as a transitional stage between the relatively unpopulated duodenum versus the densely populated large intestines.

The last factor we are going to consider as a defense against bacterial colonization in the small and large intestines is the *turn-over* of the epithelial cells. The periodic loss, or sloughing, of intestinal cells assists in washing away various infective agents that would otherwise remain adherent to intestinal cells. Of course, sloughed dead epithelial cells must be replaced. When inflammation or disease causes epithelial cells to slough faster than they are replaced, the mucosal barrier is compromised and the rest of the body is at risk of infection from invading microorganisms (See figure 1-5A and 1-5B).

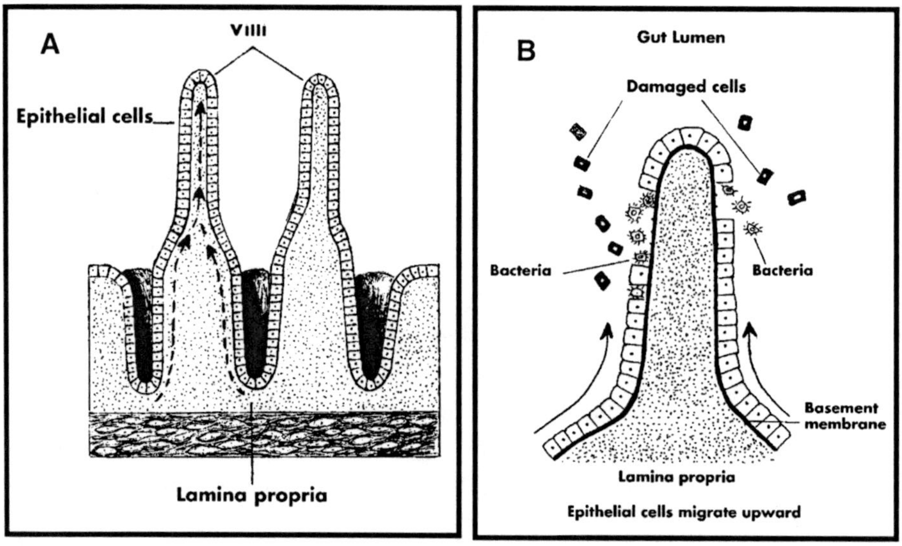

Figure 1-5. A. Illustrates the normal situation, when epithelial cells migrate from deep within gastrointestinal folds to the top of villi to replace dead, sloughed off cells that have detached from the basement membrane. Modified from Ganong WF: Review of Medical Physiology, 16th edition, 1993, Appleton and Lange, with permission of The McGraw-Hill Companies.

B. Illustrates an enlarged depiction of sloughed off epithelial cells under conditions of gastrointestinal infection or inflammation. In these situations, epithelial cells die faster than they are replaced, and bacteria can gain access to the basement membrane (and subsequently other parts of the body).

So you see that many factors — chemical, physical, and mechanical — work together in harmony inside the intestines to control bacterial populations. Without the intricate workings of the small intestines functioning in concert with each another, the small bowel becomes diseased. When bacterial populations grow out of control in the small intestines, a medical condition known as "small bowel overgrowth" occurs.

Transition to the colon (otherwise known as the large intestines)
Separating the small intestines from the large intestines (or **colon**) is a muscular region, referred to as the **ileocecal valve**. The purpose of the tightly closed ileocecal valve is to prevent backflow of microorganisms from the colon up into the small intestines. The large intestines are home to more than 350 different species of bacteria, whose numbers approximate 100 billion to 10 trillion organisms in every gram of dry feces. Large populations of *Bacteroides*, bifidobacteria, and eubacteria reside in the large intestines. Probably the most striking feature of the bacteria that live in the large intestines is that over 99% of them are **obligate anaerobes** — meaning they can grow and proliferate *only* in the *absence* of oxygen. Anaerobic cocci like peptococci and peptostreptococci, as well as clostridia, enterococci, and enterobacteriaceae consider the large intestines their home (Linskins et al., 2001). As in earlier regions of the digestive tract, mucus is secreted in the colon and helps to protect the bowel from abrasion and from bacteria that could otherwise threaten to invade the body. With such a large number of diverse microorganisms residing in the colon, bacterial growth is largely dependent upon availability of nutrients.

Despite the extensive digestive and absorptive capabilities of the small intestines, many nutrients do pass through the small bowel and enter the colon. Nutrients such as gastric mucus, dietary residues like fiber, digestion-resistant starches, complex sugars, food sweeteners, and to a lesser extent, proteins, amino acids and fats all get transported through the small intestines without being completely digested. These substances serve as food and energy for the billions of bacteria that live in the large intestines (Collins, 1999). One interesting feature about bacterial nutritional requirements is: the very nutrients that stimulate growth and multiplication of some organisms simultaneously suppress the activities of other bacterial species. Therefore, probably the most important factors governing bacterial composition within the large intestines are (a) the *amount* and (b) the *types* of nutrients available.

This is, of course, determined largely by dietary intake. Therefore, *nutrition* plays an important role in maintaining homeostasis in the large intestines.

Probably the most widely studied protective nutrients are those found in human milk that protect immature guts of infants. The roles of lactoferrin and iron in altering the microfloral environment have been addressed earlier in this chapter. There is also is an increasing body of evidence that suggests that free **oligosaccharides** — present in breast milk — may act as decoys for bacterial toxins and disease-causing bacteria in infants. Let me explain.

Oligosaccharides are complex sugars. Some investigators have found that these complex sugars act as scavengers, collecting, removing, and neutralizing disease-causing bacteria or bacterial toxins. In this way, oligosaccharides keep harmful products away from the intestinal wall before they cause severe gastrointestinal illness. Furthermore, by binding directly to some bacterial species, oligosaccharides actually promote clearance of **pathogenic** organisms from the body (Kunz, 2000).

Numerous oligosaccharides and glycoproteins have now been identified in human breast milk. Their ability to bind selectively to bacteria or bacterial toxins has been demonstrated in laboratory studies in many cases. Table 1-1 shows a partial listing of microorganisms or toxins whose activity is inhibited by specific oligosaccharides found in breast milk.

Table 1-1. Examples of common microorganisms and their toxins whose activity is inhibited by complex sugars found in breast milk.

Escherichia coli	(Cravito, 1991)
Campylobacter jejuni	(Newburg, 1997)
Streptococcus pneumoniae	(Anderson, 1986)
Vibrio cholera	(Laegreid, 1987)
Shigella toxin	(Newburg, 1992)
Rotavirus	(Newburg, 1998)

In order for breast milk-derived oligosaccharides to serve in a protectorate role in the gut, these complex sugars must survive transit through the gastrointestinal tract. Many studies have demonstrated that, in fact, the concentrations of oligosaccharides in feces and urine of breast-fed infants are much higher than those found in formula-fed babies. Additionally, fecal and urinary oligosaccharides from breast-fed infants resemble the types of sugars found in their mother's milk. In contrast, oligosaccharides recovered from formula-fed infants are at much lower concentrations and do not resemble those found in human breast milk. Therefore, it appears that certain oligosaccharides found in breast milk provide an additional advantage for breast-fed infants during acquisition of normal gut flora (Chaturvedi, 2001).

Numerous studies indicate that diet plays a role in the composition of bacteria that live in the large intestines of adults as well. Specifically, nondigestible food ingredients, particularly certain complex sugars, act as **substrates** to increase growth of one or more beneficial bacterial species in the intestine. A specific sugar or starch that selectively stimulates growth of "healthy" gut bacteria is known as a "**prebiotic.**" Information on this important new area of research will be covered in detail in chapter 10.

Function of Bacteria in the Colon

So far, we've seen the many hurdles bacteria must overcome in order to make it to the colon. Why do bacteria take up residence in our large intestines? What benefit is it to us? In return for the undigested food that we supply to bacteria via our diet, bacteria supply us with necessary vitamins and energy and also protect us from disease-causing invaders.

Bacteria obtain their energy by chemically breaking down sugars and proteins — a process known as **fermentation**. The primary substrates for bacterial growth are starches, complex sugars from plant cell walls, and mucus-like sugars from the gastrointestinal tract, as well as proteins, peptides, and simple sugars. In general, when it comes to using sugars as energy sources, the bacteria that live in our guts are living under starvation conditions. That is because most of these dietary sources of energy have already been extensively digested and utilized as energy sources by us in earlier portions of the gut. Since there is usually a relative scarcity of sugars to use as substrates, adding prebiotics to our diets (see chapter 10) can dramatically speed up growth of healthy gut bacteria.

> Numerous bacteria — including bifidobacteria, lactobacilli, ruminococci, eubacteria, clostridia, and *Bacteroides* – use **carbohydrates** as their preferred energy sources. These bacteria are well-adapted to degrade complex sugars, since they synthesize many glycosidase enzymes (enzymes that

> break down sugars). In contrast, however, other groups of bacteria are not able to break down complex carbohydrates directly, but instead, depend upon the fragments produced by other polysaccharide-degraders.

Unlike sugars, which are often in short supply in the colon, there is no shortage of proteins throughout the entire length of the intestines. In the large intestines, protein degradation occurs not only via enzymes secreted by the human body, but also by bacteria-secreted digestive enzymes; so bacteria actually assist us in breaking down proteins.

Many nutritional factors alter protein fermentation in the large intestines, including acidity of the environment, as well as types and number of bacteria residing there. Interestingly, not all bacteria can break down proteins as energy sources (some bacterial species can *only* use sugars for energy), and not all bacteria can degrade the same *types* of proteins — since degradative enzymes produced by various species differ widely. As a result of different dietary requirements among various bacterial species, nutrients that stimulate growth of one species often inhibit growth of another.

In return for the room and board that we provide bacteria in our large intestines, bacteria provide us with some important commodities. The predominant microbial break down products — produced as a result of bacterial fermentation in the colon — are short chain fatty acids (SCFA). Acetate, propionate, and butyrate (Legakis et al., 1982) with lesser amounts of lactate are the major SCFA produced in humans (See figure 1-6).

O ‖ $HOCCH_3$	**Acetic Acid (vinegar)**
O ‖ $HOCCH_2CH_3$	**Propionic Acid**
O ‖ $HOCCH_2CH_2CH_3$	**Butyric Acid**

Figure 1-6. Examples of the three most common short chain fatty acids produced by bacteria in the human gastrointestinal tract.

Metabolism of SCFA provides a source of energy for both humans and bacteria. Since each of us has a unique set of normal flora residing within us, the SCFA produced in our intestines is also unique to each individual — like a fingerprint. The range of SCFA produced as a result of the bacteria within varies widely from one individual to another depending upon diet and age (Edwards et al., 1994, Parrett et al., 1997).

> Differences in fecal SCFA exist between infants and adults. A relatively high level of acetic acid is recovered in fecal material from infants compared to that of adults (Rasmussen et al., 1988). There is also a predominance of acetic acid isolated from stools of breast-fed infants as compared to formula-fed babies (Siigur et al., 1993).

More precisely, the types and amounts of SCFA are determined by (a) dietary preferences, (b) differing normal flora colonization patterns, and (c) other environmental factors within the colon including complex metabolic interactions among bacteria. Since the amount and proportions of SCFA produced depends largely upon diet, the roles played by different starches have become a focus of study within the past few years. Additionally, since the types of bacteria colonizing the intestines also play a key role in the amounts and types of SCFA present, the characteristic profile of SCFA produced by each bacterial species can be used to identify the presence of various bacterial species.

> For example, most bacteroides species are capable of fermenting simple sugars and produce succinic, acetic and propionic acids as part of their metabolic pathways (Franz et al., 1979). In contrast, bifidobacteria and eubacteria produce mostly acetic and lactic acids (Jiang et al., 1997). Fusobacteria, gram negative anaerobic organisms commonly isolated from the gastrointestinal tract, are believed to produce butyric acid as their major break down product (Onderdonk, 2000).

Thus, the types and amounts of SCFA produced can act as a sort of "fingerprint" to identify various bacterial species. However, in the large intestines — where so many bacterial species co-exist — individual differences in SCFA production rarely show up. Instead, the amounts and types of various SCFA tend to appear relatively constant overall.

In addition to dietary intake of starches and the bacteria already residing in the intestine, some other factors are also known to alter SCFA production. For example, antibiotics are known to impair fermentation in the colon and lower fecal SCFA levels. This makes sense since antibiotics alter both the number of microorganisms and the types of bacterial species present in the gut. Diarrhea is also related to reduced SCFA concentrations in the large intestines. The length of time that food is present within the gut — to serve as a source of energy — certainly affects SCFA concentrations because bacterial growth and metabolic needs are greatest during diarrhea, when food transits through the gut rapidly.

SCFA are tremendous sources of energy (Roediger, 1980) for promoting growth, not only of bacteria, but also for the epithelial cells that line the colon. The gut epithelial cells get up to 70% of their energy from bacterial fermentation products (Cummings,1995). Although all three major SCFA are used by epithelial cells (acetic acid, propionic acid, and butyric acid), butyric acid is especially important. Butyric acid seems to play a role in modulating cell growth, **differentiation** (Cummings, 1995), and maintaining homeostasis within the intestine. Numerous studies have shown that butyric acid stimulates growth and activities of intestinal epithelial cells.

In contrast to acting as a growth factor, however, it has also been shown that butyric acid is capable of slowing the growth of cancerous cells. Specifically, butyric acid is a growth inhibitor of cancer cells — prolonging the doubling time of human colon cancer cell lines and slowing their growth rates (Siavoshian, 2000). Butyric acid has also been shown to facilitate cell migration and DNA repair mechanisms to prevent gastrointestinal cancer (Wilson, 2000; Jacobasch, 1999). Early evidence suggests that by regulating gene expression and slowing growth rates, SCFA protect us from colon and rectal cancer. These effects probably occur because butyric acid facilitates the actions of DNA "repair enzymes" to eliminate mutations. Additionally, butyric acid may trigger a "programmed cell death" in tumor cells, thus eliminating cancerous cells from the body entirely (Cummings, 1995).

SCFA are rapidly absorbed from our intestines and used by our bodies. They make significant contributions toward meeting our total daily energy requirements. Bacterial production of SCFA allows our bodies to recover energy that would otherwise have been lost in our stools. Acetic, propionic, and butyric acids are not only used as energy sources by the colon, but also by the liver and muscle cells. It is estimated that in normal, healthy individuals, SCFA account for up to 10% of the body's total daily energy requirements (Roediger, 1980). However, in individuals that eat very high fiber diets or those with malabsorption syndromes (in which the earlier portions of the gut fail to retrieve energy from foods), SCFA produced by bacterial fermentation may actually provide much more than 10% of the daily energy requirements.

SCFA also help to prevent overgrowth of disease-causing bacteria like salmonella species (Durant, 2000; Rabbani et al., 1999) simply by making the environment in the large intestines more acidic. As we've discussed, many bacteria cannot survive acidic conditions. While all organic acids like acetic acid, lactic acid, and butyric acid inhibit growth of pathogens by creating an acidic environment, butyric acid is believed to be the major player. Additionally, SCFA speed the rate of peristalsis to indirectly remove invading microorganisms, accelerating their transit through the digestive tract (Kailasapathy and Chin, 2000). Consistent with this, recent evidence indicates that when certain carbohydrates (like prebiotics) are ingested in large quantities and broken down into specific SCFA, overgrowth of disease-causing bacteria is prevented.

> In a study of 62 infants aged 5-12 months with diarrhea, dietary ingestion of either cooked green bananas or pectin (a prebiotic) improved gastrointestinal symptoms in 78% of infants eating bananas and 82% of those receiving pectin within 4 days of treatment. This is in contrast to improvements in only 23% of those eating a rice-based diet (Rabbani et al., 2001). (Note: In this study the term "green bananas" refers to a specific type of banana commonly found in Asia and Africa and not simply an unripened banana.) The authors of this study speculate that the reason for symptomatic improvements may be due to production of specific SCFA produced during the fermentation process of both green bananas and pectin.

Experimental studies also suggest that SCFA may have other health benefits like lowering blood sugar and blood cholesterol levels. However, beneficial effects on these parameters in humans have been modest and less apparent than the positive effects seen in animal studies (Berggren, 1996; Jenkins, 1998).

Other Ways Good Bacteria Fight Bad Bacteria in the Colon

In addition to producing SCFA that suppress growth of unwanted bacterial species in the colon, "healthy" bacteria also maintain the critical balance of flora in favor of the "good guys" by producing antimicrobial substances such as peroxides or bacteriocins — toxins that kill other bacteria. For example, various lactobacillus species produce hydrogen peroxide, carbon dioxide, and diacetyl, which are detrimental to food-borne pathogens (Kailasapathy and Chin, 2000). Also, lactobacilli produce a wide variety of bacteriocins such as nisin, lactobrevin, acidophilin, acidolin, lactobacillin, lactocidin, and lactolin. These bacterial toxins actively kill numerous species of bacteria (Kailasapathy and Chin, 2000).

Another example of a toxin produced by "good bacteria" directed against "bad bacteria" is the toxin produced by *Bacteroides*. Bacteroides organisms are the major gram negative **obligate** anaerobic bacilli found in the colon. Bacterial toxins produced by these microorganisms are believed to selectively destroy disease-causing *Clostridium difficile*. Many people suffering from life-threatening, chronic, persistent *Clostridium difficile*-associated diarrhea have been cured when bacteroides species were replaced in their colons (Borody, 2000).

It is speculated that normal gut flora serve as a final defense against invading disease-causing organisms in other ways, too. For example, gastrointestinal normal flora compete with other bacteria for nutrients and for binding sites on the intestinal wall. To understand how this works, think, for a moment, about a football stadium that holds 60,000 fans. If more than 60,000 fans show up for Sunday afternoon kick-off, some of the fans won't get a seat and will have to leave. The same thing happens in the gut. If there is an excess of "healthy" bacteria in the gut, the "good bacteria" simply "crowd out" disease-causing microorganisms, thereby preventing attachment of pathogenic bacteria by a process known as "competitive exclusion" (Kailasapathy and Chin, 2000) .

Other Benefits of Gut Flora

Gut bacteria provide us with other benefits, too. Some bacteria neutralize dietary carcinogens such as nitrosamines, which are produced when high protein diets are eaten (Kailasapathy and Chin, 2000). Additionally, bacterial flora in the colon are involved in synthesizing both hormone and vitamin precursors. One example is vitamin B12. Interestingly, vitamin B12 is not found in any plant sources. Instead, it is produced almost entirely by gut bacteria. Vitamin B12 is essential for red blood cell function and is also required for nerve activities. A deficiency of vitamin B12 leads to diseases like anemia and painful nerve disorders.

Thus, the bacteria in our large intestines are much more than simply inert parasites. Instead, the normal flora living in our intestines actually help us in many ways: by creating energy sources for epithelial cells, by helping us to retrieve energy that would otherwise be lost, by reducing overgrowth of disease-causing bacteria, by inactivating carcinogens, and by manufacturing vitamins. In many ways, the bacteria in our colons could actually be considered a "necessary body organ."

Common Bacteria in the Colon

With all the different bacterial organisms found in the digestive tract, it has simply not been possible to determine the impact and functions of all species individually. However, roles for some of the predominant microorganisms have been described. In fact, it has been suggested that really only 10 or so **genera** probably predominate in the normal human gut. Some of their names are: *Bacteroides, Lactobacillus, Clostridium, Fusobacterium, Bifidobacterium, Eubacterium, Peptococcus, Peptostreptococcus, Escherichia,* and *Veionella* (Isolauri et al., 2002). The last section of this chapter will be an introduction into the names and activities of a few of the more widely studied bacteria residing in the human digestive tract so you can become familiar with the key players.

Gram negative anaerobic rods

Bacteria that fall into the bacteroides genus are the major gram-negative obligate anaerobic rod-shaped organisms in the large intestines and in the feces of humans. As mentioned earlier, bacteroides organisms produce one or more bacteriocins, or toxins, that inhibit growth of other bacterial species. Bacteriocins are hardy proteins — some can withstand very acidic or extremely alkaline conditions — and can survive the degrading activities of a variety of enzymes (Riley and Mee, 1985). Another gram-negative anaerobic bacteria, *Fusobacterium*, is also commonly isolated from the colon. These organisms produce butyric acid as a major metabolite. As we discussed earlier, butyric acid is believed to provide us with numerous benefits, including growth control of many **facultative** types of bacteria.

Non-spore-forming gram positive rods

The major non-**spore** forming, gram-positive, rod-shaped bacteria include *Eubacterium*, *Lactobacillus*, and *Bifidobacterium*. These three species are capable of digesting a variety of substances including cellulose, mucin, polysaccharides, and proteins. Like *Fusobacterium*, the major metabolic product produced by *Eubacterium* is butyric acid, while lactic acid is the most abundant byproduct of lactobacilli and bifidobacterial metabolism. The short chain fatty acids produced by these bacteria create an acidic environment in the intestines, which provides antimicrobial effects. These species also produce peroxides and **bacteriocins** which eliminate disease-causing bacteria. For example, *Lactobacillus* strain GG, originally isolated from feces of a healthy individual, produces a potent inhibitory substance with antimicrobial activity against a wide variety of bacteria including clostridia, bacteroides, bifidobacteria, pseudomonads, staphylococci, streptococci, and *Escherichia coli* (Silva et al., 1987). Another mechanism by which lactobacilli and bifidobacteria control overgrowth of disease-causing organisms involves their ability to attach to the epithelial cells that line the interior of the intestines. Through competitive exclusion, these bacteria inhibit pathogenic bacteria from binding to the intestinal walls (Kailasapathy and Chin, 2000). Furthermore, the very process of these bacteria attaching to the intestinal epithelium, as we will see in subsequent chapters, stimulates the immune system, which also plays a role in eliminating harmful bacteria.

Many believe that these organisms are essential for good intestinal health (Simon and Gorbach, 1984). In fact, these species are frequently used as dietary supplements, much like vitamins. When "healthy" bacteria are used as supplements, they are referred to as "**probiotics**." [Contrast the term "probiotic" (for life) with the word "antibiotic" (against life).] Most probiotic studies described throughout the remainder of this book have used either lactobacilli or bifidobacteria to successfully prevent or treat a variety of diseases — ranging from illnesses within the gastrointestinal tract, to urinary and genital infections, to allergies and asthma.

Gram positive cocci

Peptostreptococci and enterococci are important gram-positive members of the large intestinal flora. There are approximately 10 billion of these organisms in every gram of feces. All strains are resistant to acidic environments and all produce lactic acid as a major metabolic byproduct (Onderdonk, 2000). Until recently, enterococci were considered to be benign members of fecal flora because of their uniform presence in all fecal matter and their resistance to adverse environmental conditions. However, the observance of vancomycin-resistant strains of enterococci has caused hospitals to implement special infectious control measures to contain infections and prevent further drug-resistant strains from developing (D'Agata, 2002) .

Spore-forming gram positive rods

Clostridial species are also commonly isolated from the large intestines, but their numbers rarely exceed 100 million to 1 trillion organisms per gram of fecal matter. *Clostridium* are gram-positive spore-forming rod-shaped bacteria. *Clostridium perfringes, Clostridium bifermentans,* and *Clostridium ramosum* are the most common species isolated from humans. The bacteria themselves are harmless. They are, however, capable of producing a variety of toxins that can damage the gastrointestinal tract. Although up to 8% of adults carry *Clostridium difficile* (one member of the *Clostridium* family) without suffering from ill effects, *Clostridium difficile* is the most important disease-causing anaerobic microorganism acquired in hospital settings (Onderdonk, 2000; Kelly et al., 1994). Typically, in healthy individuals, there is no problem being a "carrier" of this organism, that is, unless environmental changes occur within the gastrointestinal tract. This commonly happens during or after antibiotic therapy.

When there is a sufficient number of "good bacteria," in the gut, the growth of *Clostridium difficile* is suppressed and this microorganism does not flourish. However, if the environment becomes favorable — or if too many "good bacteria" have been killed by antibiotic therapy — *Clostridium difficile* proliferates and produces toxins that cause abdominal cramps, bloody and mucus-filled diarrhea, fever, weight loss, and yellow plaques on the intestinal wall, a condition referred to as **pseudomembranous colitis**. Failure to obtain prompt treatment when *Clostridium difficile* overgrows can lead to toxic megacolon, hemesis, and even death.

Coliforms

The most widely studied group of bacteria residing in the large intestines is the enterobacteriaceae, which includes *Escherichia coli (E. coli).* Although there are various bacteria within this group, they are often referred to collectively as coliforms. It is these bacteria that are closely monitored by water treatment facilities to ensure pure drinking water. The number of enterobacteriaceae in the colon varies widely from person to person. Normal ranges of this species run from less than 100 organisms to 1 billion organisms in every gram of feces (Onderdonk, 2000).

Normally, these bacteria only cause disease when they get outside the intestinal tract. Examples of infections caused by enterobacteriaceae include those of the abdominal cavity that occur following injury to the intestines, pelvic inflammatory infections, urinary tract infections, or infections in newborn infants. In recent years, the spread of disease-causing *E. coli* of the 0157:H7 genus has caused considerable concern to the general public. It is this genus that caused several deaths due to contaminated foodstuffs in restaurants during the past decade. However, under normal circumstances, within the confines of the intestinal tract, the total number of enterobacteriaceae is kept under control by butyric acid produced by other microbial species. Fortunately, these organisms typically do not migrate, but tend to remain relatively localized in the digestive tract (Onderdonk, 2000).

Conclusion

While there are billions of microorganisms in the digestive tract that contribute to our overall good health and well-being, the relationships between various species of bacteria in the gastrointestinal system are not well understood. Even though the potential for rapid growth is present within the large intestines, external factors limit the actual rates of bacterial propagation under normal circumstances. Limiting factors include (a) the acidic environment of the stomach which eliminates all but the most hardy bacterial species, (b) competition among various microorganisms for nutrients, (c) SCFA which suppress the growth of numerous bacterial species, (d) toxins produced by one species directed at another, and (e) competition among bacteria for a fixed number of binding sites on the intestinal walls.

It is also clear, however, that host factors certainly contribute to the health of the normal gastrointestinal tract. For example, bile acids have been shown to be a potent control mechanism for hindering overgrowth of *Clostridium*. In this chapter, we have focused on the roles of the normal gastrointestinal flora and the factors that prevent overgrowth of bacteria within our digestive system. The next chapter explores some of the medical issues that arise when things within the gastrointestinal tract don't quite function as they should, leading to imbalances between the "good bacteria" and the "bad bacteria."

Additionally, our immune systems must surely play a role in controlling propagation of microorganisms and preventing disease. The roles of the human immune system and its functions within the gastrointestinal tract are not fully understood. Why does the body not react against bacterial species in the gut and eliminate them as it would if the same species were found in the blood? What factors keep microorganisms confined to the gut and prevent their translocation to other organs? How do bacteria, in rare circumstances, gain access to other sites within the body? Relationships between the gastrointestinal tract and the immune system have not yet been fully explained. Although we don't have all the answers, the current state of our understanding of this complex relationship is described in more detail in chapters 3 and 4.

Notes

Notes

References

Anderson B, Porras O, Hanson LA, et al. Inhibition of attachment of *Streptococcus pneumoniae* and *Haemophilus influenzae* by human milk and receptor oligosaccharides. J Infect Dis. 1986; 153:232-237.

Balmer SE, Scott PH, Wharton BA Diet and faecal flora of newborn: Casein and whey proteins. Arch Dis Child. 1989a;64:1678-1684.

Balmer SE, Scott PH, Wharton BA. Diet and faecal flora in the newborn: Lactoferrin. Arch Dis Child. 1989b;64(12):1685-1690.

Balmer SE and Wharton BA. Diet and faecal flora of newborn: Breast milk and infant formula. Arch Dis Child. 1989c:64:1672-1677.

Bell MJ, Rudinsky M, Brotherton T, et al. Gastrointestinal microecology in the critically ill neonate. J Pediatr Surg. 1984;19:745-751.

Bennet R, Eriksson M, Nord CE. Fecal bacterial microflora of newborn infants during intensive care management and treatment with five antibiotic regimens. Pediatr Infect Dis J. 1986; 5:533-538.

Bennet R and Nord CE. Development of faecal anaerobic microflora after cesarean section and treatment in newborn infants. Infection. 1987;15:332-336.

Bentley DW, Nichols RL, Condran RE, et al. The microflora of the human ileum and intraabdominal colon: Results of direct needle aspiration at surgery and evaluation of the technique. J Lab Clin Med. 1972;79(3):421-429.

Berggren AM, Nyman EM, Lundquist I, et al. Influence of orally and rectally administered propionate on cholesterol and glucose metabolism in obese rats. Br J Nutr. 1996;76:287-294.

Boedeker EC. Adherent bacteria: Breaching the mucosal barrier? Gastroenterology. 1994;106:255-257.

Borody TJ. "Flora Power"— fecal bacteria cure chronic *C. difficile* diarrhea. Am J Gastroenterol. 2000;95:3028-3029.

Bullen L, Tearle PV. Bifidobacteria in the intestinal tract of infants: An *in vitro* study. J Med Microbiol. 1976; 9:335-342.

Chaturvedi P, Warren CD, Buescher CR, et al. Survival of human milk oligosaccharides in the intestine of infants. Adv Exp Med Biol. 2001; 501:315-323.

Collins MD and Gibson GR. Probiotics, prebiotics, and synbiotics: Approaches for modulating the microbial ecology of the gut. Am J Clin Nutr 1999; 69:1052S-1057S.

Cravito A, Tello A, Villafan H, et al. Inhibition of localized adhesion of enteropathic *Escherichia coli* to Hep-2 cells by immunoglobulin and oligosaccharide fractions of human colostrum and breast milk. J Infect Dis. 1991;163:1247-1255.

Cummings JH. Short Chain Fatty Acids. In: Gibson GR and Macfarlane GT, eds. Human colonic bacteria: Role in nutrition, physiology, and pathology. CRC Press, Boca Raton, FL, 1995.

Dai D and Walker WA. Protective nutrients and bacterial colonization in the immature human gut. Adv. Pediatr. 1999; 46:353-382.

D'Agata EM, Horn MA, Webb GF. The impact of persistent gastrointestinal colonization on the transmission dynamics of vancomycin-resistant enterococci. J Infect Dis. 2002;185:766-773.

Durant JA, Corrier DE, Ricke SC. Short-chain volatile fatty acids modulate the expression of the hilA and invF genes of *Salmonella typhimurium.* J Food Prot. 2000;63:573-578.

Edwards CA, Parrett AM, Balmer SE, et al. Faecal short chain fatty acids in breast-fed and formula-fed babies. Acta Paediatr. 1994;83:459-462.

Frantz JC and McCallum RE. Growth yields and fermentation balance of *Bacteroides fragilis* cultured in glucose-enriched medium. J Bacteriol. 1979;137:1263-1270.

Gorbach SL, Nahas L, Lerner PI. Studies of intestinal microflora. I. Effects of diet, age, and periodic sampling on numbers of fecal microorganisms in man. Gastroenterology. 1967a;53:845-855.

Gorbach SL, Plaut AG, Nahas L. et al. Studies of intestinal microflora. II. Microorganisms of the small intestine and their relations to oral and fecal flora. Gastroenterology. 1967b;53:856-867.

Gorbach SL. Population control in the small bowel. Gut. 1967c Dec;8(6):530-532.

Gronlund M-M, Lehtonen O-P, Eerola E, et al. Fecal microflora in healthy infants born by different methods of delivery: Permanent changes in intestinal flora after cesarean delivery. J Pediatr Gastroenterol Nutr. 1999; 28:19-25.

Guan Q, Li C, Schmidt EJ, et al. Preparation and characterization of cholic acid-derived antimicrobial agents with controlled stabilities. Org Lett. 2000;2:2837-2840.

Gyorgy P, Jeanloz RW, von Nicolai H, et al. Undialyzable growth factors for *Lactobacillus bifidus* var. pennsylvanicus. Eur J Biochem. 1974; 43:29-33.

Isolauri E, Kirjavainen PV, and Salminen S. Probiotics: A role in the treatment of intestinal infection and inflammation? Gut. 2002; 50:iii54-iii59.

Jacobasch G, Schmiedl D, Kruschewski M, Schmehl K. Dietary resistant starch and chronic inflammatory bowel diseases. Int J Colorectal Dis. 1999;14:201-211.

Jenkins DJ, Vuksan V, Kendall CW, et al. Physiological effects of resistant starches on fecal bulk, short chain fatty acids, blood lipids and glycemic index. J Am Coll Nutr. 1998;17:609-616.

Jiang T and Savaiano DA. Modification of colonic fermentation by bifidobacteria and pH *in vitro*. Impact on lactose metabolism, short-chain fatty acid, and lactate production. Dig Dis Sci. 1997;42:2370-2377.

Levy J. Immunonutrition: The pediatric experience. Nutrition. 1998;14:641-647.

Linskens RK, Huijsdens XW, Savelkoul PH, et al. The bacterial flora in inflammatory bowel disease: Current insights in pathogenesis and the influence of antibiotics and probiotics. Scand J Gastroenterol Suppl. 2001;234:29-40.

Kailasapathy K and Chin J. Survival and therapeutic potential of probiotic organisms with references to *Lactobacillus acidophilus* and Bifidobacterium sp. Immunol Cell Biol. 2000;78:80-8.

Kelly CP, Pothoulakis C, LaMont JT. *Clostridium difficile* colitis. N Engl J Med 1994;330:257-262.

Kirjavainen PV and Gibson GR. Healthy gut microflora and allergy: Factors influencing development of the microbiotia. Ann Med. 1999; 31:288-292.

Kocoshis SA, Schletewitz K, Lovelace G, et al. Duodenal bile acids among children: Keto derivatives and aerobic small bowel bacterial overgrowth. J Pediatr Gastroenterol Nutr. 1987; 6:686-696.

Kunz C, Rudloff S, Baier W, et al. Oligosaccharides in human milk: Structural, functional, and metabolic aspects. Annu Rev Nutr. 2000; 20:699-722.

Laegreid A, Kolsto Otnaess AB. Trace amounts of ganglioside GM1 in human milk inhibit enterotoxins from *Vibrio cholerae* and *Escherichia coli*. Life Sci. 1987;40:55-62.

Legakis NJ, Xanthopoulou K, Ioannidou H, et al. Direct quantitative determination of acidic end products in clinical specimens for presumptive diagnosis of anaerobic infections. J Ann Microbiol (Paris). 1982;133:281-290.

Li C, Lewis MR, Gilbert AB, et al. Antimicrobial activities of amine- and guanidine-functionalized cholic acid. Antimicrob Agents Chemother. 1999;43:1347-1349.

Long SS and Swenson RM. Development of anaerobic fecal flora in healthy newborn infants. J Pediatr. 1977;91:298-301.

Neut C, Bezirtzoglou E, Romond C, et al. Bacterial colonization of the large intestine in newborns delivered by cesarean section. Zentralbl Bakteriol Mikrobiol Hyg. 1987; 266:330-337.

Newburg DS, Ashkenazi S, Cleary TG. Human milk contains the Shiga toxin and Shiga-like toxin receptor glycolipid Gb3. J Infect Dis 1992;166:832-836.

Newburg DS. Do the binding properties of oligosaccharides in milk protect human infants from gastrointestinal bacteria? J Nutr. 1997;127:980S-984S.

Newburg DS, Peterson JA, Ruiz-Palaios GM. Role of human-milk lactadherin in protection against symptomatic rotavirus infection. Lancet. 1998;351:1160-1164.

Onderdonk, AB. Intestinal microflora and inflammatory bowel disease. In Kirsner JB (ed.) Inflammatory Bowel Disease. Philadelphia, PA, WB Saunders Co, 2000.

Pahwa A, Mathur BN. Assessment of bifidus containing infant formula part-II. Implantation of *Bifidobacterium bifidum.* Indian J Dairy Sci. 1987;40:364-367.

Parrett AM and Edwards CA. *In vitro* fermentation of carbohydrate by breast fed and formula fed infants. Arch Dis Child. 1997;76:249-253.

Petschow BW and Talbott RD. Response of bifidobacterium species to growth promoters in human and cow milk. Pediatr Res. 1991;29:208-213.

Quigley ME and Kelly SM. Structure, function, and metabolism of host mucus glycoproteins. In: Gibson GR and Macfarlane GT, eds. Human colonic bacteria: Role in nutrition, physiology, and pathology, CRC Press, Boca Raton, FL 1995.

Rabbani GH, Albert MJ, Hamidur Rahman AS, et al. Short-chain fatty acids improve clinical, pathologic, and microbiologic features of experimental shigellosis. J Infect Dis. 1999;179:390-397.

Rabbani GH, Teka T, Zaman B, et al. Clinical studies in persistent diarrhea: Dietary management with green banana or pectin in Bangladeshi children. Gastroenterology. 2001;121:554-60.

Rasmussen HS, Holtug K, Ynggard C, et al. Faecal concentrations and production rates of short chain fatty acids in normal neonates. Acta Paediatr Scand. 1988;77:365-368.

Riley TV and Mee BJ. A comparative study of three bacteriocins of *Bacteroides fragilis*. Microbios. 1985;43:115-133.

Roberts AK, Chierii R, Sawatzki G, et al. Supplementation of an adapted formula with bovine lactoferrin1: Effect on the infant faecal flora. Acta Pediatr. 1992; 81:119-124.

Roediger WE. Role of anaerobic bacteria in the metabolic welfare of the colonic mucosa in man. Gut. 1980;21:793-798.

Rubinstein E, Mark Z, Haspel et al. Antibacterial activity of pancreatic fluid. Gastroenterology. 1985;88:926-32.

Sarker SA and Gyr K. Non-immunological defense mechanisms of the gut. Gut. 1992; 33:987-993.

Savage DC. Microbial ecology of the gastrointestinal tract. Ann Rev Microbiol. 1977;31:107-133.

Sepp E, Julge K, Naaber P, et al. Intestinal microflora of Estonian and Swedish infants. Acta Paediatr. 1997;86:956-961.

Siavoshian S, Segain JP, Kornprobst M, et al. Butyrate and trichostatin A effects on the proliferation/differentiation of human intestinal epithelial cells: Induction of cyclin D3 and p21 expression. Gut. 2000;46:507-514.

Silva M, Jacobus NV, Deneke C, et al. Antimicrobial substance from a human Lactobacillus strain. Antimicrob Agents Chemother. 1987;31:1231-1233.

Simon GL and Gorbach SL. Intestinal flora in health and disease. Gastroenterol. 1984;86:174-193.

Siigur U, Ormisson A, Tamm A. Faecal short-chain fatty acids in breast-fed and bottle-fed infants. Acta Paediatr. 1993;82:536-538.

Stark PL and Lee A. The microbial ecology of the large bowel of breast-fed and formula-fed infants during the first year of life. J Med Microbiol. 1982; 15:189-203.

Van Thiel DH, Finkel R, Friedlander L, et al. The association of IgA deficiency but not IgG or IgM deficiency with a reduced patient and graft survival following liver translocation. J Trans. 1992;54:269-273.

Wilson AJ and Gibson PR. Role of urokinase and its receptor in basal and stimulated colonic epithelial cell migration *in vitro*. Gut. 47:105-111.

Yoshioka H, Iseki K, Fujita K. Development and difference of intestinal flora in the neonatal period in breast-fed and bottle-fed infants. Pediatrics. 1983:72:317-321.

Chapter 2

Was it Something I Ate? When Digestive Functions Go Amiss

In the last chapter, we learned how the gastrointestinal tract is supposed to work. Additionally, I introduced some of the bacterial species that are important pieces of the overall puzzle. Now that you know how the system works when the players are all working together, let's discuss what can go wrong in the digestive tract and consider how overall health can be adversely affected. In this chapter, we are going to discuss some problems that occur within the digestive tract — and how bacterial flora fit into the outcome. Certainly we will not be covering everything that can go wrong with the gastrointestinal tract. Instead, we will be focusing primarily on digestive abnormalities that cause an imbalance of normal flora in the digestive tract and the associated consequences. Some of the factors we will consider include: inadequate gastric acid secretion, slow gastrointestinal motility, and inadequate production of digestive enzymes. We will also consider some of the many ways by which an imbalance between "good" and "bad" gut bacteria trigger diarrhea and other inflammatory diseases of the large intestine.

This chapter introduces what *can* go wrong in the gastrointestinal tract, causing an imbalance of gut flora. In many ways, this chapter should whet your appetite for later chapters when we discuss in detail *how* probiotics can often fix these problems.

Mouth

Let's begin our discussion with the mouth. Have you ever given any thought to the nasty taste in your mouth after you awaken from a nap or to the gritty feeling on your teeth every morning? If you're like most people, you probably don't spend too much time thinking about *why* you have morning breath. Instead, chances are, you get up, brush your teeth, and forget about it for the rest of the day — unless you have onions for lunch, but that's a different story...

What's the reason for morning breath? You guessed it! Bacteria! Bacteria grow and flourish in your mouth during the night. Thanks to Crest® and Listerine®, morning breath isn't too hard to fix, but another consequence of bacterial activities — dental caries or cavities — also occurs as a result of bacteria in the mouth. I am reminded of a dental visit I had last year. I consider myself as having relatively good oral hygiene, so I was surprised to find out that I had a cavity in one of my back teeth. Interestingly, when I came home from the dental appointment, I examined my toothbrush. It turns out, after several years of wear and tear, bristles on one edge of my toothbrush had actually been shaved off and completely worn away! The spot where the cavity formed was literally not being brushed at all. As a result, bacteria or "plaque" had, over time, worn away at the tooth causing a cavity.

When you don't take good care of your mouth, bacteria cling to your teeth and form a film known as dental plaque. Plaque can be defined as a complex microbial community which causes tooth decay and cavities. Some 260 different species of bacteria have been cultivated from the mouth of humans. It has been said that "Dental caries [are] the single most common chronic disease of childhood, with a rate five times greater than that seen for...asthma (Becker et al., 2002)."

Although dentists and researchers don't agree about which bacteria actually *cause* cavities, some likely candidates are actinomyces species and *Streptococcus mutans*. Recently, a handful of dental investigators conducted two different clinical trials to evaluate whether probiotics or "healthy" bacteria had any effect on cavity formation. What they found was *Lactobacillus rhamnosus* GG prevented *Streptococcus mutans* from adhering to teeth (Wei et al., 2002) and prevented dental cavities (more details about this in chapter 11) (Nase et al., 2001).

You may be asking, if bacteria *cause* cavities, how can you *prevent* cavities by *giving* bacteria? Well, it seems that *Lactobacillus* GG is a unique species of bacteria and may be able to do this in several ways. First, *Lactobacillus* GG competes with streptococci for binding sites on teeth. Secondly, *Lactobacillus* GG produces antibacterial substances that kill *Streptococci mutans*. Thirdly, *Lactobacillus* GG has an additional biochemical advantage over many other species of bacteria — this species does not use lactose as an energy source. You see, lactose is converted by many bacteria to lactic acid, a relatively strong acid that dissolves tooth enamel. In fact, lactic acid plays a well-documented role in the formation of dental cavities (Becker et al., 2002). So there are at least three very good reasons why *Lactobacillus* GG can prevent cavities rather than cause them. Fortunately, for good oral hygiene, *Lactobacillus* GG can be administered relatively easily — simply by adding bacterial supplements to milk-containing products.

Although *Lactobacillus* GG appears to have positive effects on oral health, it is important to understand that these results are preliminary. However, investigators from two recent clinical trials assert, "The consumption of *Lactobacillus* GG-containing milk might be considered as a new vehicle for improving... oral health" (Nase et al., 2001)".

Overall, the results from these studies point to the importance of having enough "good bacteria" to counteract the harmful effects of the "bad" bacteria, even in the mouth. As I write this, a situation that involved my son several years ago comes to mind. At the time, my two year old son was very sick with a gastrointestinal infection that was not responding to conventional medical therapy. He had been on extremely potent antibiotics for nine months. During the course of his therapy, he developed the worst case of bad breath I have ever encountered. It didn't matter if we brushed his teeth or not, his breath had the stench of a dirty diaper, and he developed a yellow stain on his teeth that wasn't removable with tooth brushing! I took him to several dentists and also asked all the physician specialists that he was seeing, "What is going on? Why does my two-year old have such bad breath?" None of the dentists or doctors had any idea. Interestingly, within 10 days of starting a probiotic and discontinuing the antibiotics, his breath odor cleared up! (And incidentally, I found a dentist who was able to remove the stains from his teeth.) It was an imbalance of normal flora in his mouth that was causing the foul breath smell. So, as you can see, antibiotics disrupt normal flora in the mouth and can contribute to bad breath. Likewise, as shown in results of clinical trials, imbalances in normal mouth flora can also contribute to tooth cavities.

Stomach

Gastric Acid

As we learned in chapter 1, stomach acids are a major line of defense against disease-causing invading microorganisms. When the environment of the stomach is acidic (pH<3.0), bacteria that enter the digestive tract are killed within 15 minutes. This keeps the number of bacteria that survive transit through the stomach at relatively low levels.

Unfortunately, some folks cannot produce adequate amounts of stomach acid. This condition is known as **achlorhydria**. Other folks don't have adequate gastric acid secretion to suppress bacterial growth because they regularly use antacids or other drugs that suppress stomach acids. The obvious question is, if stomach acids are important for eliminating bacterial invaders from the intestine, what happens to gut normal flora when this defense mechanism is no longer in place?

The answer to that question is not completely apparent. However, from isolated studies during the past century, we can presume that there is, at the very least, an increased risk of gastrointestinal infections by bacterial or yeast microorganisms when inadequate amounts of stomach acids are produced. In 1934, a well known British gastroenterologist, Sir Arthur Hurst, stated "Bacillary and amoebic dysentery occur much more commonly in people with achlorhydria" (Sarker and Gyr, 1992). More recently, studies also found that individuals susceptible to *Clostridium difficile* infection of the gut — a bacterial infection that can cause fatal diarrhea — may be susceptible due to inadequate production of stomach acids (Gurian et al., 1982). It is also documented that when stomach acids are neutralized by various prescription or nonprescription medications, there is an increased risk of gastrointestinal infections caused by cholera, *Escherichia coli*, Shigella, *Campylobacter jejuni*, and fungi (Sarker and Gyr, 1992).

Other factors can lower the amount of gastric acid secretion including: fever, aging, and prior surgery. Fevers, or elevated body temperatures, reduce gastric acid secretion. As a result, illnesses with prolonged fevers cause individuals to be more susceptible to bacterial illnesses within the digestive tract. The very process of aging is accompanied by a decline in gastric acid secretion. Studies have found even healthy elderly persons have streptococci, staphylococci, and haemophilus species living in their stomachs (Husebye et al., 1992). Sometimes, surgical removal of part of the stomach also results in low acid production. It is well known that low acid secretion is associated with overgrowth of bacteria, including Bacteroides.

When there is inadequate stomach acid, bacteria flourish instead of being quickly eliminated. Frequently, these bacteria take up permanent residence, irritating lower portions of the digestive tract like the small intestines. This can lead to a situation known as "small bowel overgrowth". Additionally, low gastric acid levels can contribute to **diverticulitis**, which is inflammation in weakened areas of the intestinal tract where pouches form. Low levels of stomach acid secretion allow bacteria to overgrow in stagnant, food-containing diverticular pouches. These bacteria produce large amounts of gas, which causes flatulence and gives the feeling of being bloated. When folks have the feeling of fullness in their stomach, they tend to stop eating. When one stops eating on a chronic basis, malnutrition occurs. Malnutrition associated with diverticulitis can also be a direct result of bacterial overgrowth, since bacteria compete with the human body for nutrients, especially vitamin B12. In these situations, malabsorption also occurs. Unfortunately, from a traditional medical perspective, often the only way to manage these individuals is by rotating various antibiotics to control bacterial flora. However, new research is illustrating that probiotics may correct bacterial imbalances associated with these conditions. Probiotics, for numerous reasons, are a much better long-term solution for controlling bacterial overgrowth since they actually *correct* the problem — that of imbalanced gut bacteria — rather than just *manage the symptoms* as antibiotics do.

H. pylori

Although infections in the stomach are normally uncommon — probably due to the sterilizing activities of normal stomach acids — an important exception exists. *Helicobacter pylori* (*H. pylori*) is a bacterium that has adapted to the gastric environment. During the past two decades, it has become increasingly apparent that *H. pylori* is responsible for most cases of peptic ulcer disease. This bacterium is found in 100% of patients with duodenal ulcers, 70% of patients with gastric ulcers, and up to 30% of children suffering from abdominal pains and vomiting (Sarker and Gyr, 1992). As a result, treatment regimens for peptic ulcer disease now focus upon eliminating *H. pylori*.

There seems to be a correlation between mucus, gastric ulcers, and *H. pylori*. Defects in mucus production have been seen in ulcerated patients. In the stomach, *H. pylori* lives in the mucus layer, close to the epithelial wall. Some investigators have suggested that *H. pylori* is capable of secreting several enzymes and chemicals that destroy the mucus layer; and some researchers have suggested that the bacterium itself may inhibit intestinal mucus secretion. In both experimental animals and human beings, there is also correlation between increased levels of gastrointestinal *H. pylori* and significantly decreased amounts of stomach acid production (Sarker and Gyr, 1992). But, even with these correlations, it has not yet been determined which comes first. Just like the old "chicken and the egg" scenario, which is the *cause* and which is the *effect*? Does *H. pylori* inhibit mucus and stomach acid secretion? Or, does inadequate production of mucus and stomach acid make one more susceptible to infection by *H. pylori*? Further investigations into these areas are needed.

What we do know, from laboratory experiments, is that mice inoculated with *H. pylori* end up with gastric erosions, inflammation, and stomach ulcers. Likewise, most gastrointestinal ulcers in humans heal when *H. pylori* has been eliminated by simultaneous treatment with several potent antibiotics. Of note, when the number of lactobacilli increases in the gastrointestinal tract the number of *H. pylori* decreases (Isogai et al., 1997). These data illustrate two important points. First, we again see the importance of maintaining a balance between "healthy" bacteria and aggressive, disease-causing bacteria. In this case, when the "bad" *H. pylori* bacteria overgrow, gastrointestinal ulcers occur. Secondly, since lactobacilli suppress the growth of *H. pylori*, it may be possible to treat and prevent peptic ulcer disease with probiotics instead of relying upon antibiotics to eliminate this aggressive bacteria from the gastrointestinal tract.

Small Intestines

Peristalsis

One of the most effective mechanisms for ridding the digestive system of unwanted bacterial invaders is the peristaltic movements of the small intestines. Contractions of muscles surrounding the gastrointestinal tract move the contents of the digestive system at a rate of 2.5-3 inches every minute. As a result, this homeostatic mechanism gets rid of microorganisms that managed to escape other barriers higher in the gastrointestinal tract. Sometimes, peristaltic contractions slow down. Under circumstances of slowed gastrointestinal motility, bacterial organisms sometimes overgrow. Drugs, like morphine and other narcotics, as well as various diseases, including diabetes, can slow gastrointestinal motility and permit bacterial overgrowth in the small intestines. For example, in experimental rodents given the drugs atropine or morphine — two drugs that slow gastrointestinal contractions so much that constipation frequently occurs — the balance of gut flora is substantially altered (Isogai et al., 1997; Summers and Kent, 1970). On the other hand, experiments have shown drugs that speed up the gastrointestinal tract reduce bacterial populations in the small intestines (Summers and Kent, 1970).

Altered gastrointestinal motility doesn't just affect bacterial flora in experimental animals. It is well documented to occur in humans also. Often, diabetic individuals suffer from slowed motility and small bowel bacterial overgrowth. Likewise, thermal injury, peritonitis, and ischemia/reperfusion disorders all have the potential to cause bacterial overgrowth in the small bowel (Spitz et al., 1994). Additionally, medications like narcotic pain relievers, atropine-like drugs, or drugs with anticholinergic side effects (dry eyes, dry mouth, fever, constipation, urinary retention) can have constipating side effects due to reduced peristaltic contractions. Any time there is slowed or disordered gastrointestinal movements, bacteria have a tendency to overgrow in the small bowel (Vantrappen et al., 1986; Vantrappen et al., 1977). Although there are normally billions of bacteria in our intestines, when the wrong species overgrow, gastrointestinal infections and painful inflammatory conditions like diverticulitis may result. On the other hand, experimental data shows that probiotics may selectively prevent and alleviate medical conditions associated with small bowel overgrowth (more about this in chapter 11).

Pancreatic dysfunction

Other health problems arise when insufficient amounts of pancreatic enzymes are secreted into the intestines. As you recall from chapter 1, pancreatic enzymes are required for adequate digestion of proteins, sugars, and fats. Normally, we think of these digestive activities as pertaining to dietary foods. However, we also know that pancreatic enzymes degrade bacteria as well. Pancreatic juices protect us from illness by degrading harmful bacterial toxins like cholera toxins. These same pancreatic enzymes also damage the protective outer layer of bacteria and destroy species of *Escherichia coli*, *Klebsiella pneumoniae,* and *Shigella* (Rubenstein et al., 1985; Sarker and Gyr, 1992).

In the absence of sufficient pancreatic secretions, malnutrition can occur. In children that are malnourished, it is not uncommon for the small intestines to experience overgrowth of various bacterial species (Mata et al., 1972). Sometimes this overgrowth causes gastrointestinal diseases, but did you know that allergic illnesses like food allergies and even eczema or asthma also occur when abnormal species of bacteria are permitted to overgrow due to insufficient pancreatic enzymes? Some food allergists report that patients get relief from allergy symptoms when pancreatic enzyme supplements are prescribed (Raithel et al., 2002). I will briefly explain the thought process behind this here, but this topic is covered in much greater detail in chapter 7 where the effects of the immune system are also taken into account.

Normally epithelial cells in the intestines are lined up very tightly, next to one another with minimal space between the cells. The minute spaces between cells are referred to as **tight junctions**. Typically, very few molecules are able to permeate through tight junctions because they are so small in size, only about 5 nanometers in radius (Spitz et al., 1994). How big is that? Only big enough to allow passage of proteins that contain 11 amino acids or fewer. Epithelial cells are like a picket fence. Just like a fence keeps bad people from entering the yard, a major job of the gut's epithelial cells is to protect the body from invaders, preventing undigested dietary components and disease-causing bacteria from entering the body.

Under optimal circumstances, the integrity of the epithelial cell wall remains intact — large, undigested foods and harmful bacteria get eliminated via the feces because they do not breach the security provided by the epithelial cells. The pancreas plays its own security role, too, by secreting pancreatic digestive enzymes that break down food particles into very small pieces. In this way, the combination of the epithelial cell "picket fence" and the pancreatic digestive enzymes act as a security system of sorts, preventing large undigested food particles from crossing the intestinal cell wall and being absorbed into the blood stream. When the system works properly and food particles are broken down into tiny pieces, often into individual amino acids, these may be safely absorbed into the blood stream by fitting through the tight junctions found between individual epithelial cells (See figure 2-1A).

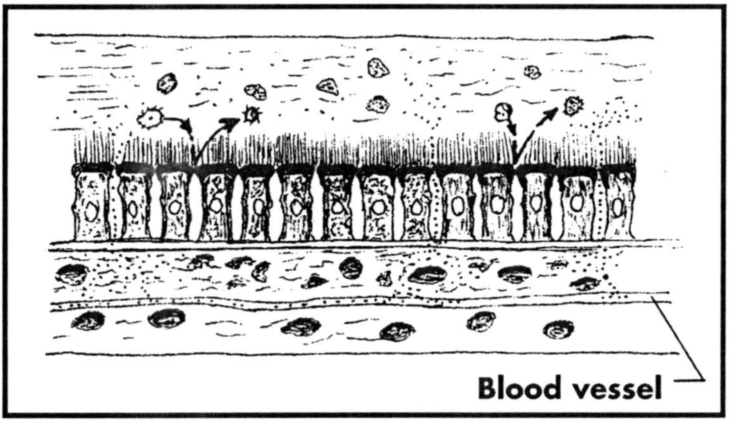

Figure 2-1A. Epithelial cells lining gastrointestinal tract are intact. Note small food particles (represented by small dots) easily pass through tight junctions and are absorbed into blood stream, while large food particles are "repelled" from the intestinal wall and are retained inside the gastrointestinal tract.

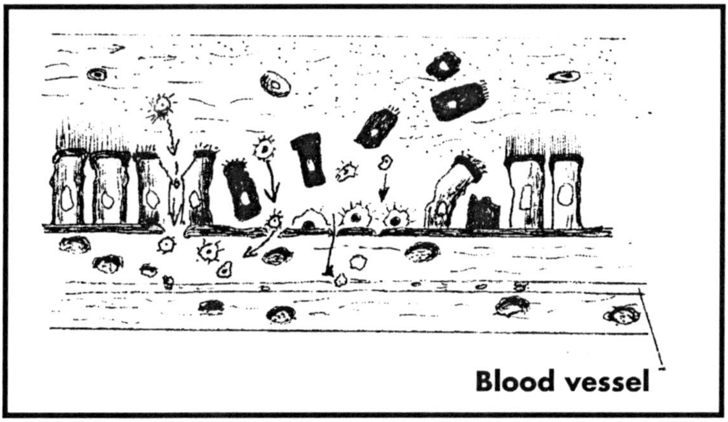

Figure 2-1B. When there is insufficient pancreatic enzyme activity, food particles aren't broken down and bacteria, that otherwise would have been eliminated, survive. When the bacteria overgrow and irritate the epithelial lining of the digestive tract, epithelial cells die. Unfortunately, this compromises the integrity of the epithelial barrier. Now, bacteria can gain access to the blood stream and can cause infections in other parts of the body. Large food particles get absorbed into the blood stream. In blood vessels, the immune system reacts aggressively to food "invaders." Food allergies result.

Now, contrast the optimal scenario described above with a situation where there is a deficit of pancreatic enzymes. With inadequate production of pancreatic enzymes to sufficiently break down food particles and suppress growth of bacteria, a situation known as "small bowel overgrowth" can occur. If the bacteria that are overgrowing are relatively aggressive and harmful in nature, they or their toxins can directly alter the integrity and stability of the epithelial "wall" that normally lines the gut. As a result, epithelial cells begin to die and slough off the intestinal wall more rapidly than they can be replaced. This gives aggressive bacteria or large food particles access to the rest of the body. Now, instead of having a tight security system, the gate to the picket fence is wide open, practically inviting invaders into the house (See figure 2-1B)! This phenomena is commonly referred to as "leaky gut syndrome", because that's exactly what happens. A handful of different factors can impair the integrity of the epithelial tight junctions making them "leaky". The obvious factors worth mentioning here are toxins produced by *Vibrio cholerae*, *Clostridium difficile*, *Escherichia coli*, and other disease-causing bacteria. Some chemicals that direct activities of the immune system, called **cytokines**, can also decrease the barrier function of the tight junctions (Groot, 1998; Clinicians, see this paper for an excellent review of transport functions in the intestinal epithelium). Leaky tight junctions cause diarrhea and can lead to allergies. Read on to find out how.

Via a "leaky gut", not only can bacteria themselves begin to invade and potentially cause infection throughout the body, but smaller security violations can also occur. Since a pancreatic deficiency is the underlying factor for this scenario, food particles are not getting degraded as well as they should be. Now, through the "leaks" due to lost epithelial cells, large proteins get absorbed into the blood stream. The problem is, once in the blood stream, the body's immune system doesn't recognize the invaders as friendly! The immune system isn't accustomed to seeing such large proteins — it is used to very small proteins or simple amino acids only. In response to what the immune system perceives as an invasion, an attack is mounted. Immune cells and antibodies are sent out to inactivate and neutralize the invaders. Widespread activation of the immune system can lead to inflammation, severe allergies, asthma, eczema, and even a life-threatening allergic response known as **anaphylaxis**.

For decades, there has been a consistent association between pancreatic insufficiency and allergic diseases. Likewise, there is a consistent correlation between abnormal gut flora and allergic diseases. As investigators learn more, it is becoming increasing apparent that there may be two ways to prevent or treat some allergic diseases: use pancreatic enzyme supplements and/or repopulate the digestive tract with "gastrointestinal tract-friendly" bacteria using probiotics (more on these topics in chapter 8).

Role of IgA Antibodies

As I alluded to earlier, breakdown of the intestinal barrier by agents that cause inflammation, like bacteria or bacterial toxins, can cause disordered inflammation throughout the entire body. Indeed, increased intestinal "leakiness" has been associated with failure of numerous organs, trauma, severe infections, and even death. Under normal conditions, the majority of bacteria living in our intestines completely lack contact with gut epithelial cells due to coordinated efforts of mucus, peristalsis, and IgA antibodies that line the inside of our intestines. The main job of IgA is to coat bacteria and prevent bacteria from adhering to epithelial cells. Unfortunately, some individuals are genetically deficient in IgA. Those who have an IgA deficiency are susceptible to gut-derived sepsis — that is they have an increased tendency of suffering from bacterial infections in their blood — infections caused by bacteria that originated in their own intestines, but gained access to other parts of the body through a deficient "mucosal barrier" (Spitz et al., 1994). Some immunosuppressant drugs like prednisone or dexamethasone can also decrease IgA levels, increasing the likelihood of increased intestinal "leakiness" and all the associated complications that go along with it.

Colon

Of course, by now you are beginning to gain an appreciation of the enormously complex ecosystem of gut bacteria. The roles of normal intestinal flora as they are beginning to be understood, were discussed in the previous chapter. Obviously, then, if the balance between the various species living in the gut is altered in any way and shifted out of balance, disease can result. How does gut flora get thrown out of balance? Well, it can occur in a variety of ways. Most commonly there is either (a) a history of antibiotic use that disrupted the delicate balance of intestinal flora or (b) the presence of too few "healthy" gut bacteria allowing "aggressive, disease-causing" bacteria to overpopulate the intestines.

There is considerable evidence that links lesser-than-optimal levels of gut bacterial flora with an increased susceptibility to infections. This has been demonstrated in experimental situations where mice become substantially more susceptible to *Salmonella* infections when their gut flora has been wiped out by antibiotics (Bohnhoff et al., 1964). Elimination of certain microorganisms, like Bacteroides, for example, causes animals to be more susceptible to gut bacterial infections. In human tourists, use of antibiotics did not prevent infection with *Salmonella* because the antibiotics wiped out many species of normal gut flora that would otherwise have kept *Salmonella* in check (Mentzing and Ringertz, 1968). These results suggest that, at times, antibiotics may do more harm than good.

The most obvious signs and symptoms of imbalanced gut flora in the colon are diarrhea, inflammation, and abdominal pain. In fact, it is estimated that intestinal infections cause four billion cases of diarrhea each year, and diarrhea is responsible for 3-4 million deaths annually. Many different factors can cause diarrheal disturbances in the colon, and I won't go into detail here since we will cover the topic of diarrhea at great length in chapter 5. However, clinicians should be aware that diarrhea is certainly not the only manifestation of an imbalanced gut normal flora. Other signs and symptoms of gastrointestinal **dysbiosis** may also be apparent, especially if the condition has not been adequately treated and persists for long periods of time. Dehydration, electrolyte imbalances (leading to heart problems), blood or mucus in the stools, malnutrition or anemia can all result from untreated gastrointestinal disturbances and can lead to life-threatening complications.

You may be wondering at this point *how* exactly does altered bacterial gut flora cause diarrhea and inflammation? With the billions of bacteria that live in the large intestines, how do the intestines know that there is an imbalance of bacterial species? When there is an imbalance between "healthy" bacteria and "aggressive" species, the harmful bacteria or their toxins can cause diarrhea in several ways. Although the details by which various bacterial species cause diarrhea differ, the end result is the same: water is lost from the body, pulled into the intestines, and eliminated from the body in the form of diarrhea.

As our first example, I will describe how some bacterial toxins, like those of *Vibrio cholerae* and *Escherichia coli* activate intestinal secretory mechanisms in epithelial cells. Keep in mind that under ideal circumstances these microorganisms would have already been destroyed before they reached the large intestines — or — their growth and activities would be held in check by other species of bacteria. But, when *Vibrio cholerae* or certain subspecies of *Escherichia coli* are growing and proliferating aggressively in the large intestines, they release toxins. These toxins bind to a specific protein site (known as a **receptor**) on epithelial cells. Binding to this receptor activates a cascade of chemical "messengers" inside epithelial cells, triggering specific channels to open on the intestinal wall (Farthing, 2002). The channels that open conduct chloride ions. When chloride channels are open, chloride ions (Cl^-) leave epithelial cells and move into the **lumen** of the intestines. As you may recall from high school chemistry class, chloride has a negative charge associated with it. In order to remain electrically neutral, sodium ions (Na^+) also begin to leak out of the epithelial cells into the lumen of the intestine to combine with the chloride ions. The combination of Na^+ with Cl^- leads to NaCl, which many of us recognize as regular, old table salt!

$$Na^+ + Cl^- \leftrightarrow NaCl \text{ (table salt)}$$

Salt, of course, has a high capacity to absorb water, so elevated salt concentrations in our intestines, pull water out of our bodies and into our intestines. Thus, as a result of bacterial toxins binding to the intestinal wall, large amounts of water are lost by the body — in the form of diarrhea (See figure 2-2).

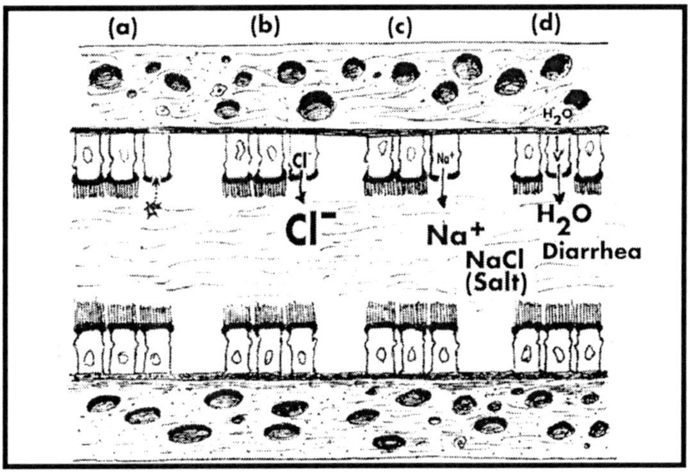

Figure 2-2. (a) Bacterial toxins bind to chloride channels (or pores) on epithelial cells. (b) The toxins cause the channels to open, allowing chloride ions to leak into the gut. (c) Sodium also begins leaking out of cells, into the gut, in order to "neutralize" chloride. The combination of sodium with chloride forms salt. (d) Salt absorbs water, so water gets "pulled" out of the body into the intestines, causing diarrhea.

Another way an imbalance of gut bacteria or **dysbiosis** causes diarrhea is by altering protein synthesis mechanisms inside intestinal epithelial cells. Depending upon the type of protein that is either (a) no longer being manufactured or (b) being made in excess, diarrhea can result. Different types of bacteria can alter protein synthesis in different ways. One type of toxin, termed a Shiga toxin, is produced by the bacterium *Shigella dysenteriae*. Shiga toxins bind to **ribosomes** inside intestinal epithelial cells. Ribosomes are **organelles** located inside epithelial cells, whose primary job is to make proteins. When Shiga toxins bind to ribosomes, all protein synthesis inside the cells comes to a screeching halt, leading to death of the cells that line the intestinal tract. When the epithelial cells die, fluids begin to be lost from the body, and ultimately diarrhea occurs. On the other hand, a toxin from another species of bacteria — staphylococci — causes diarrhea by *increasing* protein synthesis — especially synthesis of pro-inflammatory chemicals like **interferon-γ**. As we will see in the next chapter, there are different types of interferons; these small molecules are important chemicals that act as communication mechanisms between gut bacteria and the human immune system. In this example, streptococci stimulates synthesis of interferon-γ, a chemical that causes inflammation in the gut. Gut inflammation causes epithelial cells to die, and again, body fluids are lost into the intestines and diarrhea results.

A growing number of other bacteria like *Clostridium difficile, Escherichia coli*, or *Bacteroides fragilis* are now recognized as producing toxins that alter the cytoskeletal system within epithelial cells. The **cytoskeleton** can be thought of as a scaffold or structural support system inside epithelial cells. It is made up of various proteins whose jobs are varied. Some of the most important roles played by the cytoskeleton — at least as far as our discussion is concerned are: (1) maintaining cell shape (2) promoting adhesion to the basement membrane (3) and maintaining tight junctions between cells. *Clostridium difficile, Escherichia coli*, and *Bacteroides fragils* all secrete toxins that ultimately inactivate specific enzymes that regulate cytoskeletal functions (these enzymes are part of a large family of proteins known as Rho GTPases). When the cytoskeleton of epithelial cells breaks down, the cells lose their characteristic shape, round up, and die. Understandably, as cells die, the tight junctions normally found between cells are disrupted. The intestinal wall becomes "leaky" and body fluids are lost into the intestines. Diarrhea is the obvious result (Fasano et al., 2002; for a great review and more details, clinicians can refer to Sears, 2002). This "gut leakiness" is also referred to as "increased gastrointestinal permeability".

Gastrointestinal permeability is increased in folks that have certain diseases of the colon, including Crohn's disease. This has led to the "increased permeability hypothesis" of Crohn's disease — that is, increased intestinal permeability *precedes the onset of Crohn's disease* and increased intestinal permeability *triggers reactivation of inactive Crohn's disease.* The relationship between intestinal permeability and Crohn's disease has been documented in several studies (Irvine and Marshall, 2000; Arnott et al., 2000; D'Inca et al., 1999; Wyatt et al., 1993). Since an imbalance of gut flora/infectious bacteria increases intestinal permeability and since those with Crohn's disease suffer from increased gastrointestinal permeability, there is reason to suspect that individuals with altered bacterial flora may be more likely to suffer from Crohn's disease. Alternatively, individuals afflicted by Crohn's disease may find relief by ingesting healthy bacteria that correct the underlying gut bacterial dysbiosis. Some researchers have specifically suggested that individuals with Crohn's disease may have "gastrointestinal leakiness" due to the presence of harmful bacteria secreting enzymes that degrade the protective mucus layers in the gut (Quigley and Kelly, 1995). We will discuss four different dysbiosis theories of Crohn's disease in chapter 6.

In the preceding paragraphs, I've used Crohn's disease as one example of a medical condition that arises from a dysbiosis of gut bacteria. However, certainly, Crohn's disease does not stand alone in this respect. Another example of an inflammatory bowel condition that causes diarrhea is seen in patients with a prior history of ulcerative colitis who have had the diseased portion of their intestines removed. Unfortunately, in about 50% of these people, inflammation reoccurs, this time within an area termed the ileal pouch, a condition termed **pouchitis**. In addition to diarrhea and fecal incontinence, pouchitis also causes rectal bleeding, abdominal cramping, a low fever, and joint pains to occur. Traditionally, treatments for pouchitis have relied mostly upon anti-inflammatory agents like steroids to prevent inflammation or antibiotics to suppress activities of "bad" bacteria. The beneficial effects that occur from antibiotic treatments point a direct finger to bacterial dysbiosis as the underlying cause for the inflammation seen in pouchitis. In fact, recent studies indicate that when the gut flora imbalance is corrected by treatment with "healthy" gut bacteria (probiotics), the signs and symptoms of pouchitis are alleviated (see chapter 6 for more details).

Conclusion

To summarize, in this chapter we have learned that sometimes things don't go quite the way they should within the digestive system. When this happens, illness or medical conditions can result. Interestingly, sometimes, these illnesses aren't just limited to the gastrointestinal tract, but can also involve other parts of the body (ie. allergies, eczema, etc.).

You can remember the bottom line of this chapter in terms of offense and defense. Whenever activities of offensive, harmful bacteria overshadow the defensive factors like stomach acids, mucus, pancreatic secretions, and peristaltic actions, there is potential for disease or illness. In the next two chapters, we will learn how gut bacteria communicate with our immune systems to "program" our immune systems for appropriate responses throughout our entire lives. We will also consider how bacterial dysbiosis, especially early in life, leads to inappropriate immunological "programming" and contributes to diseases like allergies and inflammatory bowel disease.

Notes

Notes

References

Arnott ID, Kingstone K, Ghosh S. Abnormal intestinal permeability predicts relapse in inactive Crohns disease. Scand J gastroenterol. 2000;35:1163-1169.

Becker MR, Paster BJ, Leys EJ, et al. Molecular analysis of bacterial species associated with childhood caries. J Clin Microbiol. 2002;40:1001-1009.

D'Inca R, Di Leo V, Corrao G, et al. Intestinal permeability test as a predictor of clinical course in Crohn's disease. Am J Gastroenterol. 1999;94:2956-2960.

Farthing MJG. Novel targets for the control of secretory diarrhoea. Gut. 2002;50:III15-18.

Fasano A. Toxins and the gut: Role in human disease. Gut. 2002;50:III9-III14.

Groot JA. Correlation between electrophysiological phenomena and transport of macromolecules in intestinal epithelium. Vet Q. 1998;20 Suppl 3:S45-49.

Gurian L, Ward TT, Maton RM. Possible food borne transmission in a case of pseudomembranous colitis due to *Clostridium difficile*. Influence of gastrointestinal secretions on *Clostridium difficile* infection. Gastroenterology. 1982;83:465-469.

Hohnhoff M, Miller P, Martin WR. Resistance of the mouse's intestinal tract to experimental Salmonella infection. J Exp Med. 1964;120:805-816.

Huseby E, Skar V, Hoverstad T, et al. Fasting hypochlorhydria with Gram positive gastric flora is highly prevalent in healthy old people. Gut. 1992;33:1331-1337.

Irvine EJ and Marshall JK. Increased intestinal permeability precedes relapse in inactive Crohn's disease in a subject with familial risk. Gastroenterol. 2000;119:1740-1744.

Isogai H, Isogai E, Hayashi S, et al. Experimental *Helicobacter pylori* infection in association with other bacteria. Microbiol Immunol. 1997;41:361-365.

Matta LJ, Jimenez F, Cordon M, et al. Gastrointestinal flora of children with protein-calorie malnutrition. Am J Clin Nutr. 1972:25:1118-1126.

Mentzing LO and Ringertz O. Salmonella infection in tourists. Prophylaxis against Salmonellosis. Acta Path. Microbiol. Scandinav. 1968;74:405-413.

Nase L, Hatakka K, Savilaht E, et al. Effect of Long-Term Consumption of a Probiotic Bacterium, *Lactobacillus rhamnosus* GG, in Milk on Dental Caries and Caries Risk in Children. Caries Res. 2001; 35:412-420.

Quigley ME and Kelly SM. Structure, Function, and Metabolism of Host Mucus Glycoproteins. In: Gibson CR and MacFarlance GT, eds. Human colonic bacteria: Role in nutrition, physiology, and pathology. CRC Press, Boca Raton, FL, 1995.

Raithel M, Weidenhiller M, Schwab D. Pancreatic enzymes: A new group of antiallergic drugs? Inflamm Res. 2002;51:S13-S14.

Rubinstein E, Mark Z, Haspel J, et al. Antibacterial activity of pancreatic fluid. Gastroenterology. 1985;88:926-32.

Sarker SA and Gyr K. Non-immunological defence mechanisms of the gut. Gut. 1992;33:987-993.

Sears CL. Molecular physiology and pathophysiology of tight junctions. Assault of the tight junction by enteric pathogens. Am J Physiol Gastrointest Liver Physiol. 2000;279:G1127-G1134.

Spitz J, Hecht G, Taveras M, et al. The effect of dexamethasone administration on rat intestinal permeability: The role of bacterial adherence. Gastroenterology. 1994;106:35-41.

Summers RW and Kent TH. Effects of altered propulsion on rat small intestinal flora. Gastroenterol. 1970;59:740-744.

Vantrappen G, Janssens J, Coremans G, et al. Gastrointestinal motility disorders. Dig Dis Sci. 1986;31:5S-25S.

Vantrappen G, Janssens J, Hellemans J, et al. The interdigestive motor complex of normal subjects and patients with bacterial overgrowth of the small intestine. J Clin Investig. 1977;59:1158-116.

Wei H, Loimaranta V, Tenovuo J, et al. Stability and activity of specific antibodies against *Streptococcus mutans* and *Streptococcus sobrinus* in bovine milk fermented with *Lactobacillus rhamnosus* strain GG or treated at ultra-high temperature. Oral Microbiol Immunol. 2002; 17:9-15.

Wyatt J, Vogelsang H, Hubi W, et al. Intestinal permeability and the prediction of relapse in Crohn's disease. Lancet. 1993;341:1437-1439.

Chapter 3

Bacterial Instant Messaging
The Gut as an Immune Organ

The gut as an immune organ...now, that's an interesting thought! When we think about "immunity", we are all familiar with vaccinations for infants and the tetanus shot we get when we step on a rusty nail. But, what does the gut, the body's garbage can for food, body waste, and bacteria have to do with conferring immunity to disease? And what happens when it fails to do its job appropriately? These are some of the things we will be exploring in the next two chapters.

Within the past few decades, there has been a dramatic increase in immune-related medical conditions. The incidence of allergies (food allergies, topical eczema, asthma, allergic rhinitis), autoimmune disorders (diabetes, arthritis), and inflammatory diseases (Crohn's disease, ulcerative colitis) has exploded in Western societies during the past 50 years. In fact, researchers speculate that one out of every three children born in industrialized countries will develop an allergic disorder (Alm et al., 1999). While genetics certainly plays a part in most diseases, the dramatic increase in allergic and inflammatory disorders since the late 1950s suggests other risk factors must play a significant role. Most researchers believe environmental factors are probably involved. Two big environmental differences distinguishing today's Western society from societies of the past involve (1) improvements in hygienic standards and (2) unbalanced nutrition due to fast foods and harried lifestyles. Most of our discussion in this and the subsequent chapter will concern the way in which these factors contribute to the increase in allergic and inflammatory diseases, focusing on the role the gastrointestinal tract plays as an immune organ.

Do Diet and Nutrition Play a Role in Allergies and Inflammation?

Compared to the previous 5,000 years of civilization, there has been a dramatic change in hygiene during the past 60 years. Data gathered during the last decade from cultures that are less concerned about "germs" than we are in the Western world illustrate, without a doubt, that those who reserve the use of antibiotics to life-threatening infections only, those who refuse vaccinations, and those who eat diets of fermented vegetables and organic foods have dramatically fewer allergic disorders than the rest of the modernized world (Alm et al., 1999). This indicates that *exposure* to various types of bacteria — through dietary sources and by actually getting sick and letting the immune system do its job — makes a dramatic impact on the development of allergic diseases.

Contrast the life style just described above with the way most of us live in the Western world. Take a moment to consider all the ways we avoid exposure to bacteria: antimicrobial soaps to reduce normal bacterial flora on our skin, vaccinations to minimize the many infections to which we are exposed, antibiotic drugs to compensate for the immune responses that our bodies would otherwise mount against disease-causing invaders.

Think also about the ways nutritional practices have changed. In the not-too-distant past, the human diet contained several thousand-fold more bacteria than it does today. This is because, in the past, more fermented and dried foods were consumed. Most of us probably catch our meals on the run or eat pre-packaged, sterilized foods as opposed to eating fresh or fermented organic meats, fruits, and vegetables. Our diets today don't contain anywhere near the amount of bacteria that our parents' or grandparents' diets did. It is likely that these two components — hygiene and nutrition — may be responsible for a decline in immune stimulation or lack of "priming" within the immune system early in life.

For thousands of years, our bodies have cohabited perfectly well with bacteria, especially the bacteria in our gastrointestinal tracts. In fact, the bacteria that live in our digestive system provide important cues to the immune system, and when those cues are gone or disrupted, the immune system responds in an unpredictable fashion. Lack of "priming" or lack of immune system stimulation, especially during infancy and early childhood may disrupt the way that the digestive and immune systems "view" disease-causing bacteria. These disruptions may contribute to illnesses later in life. Indeed, several studies now support the idea that *normal gut flora is the most important source of immune stimulation*, providing all the signals needed for the immune system to mature in a healthy fashion.

Yes, the idea that the gastrointestinal tract is not only a digestive organ, but also an immune organ surprises many folks. In fact, most are unaware that the gastrointestinal tract is the *largest* immune organ in the body. The gut provides immunological surveillance signals at the **mucosa-lumen** interface of the digestive tract. These mechanisms, while not well understood, are essential for ensuring that appropriate reactions are made against disease-causing substances, while, at the same time, tolerating normal foods and normal intestinal flora — a process referred to as "**oral tolerance**". The cells of the immune system and the epithelial cells that line the intestinal wall communicate information regarding colonizing bacteria. As we currently understand it, interactions of gut bacterial flora with epithelial and immune cells regulate immune development. Furthermore, *normal gut bacteria acquired in infancy are likely to be the most important determinants of allergies and diseases of chronic inflammation later in life.* As a result, we need to assure that healthy gut flora is acquired early in life so that the immune system matures properly in order to avoid passing down a life-time of allergic and inflammatory diseases to our children.

Basic Immunological Principles

Before we begin talking about the role of the digestive tract as an immune organ, we need to introduce some of the basic players within the immune system. **Immunology** — the study of the immune system — is still a relatively new science. In the late 18th century, Edward Jenner discovered that inoculation of humans with cowpox — a process he called *vaccination* — provided protection against human smallpox, an often deadly disease. Although Jenner's experiment was successful, vaccination was not widely accepted for two more centuries. It wasn't until the late 19th century, when Robert Koch proved that infectious diseases were caused by microorganisms — each microorganism responsible for a different disease, that vaccination became a standard practice.

The small steps forward in immunology, pioneered by Jenner and Koch, led researchers to search for the *mechanisms* by which we are protected against disease. In 1890, substances called **antibodies** (or **immunoglobulins**, often abbreviated as **Ig**) were discovered in the blood of vaccinated individuals. Antibodies are specific molecules that bind and neutralize invading substances and assist scavenger cells in destruction of "foreign substances". (Scavenger cells destroy microorganisms by a process known as **phagocytosis**.) There are five distinct types of antibodies with specialized functions: IgM, IgG, IgA, IgE, and IgD. In general terms, IgM protects the blood stream, IgG protects the blood stream and tissues, IgA protects the gut, and IgE is involved in causing allergic responses, but the function of IgD is unknown. Of course, this is tremendously oversimplified, but if it helps you to recall their activities, remember this acronym: IgG — good; IgE — evil.

Antibodies were identified largely as a result of the discovery of **macrophages**, specific **phagocytic** cells that engulf and digest bacteria and other "foreign" molecules. By binding to foreign materials, antibodies assist macrophages in eliminating invading substances.

After their discovery, it soon became apparent that antibodies are produced against a wide range of substances. Any substance that stimulates the production of antibodies is now referred to as an **antigen**. In the 1960s, James Gowans identified **lymphocytes**, white blood cells that play a role in stimulating immune responses. Lymphocytes can be broadly broken down into two different types: **B lymphocytes** which produce antibodies and **T lymphocytes** which either kill bacteria, activate other immune cells, or both. T lymphocytes are further characterized on the basis of their specific functions or by virtue of the chemicals they secrete. It is these chemical mediators — known as **cytokines** — that "communicate" with the epithelial cells of the gut, a process known as "cross-talk".

Cytokines are small molecules, found in miniscule concentrations in our blood stream, that affect the behavior of other cells, especially, cells of the gut and immune system. It appears that the immune system — especially allergic and inflammatory components of the immune system -- rely heavily on signals from cytokines. Cytokines are divided into several different families which are sometimes referred to as **interleukins** (abbreviated as **IL**), **interferons** (abbreviated as **IFN**), or tumor necrosis factors (abbreviated as TNF). There are many different types of cytokines and their names get very confusing. Although I will describe, in general terms, some of the cytokines and their activities, it is important to remember that *it is this group of chemicals that allow bacteria in the gastrointestinal tract to communicate with our immune systems*.

When bacteria are present as part of the gut's normal flora, the very presence of the bacteria stimulates white blood cells and epithelial cells to secrete cytokines. These cytokines, then, serve as signals to other components of the immune system. Cytokines can send allergic signals, inflammatory signals, or anti-allergy/anti-inflammatory signals. The type of signal that is transmitted depends upon the type of bacteria present; different species of bacteria stimulate release of different cytokines. As you are probably beginning to see, the bacteria in our gastrointestinal tract play an important role in determining the actions of the entire immune system.

In very broad terms, the actions of cytokines can be broken down into different groups: Th1 and Th2. Th1 cytokines are produced by Type-1 helper T lymphocytes, while Th2 cytokines are manufactured by Type-2 helper T lymphocytes. Examples of specific Th1 cytokines are IL-2, interferon-γ (IFN-γ), IL-12, and tumor necrosis factor-β (TNF-β). In general, we often refer to Th1 cytokines as stimulators of inflammation.

On the other hand, we often refer to Th2 cytokines as those responsible for causing allergies. Examples of Th2 cytokines include IL-4, IL-5, IL-6, IL-10, and IL-13. By the way, these aren't nearly ALL the cytokines, just a representative handful. Nor is the entire immune process nearly as cut and dried as I've made it sound. For example, there is no such thing as a "good" or "bad" cytokine. We need them all. Rather, it is the *balance of cytokines* that controls initiation of allergies/inflammation, perpetuation of allergies/inflammation, or the cessation of allergies/inflammation (Henderson, 1996). However, for our purposes, to keep things as simple as possible, we will mostly consider Th1 cytokines as being "pro-inflammatory" and Th2 cytokines as "pro-allergic" (See figure 3-1). Just remember, this is a blatant oversimplification. But, we need to keep things as simple as we can since there are more than 35 different cytokines; and just to keep things interesting, many of them go by more than one name!

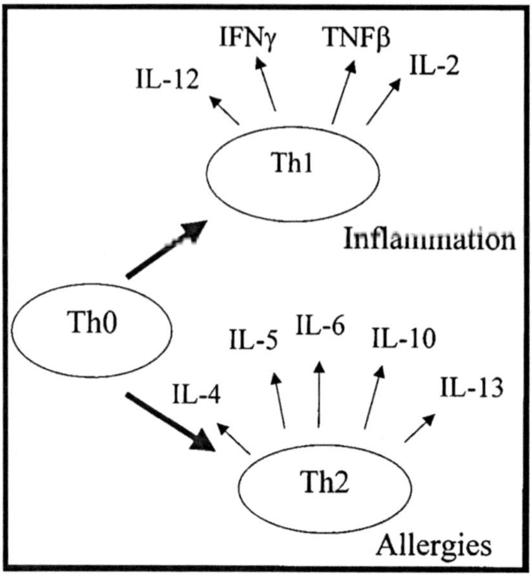

Figure 3-1. Type-0 helper lymphocytes differentiate into either Type-1 helper lymphocytes (Th1) or Type-2 helper lymphocytes (Th2). Early differentiation in infancy is largely controlled by the specific types of bacteria that are present in the gastrointestinal tract as part of the normal flora. Th2 cells tend to secrete cytokines that are inflammatory in nature, while Th1 cells secrete cytokines that favor allergies. Just to reiterate, the KEY point here is to understand that it is the *type* of bacteria in the gut that influences which cytokines are secreted. These cytokines are "communication signals" between gut bacteria and our immune systems. The *balance* and *type* of cytokines released in response to gut bacteria determine whether you are healthy, whether you have allergic tendencies, or whether your body has a tendency toward inflammatory diseases.

The reason for mentioning these cytokines will be more apparent in later chapters when we talk about inflammatory bowel disease and allergies. Pro-inflammatory cytokines are thought to underlie certain kinds of inflammatory bowel disease, while pro-allergic cytokines are involved with various allergic disorders. Interestingly, as we will discuss, particular strains of probiotic bacteria modify cytokine production. In this way, probiotics can be useful treatments for these conditions.

Understandably, for optimal health, there is a fine balance between Th1 and Th2 cytokines. Too many Th1 cytokines can perpetuate inflammatory conditions, while Th2 cytokines, when left unchecked, can lead to a variety of allergies. At birth, helper T-lymphocytes have not yet been assigned to a specific fate – meaning, there is neither Th1 nor Th2 predominance; instead, initially, the helper cells are called T0-helper cells. The *presence of gut flora* — specifically the types of bacterial species in the gut — is an important determinant of whether T0-helper cells differentiate into Th1-dominated responses or Th2-dominated responses. In infancy, there is a natural shift in favor of Th2 cytokine production. This may account for the tendency to acquire allergic diseases early in life. On the other hand, inflammatory bowel diseases are associated with increased production of Th1 cytokines.

How do bacteria stimulate our immune systems to release cytokines? Bacteria do this in a number of ways. Some bacteria produce specific chemical or protein molecules — molecules that are either part of the bacterial cell wall or secreted by the bacteria. These bacterial molecules bind directly to cells of the gut's immune tissues and either stimulate release of pro-inflammatory or anti-inflammatory cytokines, depending upon the bacterial species (Henderson et al., 1996). For example, toxins secreted by infectious bacteria (*Escherichia coli, Staphylococcus aureus, Clostridium difficile, Streptococcus pyogenes, Pseudomonas aeruginosa*, etc.) stimulate our gut's immune systems to release inflammatory cytokines. On the other hand, presence of other bacterial species, (including *Yersinia enterocolitica, Actinobacillus actinomycetemcomitans)* actually inhibits the actions of inflammatory cytokines.

Cytokines can also bind directly to bacteria and influence the bacteria's behavior. For example, TNF-α inhibits growth of *Legionella pneumophila;* and growth of *Brucella abortus* is blocked by the cytokines IL-2 and IFN-γ. On the other hand, growth of certain strains of *Escherichia coli* is stimulated by another cytokine, IL-1.

Any time bacteria and the cells of the gut's immune system are in close contact with one another, it can be assumed that they are communicating (Henderson et al., 1996). Since there are at least 10 times more bacteria in your body than human cells — you can be sure that your bacterial flora is *actively* communicating important immunological information at all times. This information is received, translated, and acted upon by a very complicated network of cytokine signalling molecules. It is the information received by bacterial communication that ultimately governs the responses of the immune system.

How the Gut Gets Involved in Immunity

The gut immune system

Admittedly, the gut's involvement in immunity is complex. Even the most renown scientists and learned physicians do not pretend to understand how all the pieces of the immune system puzzle fit together. Within the intestine, 25% of the intestinal epithelium is made up of the **gut-associated lymphoid tissues**, or **GALT** for short. Just like the network of blood vessels that transport blood throughout the body, there is also a network of lymph nodes and lymph vessels that transport water, electrolytes, and proteins from tissue fluids into the blood stream. Lymphoid tissues are the primary location where **antigens** are handed over to immune cells.

Any substance that the body regards as foreign and potentially dangerous is considered an antigen — this includes food particles, bacteria, bacterial toxins, viruses, etc. — essentially *anything* may be viewed by the immune system as an antigen. Normally, only truly harmful substances are viewed by the immune system as antigens. However, occasionally the immune system reacts inappropriately — it sees a particular substance as harmful when in actuality it does not pose a threat. Sometimes, for example, the immune system views a food substance as an allergen. The immune system mounts an attack against that particular food. As a result, a food allergy occurs. Sometimes the immune system even mounts a response against part of the body. When this happens, autoimmune illnesses like myasthenia gravis, lupus, or multiple sclerosis may result. On the other hand, the immune system may also act inappropriately by learning to "tolerate" a substance or disease-causing invader, when, in fact, the substance is extremely harmful and can cause disease.

The GALT are an important first line of defense against bacterial infections and food allergies. Various cells are involved with controlling the actions of GALT, including the epithelial cells that line the inside of the intestines, the connective layers of tissues lying beneath the gut epithelium, and various types of white blood cells including antibody-secreting cells. The cells of the GALT interact and communicate with each other in a coordinated fashion — conveying messages about bacteria encountered in the gut — to produce immune responses that affect the entire body.

As discussed in chapter 1, intestinal epithelial cells not only provide a barrier to prevent harmful bacteria from leaving the gut, they also secrete mucus. Mucus acts as a filter to prevent excessive diffusion of large molecules, but also prevents bacteria from attaching directly to the walls of the intestine. Large particles or bacteria that penetrate through the mucus-lined epithelial cells find themselves taken up by specialized lymph-associated epithelial cells — collectively known as **Peyer's Patches**. In the areas underlying Peyer's Patches are loose connective tissues — called **lamina propria** (See figure 3-2). This area is rich in blood vessels and specialized white blood cells (called CD4+ and CD8+ cells) that protect our bodies from would-be foreign invaders. Other cells types found in the lamina propria are bone marrow-like cells, nerve cells (dendrocytes), and inflammatory cells (mast cells). All of these different cell types are involved one way or another with recognizing and eliminating foreign invaders (Cebra, 1999). Collectively, these three compartments — epithelial cells, Peyer's patches, and lamina propria — make up most of the immune tissues within the gut.

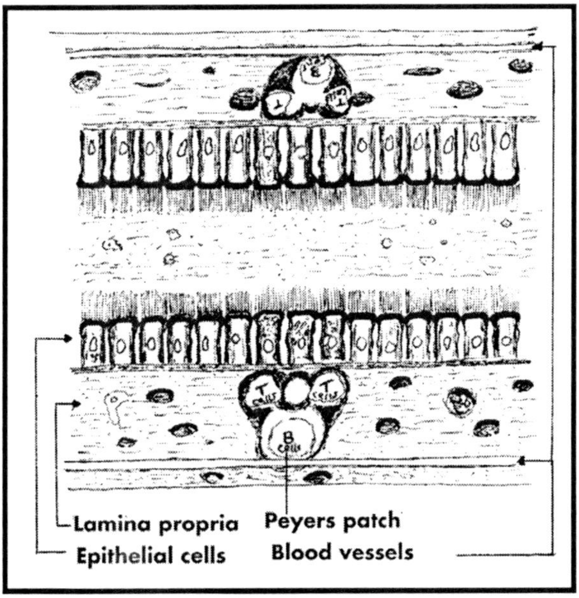

Figure 3-2. Epithelial cells rest on a basement membrane. Periodically, underneath epithelial cells, Peyer's Patches can be found. Peyer's Patches are rich in white blood cells, containing many B cells (antibody cells) and T cells that inactivate "invaders" if they penetrate through the epithelial barrier. The spongy lamina propria also contains many different cell types, including specialized immune system cells that react against foreign "invaders" whenever necessary.

Within the gut, another line of immunological defense against disease-causing bacteria is carried out by IgA-type antibodies. IgA antibodies bind directly to bacteria, preventing microorganisms from attaching to the walls of the intestine. In fact, we've learned from experiments that gut flora is absolutely *necessary* for IgA antibody cells to mature. The dramatic influence that intestinal bacteria have over the immune system is best described by comparing germ-free mice — mice that literally live in a bubble and have never been exposed to bacteria (similar to the famous "bubble-boy") — with conventional mice. Realize, of course, that germ-free mice have no gut flora. In these types of comparisons, it is apparent that the presence of digestive flora — especially *E. coli* and *Bacteroides* —are *essential* for appropriate immune function. Without their presence in the gut flora, the appropriate cytokine signalling messages don't get conveyed to our immune systems, placing us at risk of disease.

Not only is gut flora required for the maturing of IgA-secreting cells, but normal gut flora is also responsible for activating macrophages — the scavenger white blood cells that protect us from disease. Additionally, digestive flora stimulates epithelial cell growth within the gut and plays a role in the production of various cytokines (Moreau and Coste, 1993). Remember, *cytokines produced by GALT, in response to gut bacteria, are the major determinants of normal immune function versus "allergic" or "inflammatory" immune states.* So, "normal" bacterial flora is not just *involved* in immune activities, it is *absolutely required* for developing healthy immune responses.

Controlled Inflammation

Now that we understand all the components of the gut's immune system, let's discuss how all the pieces of the puzzle fit together, while also considering how normal gut flora fits into the picture.

In the intestines, immune cells are always on a heightened state of alert. Compared to immune cells in other parts of the body, various types of white blood cells — CD4+ cells, CD8+ cells and natural killer cells — never "rest". They are always at a pre-primed or activated state because they are always in contact with bacteria. This heightened state of immune activation results in *controlled inflammation* — a low level of inflammation within the gut — and this inflammation is believed to be necessary for healthy interactions at the mucosal barrier. Colonization of the gut by normal gut bacteria increases the number of white blood cells in the intestinal lymph tissues that are on a heightened state of alert. Therefore, normal flora is essential for controlled inflammation in the gut.

Under normal circumstances, when CD4+ white blood cells in the gut encounter bacteria, they respond by secreting cytokine chemical messengers like IL-12, IL-2, and IFN-γ. Additionally, IFN-γ stimulates the release of other pro-inflammatory cytokines like IL-1, IL-6, and TNF-α. The latter cytokine, TNF-α, possesses a broad spectrum of activities that can perpetuate inflammation. Specifically, TNF-α activates more macrophage scavenger cells, stimulates release of other pro-inflammatory mediators (nitrous oxide, prostacyclin, and platelet activating factor), alters adhesive properties of epithelial cells, and compromises the integrity of the epithelial barrier (See figure 3-3A).

All together, as you can imagine, the above mentioned chemicals have the potential to cause deleterious inflammation and excessive tissue injury if not kept in check. The good news is, despite a state of controlled inflammation in the gut due to the presence of gut normal flora, there are usually other cytokines that turn *off* the pro-inflammatory/damaging cytokines — namely, IL-10, and TGF-β (See figure 3-3B). Additionally, there is at least one other mechanism in place that, under normal circumstances, prevents excessive release of pro-inflammatory chemicals — activated CD4+ cells undergo an immunologically-induced programmed cell death (a phenomenon known as ***apoptosis***). Therefore, once activated, CD4+ cells normally die *before* they cause a widespread deleterious response. (Recall, CD4+ cells initiate the pro-inflammatory cascade of events responsible for physiologic inflammation within the gut.)

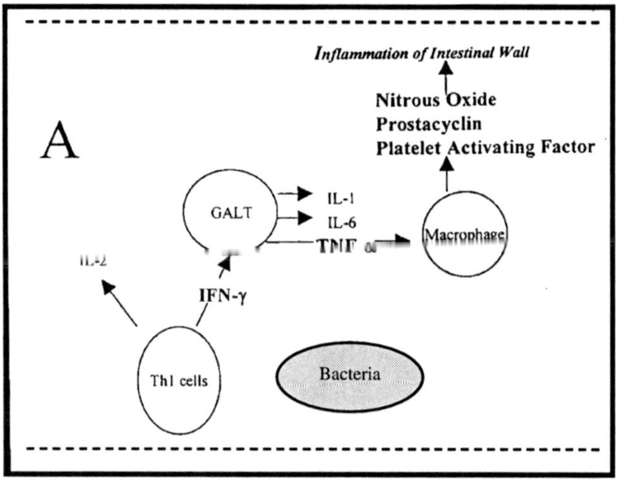

Figure 3-3A. Bacteria in the gut cause physiologic inflammation by stimulating cells of the immune system to secrete pro-inflammatory cytokines (IFN-γ and TNF-α). For example, in response to IFN-γ, GALT like macrophages, T cells, and NK cells secrete TNF-α, which activates more macrophages to release their inflammatory components. Note the wall of the intestines is illustrated by a dashed line to depict inflammation. If these were the only cytokines secreted in the gastrointestinal tract, we'd be in trouble and we'd all have chronic intestinal inflammation.

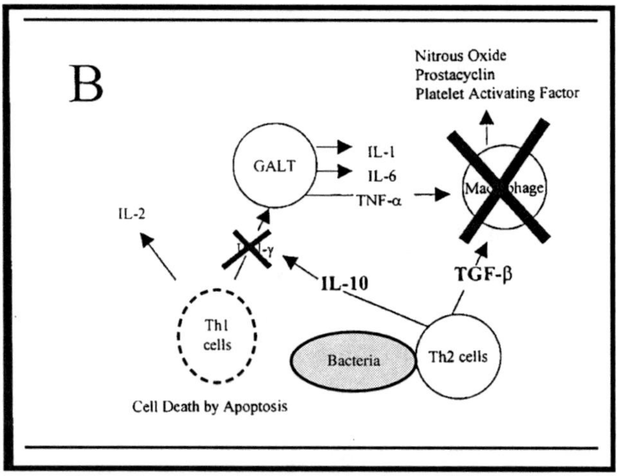

Figure 3-3B. Regulatory cytokines, IL-10 and TGF-β, are also secreted by Th-2 cells in response to gut bacteria. These cytokines "turn off" pro-inflammatory events and help maintain homeostasis and integrity of the intestinal wall. Additionally, under normal circumstances, once Th-1 cells are activated, they automatically self-destruct so they don't continue to perpetuate inflammation. These mechanisms illustrate why, under normal circumstances, physiologic inflammation doesn't get out of control.

Due to the presence of normal flora in the gut, white blood cells throughout the body are already primed and ready to be activated when a foreign, harmful antigen is encountered. As a result, a fast response can be mounted when disease-causing bacteria are confronted. It is not entirely clear *what in particular about* healthy normal flora stimulates the immune system. However, we do know that components (proteins, lipids, or sugars) on the cell walls of various strains of bifidobacteria and lactobacilli bind to GALT, which stimulates cytokine release, which then activates and recruits white blood cells to the gut. In this way, immune cells that can attack, engulf, and destroy disease-causing bacteria are already on alert and in the vicinity when a problem is encountered (Tannock, 1995).

Ridding the Gut of Some Microorganisms While Tolerating Others

Immune exclusion

Along with normal flora stimulating the gut's immune system so that immune cells are "on call" and ready to act at a moment's notice, another line of defense exists within the gastrointestinal tract. It is known as *immune exclusion.* To *exclude* harmful substances, the immune system sees that most invaders are killed, inactivated, or neutralized before an allergic or inflammatory reaction is triggered. This is accomplished largely by the special secretory antibodies — IgA immunoglobulins. IgA antibodies are abundant at mucosal surfaces especially in the gut, and these antibodies increase the likelihood that potential **pathogens** will be removed from the gut.

Recent studies have indicated that some strains of "good" bacteria enhance IgA antibody responses at mucosal surfaces. For example, administration of yogurt supplemented with *Lactobacillus acidophilus* and *Bifidobacterium* increases levels of IgA antibodies produced both in the blood stream and the gut mucosa of mice when exposed to harmful antigens like cholera toxin (Tejada-Simon et al., 1999). This means that the very *presence* of certain strains of "beneficial" bacteria stimulates and primes the immune system to respond quickly and efficiently, producing more antibodies when exposed to disease-causing bacteria.

Because IgA antibodies secreted in the gut are simply an extension of the immune system throughout the rest of the body, an immune response generated in the GALT affects immune responses in other parts of the body. Experiments in laboratory animals suggest that the ability to generate IgA responses to normal bacterial flora in the gut reduces the likelihood that these bacteria will leave the intestines and migrate to other organs of the body. This is because IgA antibodies "attack" the bacteria if they try to leave the gut and go elsewhere in the body. This further reflects the maturation of the intestine's immunologic defense mechanisms — defenses that have matured to the point of eliminating harmful bacteria that threaten to invade the body while simultaneously tolcrating the same bacteria when they remain in the gut as normal flora (Shroff et al., 1995).

Immune elimination

Although normal gut flora is an important defense barrier that prevents bacteria from leaving the gastrointestinal tract (by stimulating IgA antibody protection), sometimes gut bacteria do penetrate through epithelial cells. Another type of defense in the gut is referred to as *immune elimination.* This occurs when antigens have already penetrated and made it across the epithelial layer of the gut. Because gut-associated lymph tissues are already on alert, when harmful invasion does occur, the invaders are rapidly degraded by the lymph cells and tissues underlying the epithelial cells. Immune exclusion is a minor — but effective — pathway for removal of antigens that have penetrated the gut's epithelial layer.

Immune regulation

Yet another line of gut defense that protects against invaders involves *immune regulation.* Not all antigens that make it through the mucosal barrier are rapidly degraded by immune elimination as described above. Some antigens are presented to specialized cells of the immune system (T cells) so the antigens can be "remembered." Memory of previously encountered antigens is an important attribute of the immune system.

The immune system's memory allows for "recall" so a fast response can be mounted if a harmful antigen is encountered again. The immune system gears up for a future "attack" by preparing antibodies against the antigen in advance. *Immune regulation* also permits the immune system to "remember" a harmless antigen as simply that — harmless.

In this case, when the immune system sees the antigen again, the body simply tolerates it. As previously mentioned, the *lack* of immune response to antigens encountered by the gut's immune system — to substances remembered as harmless — is referred to as *oral tolerance*. Normally, ingested food antigens and gut flora should *not* evoke strong immune activity of either the Th1- or Th2-type. This is tolerance.

Oral tolerance mechanisms not only apply to food substances encountered by the immune system, but also to bacteria residing in the intestines. Many different factors can break down normal mechanisms of oral tolerance. When this happens, the immune system reacts inappropriately to foods leading to allergies, eczema, or asthma. Alternatively, oral tolerance can be ineffective when the presence of a harmful bacterium such as *Clostridium difficile* is tolerated as normal. Furthermore, evidence is beginning to suggest that people with inflammatory bowel diseases may lack oral tolerance to their own normal flora (Duchmann et al., 1995).

The mechanisms by which oral tolerance is acquired are complex and not fully understood. Experiments have demonstrated that in addition to genetic factors, *age* when exposed to antigens, and *duration* of antigen exposure may be involved. It is also believed that intestinal damage due to local inflammatory reactions impairs the process of oral tolerance. Immunosuppressive diseases, including malnutrition, and immunosuppressive drugs, such as prednisone, may also adversely affect the process of oral tolerance, especially during infancy when oral tolerance is just beginning to develop. Some studies have demonstrated that the absence of certain components of the immune system — like IgA deficiency — is associated with a high incidence of food allergies.

It is becoming increasingly obvious through scientific investigations that gastrointestinal flora — especially gram-negative bacteria — plays a large role in inducing and maintaining oral tolerance in laboratory animals (Moreau and Coste, 1993). In fact, not only is the *presence* of certain strains of bacteria necessary for inducing oral tolerance, but *disruptions* in the balance of normal gut flora through vomiting or diarrhea or infectious colonization with *Staphylococcus aureus* or *Clostridium perfringes impair* acquisition of oral tolerance mechanisms in neonates (Moreau and Coste, 1993). Consequently, *gut microorganisms are the earliest and largest stimulus for acquiring oral tolerance in gut associated lymph tissues.*

Conclusion

In this chapter we have learned the basics of immunology and how bacteria within the gut contribute to immune responses. We've discussed how normal gut flora heightens the state of the immune system in the gut. We've considered many ways (immunological and physiological) by which bacteria are normally prevented from leaving the gut and causing disease in other parts of the body. Perhaps, most importantly, we've introduced the idea of oral tolerance and why we tolerate certain foods and bacteria in our guts. However, sometimes things within the immune system don't work as smoothly as they should. In these instances, abnormal immune responses can cause severe inflammation or allergic manifestations to be perpetuated throughout the entire body. Many of these abnormal responses have now been definitely linked back to disturbances in gut flora.

In the next chapter we'll consider the basic relationships between gut bacteria and the mechanisms for developing inflammation and allergies. We will also consider how probiotics may be therapeutic for inflammation and allergies. Although I am introducing these abnormalities in the next chapter, certain topics like inflammatory bowel disease, as well as specific allergic illnesses will be covered in much greater detail in chapters 6 and 7. In these later chapters, we will also discuss specific probiotic therapies for dealing with these medical ailments.

Notes

Notes

References

Alm JS, Swartz J, Lilja G, et al. Atopy in children of families with an anthroposophic lifestyle. Lancet. 1999;353:1485-1488.

Cebra JJ. Influences of microbiota on intestinal immune system development. Amer J Clin Nutr. 1999;69:1046S-1051S.

Duchmann R, Kaiser I, Hermann E, et al. Tolerance exists towards resident intestinal flora but is broken in active inflammatory bowel disease (IBD). Clin Exp Immunol. 1995;102:448-455.

Henderson B, Poole S, Wilson M. Microbiol/host interactions in health and disease: Who controls the cytokine network? Immunopharmacol. 1996;35:1-21.

Moreau MC and Coste M. Immune Responses to Dietary Protein Antigens. Simopoulos AP, Corring T, Rerat A (eds) In Intestinal Flora, Immunity, Nutrition and Health, World Rev Nutr Diet. Basel, Karger, 1993, vol 74, pp22-57.

Shroff KE, Meslin K, Cebra JJ. Commensal enteric bacteria engender a self-limiting humoral mucosal immune response while permanently colonizing the gut. Infect Immunol. 1995;63:3904-3913.

Tannock GW. Role of probiotics. In: Gibson GR and Macfarlane, eds. In Human colonic bacteria: Role in nutrition, physiology, and pathology, CRC Press, Boca Raton, FL, 1995.

Tejada-Simon MV, Lee JH, Ustunol Z, et al. Ingestion of yogurt containing *Lactobacillus acidophilus* and *Bifidobacterium* to potentiate immunoglobulin A responses to cholera toxin in mice. J Dairy Sci. 1999;82:649-660.

Chapter 4

The Bacteria Balancing Act
Dysbiosis and the Immune System

We have seen that normal gut flora plays an important role in immunity, stimulating the immune system to work efficiently. But sometimes, communication between gut bacteria and the immune system fails to develop "healthy" immune responses. How does this occur and what is the result? We will explore these topics in this chapter.

As discussed in the previous chapter, the integrity of the intestinal immune system depends on many defensive strategies. These defenses (a) restrict colonization by disease-causing bacteria, (b) eliminate foreign invaders that penetrate through epithelial cells, and (c) regulate antigen-specific immune responses. In order to cause diseases, antigens must overcome this impressive array of intestinal defense mechanisms.

Inflammation

What causes it?

Crohn's disease and ulcerative colitis are two common forms of inflammatory bowel disease. Growing evidence points to **dysbiosis**, a disturbance in normal gut flora, as a major underlying factor for these illnesses. Gut inflammation can occur due to the mere *presence* of certain types of bacteria, *overgrowth* of bacteria, or *toxins* released by bacteria. Loss of **oral tolerance**, leading to overly sensitive responses towards gut bacteria, seems to play an important role. Additionally, inflammatory bowel disease could result from a predictable immune response to an unknown pathogen (we just don't know which one yet). There is also evidence that inflammatory bowel disease is caused by a lack of anti-inflammatory cytokines, namely TGF-β and IL-10 (Monteleone et al., 2002), thus allowing intestinal inflammation to be perpetuated. Furthermore, it has been shown that activated CD4+ cells don't undergo **apoptosis** as readily as they should in folks that have Crohn's disease (Monteleone et al., 2002), thus leading to a continual state of inflammation since these pro-inflammatory immune cells fail to self-destruct. Interestingly, what appears on the surface to be an "immune abnormality" may, in fact, result from faulty "immune programming" caused by gut dysbiosis.

Numerous studies have addressed the role of bacterial flora as a stimulus for inflammation. When drugs, like antibiotics, or procedures, such as surgical bypass of the intestines, alter gut flora, patients with inflammatory bowel disease often go into remission (Harper et al., 1983; Steinhart et al., 2002). Likewise, laboratory animal studies indicate that intestinal bacteria play a large role in inflammation. Experimentally-induced intestinal inflammation in rodents fails to occur — or occurs much less severely — when mice are kept in germ-free environments — or in environments where they have no gut flora (Taurog et al., 1994; Sadlack et al., 1993; Kuhn et al., 1999.

To experimentally study intestinal inflammation in rodents, scientists often use mice that cannot make either IL-2 or IL-10 — cytokines that are potent regulators of immune function. Without IL-2 or IL-10, mice develop severe intestinal inflammation. However, if these mice are kept inside a bubble — in a germ-free environment — the inflammation is either completely eliminated (in mice lacking IL-2) or dramatically reduced (in mice lacking IL-10). These experiments clearly indicate that intestinal *inflammation occurs as a result of uncontrolled immune responses to intestinal bacteria.* These studies also illustrate the importance that cytokine-signalling pathways play in communicating messages from gut bacteria to our immune systems (Kuhn et al., 1993; Sadlack et al., 1993).

Although the previously mentioned IL-2 and IL-10 experiments were initially conducted in mice, later data gathered from human studies also supports these results. It now appears that healthy individuals develop a tolerance to their own bacterial flora, but folks with inflammatory diseases lose this tolerance. As a result, in inflammatory bowel diseases, the immune system is super-sensitive and overactive towards normal gastrointestinal flora (Duchmann et al., 1995; MacDonald,

1995; Macpherson et al., 1996; Strober et al., 1998; Hendersen et al., 1996)!

While Crohn's disease and ulcerative colitis appear to be similar diseases in many respects, from an immunological point of view, there are some key differences in the types of dysregulation that underlie these conditions. For example, Crohn's disease may stem, in part, from dysregulation of CD4+ cells. (These inflammatory cells that get stimulated by gut flora just won't die!). On the other hand, ulcerative colitis seems to be associated with overactive antibody activity — perhaps production of antibodies directed against intestinal flora that should be recognized as "normal" (Monteleone et al., 2002).

In inflammatory bowel diseases, there are high levels of pro-inflammatory cytokines like IL-1, IL-6, IL-8, IL-16, TNF-α, as well as NFκβ detected. Unfortunately, NFκβ activates greater production of IL-1, IL-6, IL-8, and TNF-α. Likewise, IL-1, IL-18, and TNF-α stimulate production of more NFκβ. As a result, these pro-inflammatory cytokines continually stimulate the production of more pro-inflammatory cytokines. Thus, it is easy to see how a vicious cycle of inflammation gets perpetuated by a positive feedback loop (See figure 4-1)!

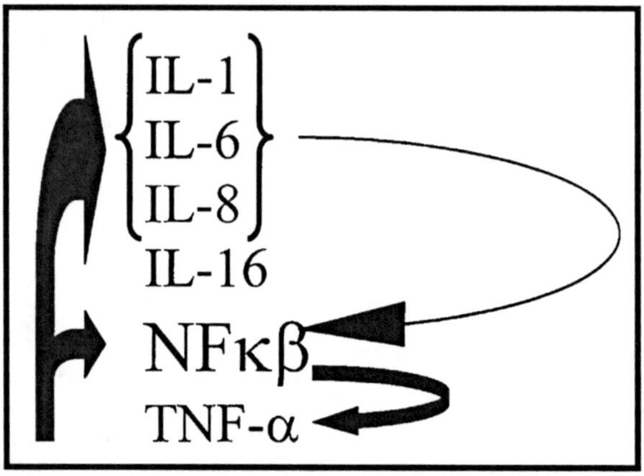

Figure 4-1. In inflammatory bowel disease, the inflammatory cytokine, NFκβ perpetuates inflammation by stimulating synthesis of other pro-inflammatory cytokines. In turn, those inflammatory cytokines produce more NFκβ, starting a vicious cycle of inflammation.

Alterations in gut bacterial composition — too much of a "harmful" species or too little of a "healthy" species — have been suggested as underlying triggers for perpetual inflammation. Some of the many possibilities include: too many *Escherichia coli, Bacteroides,* coliforms, anaerobic gram-negative cocci or bacilli, and certain strains of streptococci; or, alternatively, too few lactobacilli or bifidobacteria (Kennedy et al., 2000). When there is an imbalance of "healthy" versus "harmful" bacteria in the gut, there is less production of metabolic by-products, such as short chain fatty acids and nitric oxide, which normally inhibit disease-causing bacteria (Kennedy et al., 2000). Alternatively, with less competition among bacteria for nutrients and sites of attachment, overgrowth of certain species can provoke inflammatory responses from the immune system.

Role of increased gut permeability

Not only can a persistent infection by disease-causing bacteria result in inflammation and tissue damage, but *anything that increases intestinal permeability also perpetuates inflammation*. Invasion of epithelial cells by bacterial toxins and stimulation of epithelial cells by certain cytokines are two primary causes of increased gut permeability and accompanying inflammation. The net result of inflammation and increased gut permeability is epithelial cell death, disruption of tight junctions, and enhanced uptake of bacteria or bacterial toxins into the rest of the body (See figure 4-2). Even a brief state of gut inflammation can become self-sustaining if immune function is defective (Linskens et al., 2001). If the immune system does not respond appropriately, "physiologic inflammation" can get out of control.

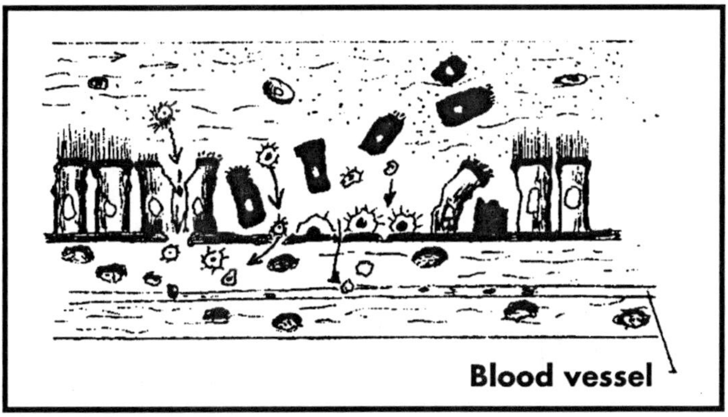

Figure 4-2. Once the epithelial cell barrier is compromised, bacteria and their toxins gain access to underlying tissues. This situation perpetuates inflammation and leads to even more intestinal damage and disease. Bacteria and their toxins now have access to other areas of the body.

Interestingly, folks who suffer from inflammatory bowel disorders are also quite susceptible to other types of inflammatory disorders, for instance, rheumatoid arthritis. There is a great deal of evidence that alterations in gut bacteria trigger inflammation throughout the entire body. In fact, even people with inflammatory diseases outside of the gut — such as folks with rheumatoid arthritis but no obvious inflammatory bowel disorders — have gastrointestinal dysbiosis compared to healthy people (Isolauri et al., 2001; Malin et al., 1996). Pro-inflammatory cytokines like IL-1, TNF-α, and even excessive amounts of IFN-γ, play pivotal roles in propagating inflammation. Thus, disruption in the gut's microbial environment — with associated imbalances in inflammatory chemical controls — disturbs mucosal integrity and causes wide-spread havoc throughout the body, even outside the gastrointestinal tract.

Experimental situations have repeatedly demonstrated that _imbalances in cytokines cause inflammation_ (Henderson et al., 1996; Isolauri et al., 2002). Since the types of bacteria in the gut largely determine the types and amounts of cytokines produced, it is reasonable to conclude that _abnormal gut flora triggers a disarray of pro-inflammatory cytokines_. Since cytokines circulate widely throughout the body, abnormal gut flora could be responsible for the large increase in inflammatory and autoimmune diseases that we have experienced in Western societies within the past several decades.

In human studies, supplementation with "healthy" bacteria reduces inflammation. Although it is not entirely clear how this occurs, several ideas have been suggested. For example, when lactobacilli are given, there is a reduction of pro-inflammatory cytokines like TNF-α. Therefore, the presence of certain bacteria may stabilize the immune barrier of the gut mucosa by restoring a balance between pro-inflammatory mediators and protective chemicals in the gut. Alternatively, another proposed mechanism for stabilizing the gut mucosa by lactobacilli and other probiotics involves production of the short chain fatty acid, butyric acid, which is produced by "healthy" bacteria (Okamoto et al., 2000). As you recall from chapter 1, butyric acid is largely beneficial in the gut. Recent experiments indicate that butyric acid decreases activities of pro-inflammatory components of the immune system (Chapman, 2001). Thus, lactobacilli and other probiotic bacteria work by several mechanisms to regulate the immune system and correct epithelial unrest and inflammation.

There is, in fact, a great deal of evidence supporting a role for "healthy" bacteria in reducing inflammation both in experimental animals and in humans. In several different animal models of inflammation, administration of different strains of *Lactobacillus* reduced intestinal inflammation (Fabia et al., 1993; Madsen et al., 1999). Likewise, giving various species of "good bacteria" to patients with inflammatory gut diseases increases IgA activities, suggesting improvements in the immunologic barrier function of the gut (Tejada-Simon et al., 1999). Other benefits of using probiotics to treat inflammatory diseases are: resolution of inflammatory symptoms and a decreased need for drugs like steroids to control inflammation (Kennedy et al., 2000). When probiotics have been used to prevent flare-ups of inflammatory diseases like Crohn's disease, ulcerative colitis, and pouchitis, the results have been dramatic (Gionchetti et al., 2000; Gupta et al., 2000; Kennedy et al., 2000; Kruis et al., 1997; Rembacken et al., 1999). In fact, bacterial therapy for inflammatory gut diseases is as effective, and sometimes even more effective, than prescription drugs commonly used to maintain remission of inflammatory symptoms (Kruis et al., 1997; Rembacken et al., 1999). In chapter 5, we will discuss in much greater detail the role of probiotics as treatments for inflammatory bowel disorders.

Allergic Diseases

As mentioned in chapter 3, appropriate priming of the intestinal immune system early in infancy is necessary for oral tolerance — the *nonresponsiveness* to non-disease-causing antigens encountered in the gut. Oral tolerance is considered to result from both (a) immune exclusion and (b) simultaneous suppression of systemic immune responses. These seemingly opposing actions, quite possibly, are attributed to effects of TGF-β. Inadequate neonatal production of TGF-β may promote food allergies (Isolauri et al., 2001).

Normal gut flora promotes anti-allergenic processes by (1) stimulating Th1 immune activities in preference to Th2, (2) stimulating production of a cytokine known as transforming growth factor-β (TGF-β) which regulates production of other cytokines and (3) stimulating IgA antibodies that defend the intestinal mucosa.

In the event of gut inflammation, altered <u>rates</u> and <u>routes</u> by which dietary antigens become associated with **GALT** (gut-associated lymph tissues) can contribute to loss of oral tolerance. Oral tolerance can also be lost when intestinal permeability increases. Certainly, as we already know, inflammation and associated intestinal permeability can occur due to the presence of bacteria, viruses, or food particles. When insufficient pancreatic digestive enzymes are secreted, the normal way of handling dietary proteins is impaired. This can also cause inflammation which, in turn, triggers faulty immune responses and leads to allergy sensitization. Thus, food allergies often result when GALT fail to achieve or maintain oral tolerance (Isolauri et al., 2001).

Laboratory experiments have used germ-free mice (mice never exposed to bacteria, hence having no bacteria in their guts) to study mechanisms of oral tolerance. These mice are more likely to develop food allergies than normal mice. Germ-free mice produce high levels of systemic IgE antibodies when exposed to certain foods. However, if normal bacterial flora is introduced into the guts of these germ-free mice *at neonatal stages of life*, the very *presence* of the microorganisms *corrects* the overactive allergic responses to foods (Sudo et al., 1997). Interestingly, introduction of normal flora *only* prevents allergic responses if bacterial flora is introduced while mice are still neonates. If normal gut flora is introduced to these mice later in life, the normal flora doesn't protect from allergies; allergic responses still develop when normal gut flora is replaced once mice age beyond the neonatal time period. These results seem to indicate that gut flora directs regulation of both local and systemic immune responses. Furthermore, these findings indicate that *to avoid allergic reactions later in life, a healthy balance of gut flora is necessary from an early age* for appropriate maturation of GALT.

In agreement with experiments in laboratory mice, studies in human infants also indicate that the *type* of bacteria colonizing the intestines of newborns and the *timing* of that colonization modulates naive immune responses. Infants that have *Bacteroides fragilis* in their intestines at one month of age are significantly more likely to have mature immune responses — IgA and IgM-secreting cells — by two months of age than are infants colonized with bifidobacteria or lactobacilli. It seems that colonization by *Bacteroides* — at a critical point early in life — has important immuno-stimulating and immuno-stabilizing effects in infants. These results indicate that both the *type* of bacteria in the newborn and the *timing* of acquisition are important factors in immune system maturation (Gronlund et al., 2000).

Several studies recently examined the differences in gut flora between Estonian and Swedish children. The environment in which Estonian children are reared still resembles that of the "unsanitary, old world" while Swedish children grow up under more "sterile, modernized" conditions. The major differences in intestinal flora between these two groups of children were: high counts of lactobacilli and eubacteria (healthy bacteria) in stools of Estonian children, but increased numbers of clostridia (disease-causing bacteria) in infants reared in Sweden (Sepp et al., 1997).

These children were also evaluated for relationships between gut flora and allergies. There is a low incidence of allergic diseases in Estonia, but a high prevalence of such illnesses in Sweden. *Both* Estonian and Swedish children afflicted by milk or egg allergies lack normal levels of gut lactobacilli (healthy bacteria), as compared to healthy children (Sepp et al., 1997). In addition, allergic children are colonized by higher amounts of aerobic microorganisms like coliforms and *Staphylococcus aureus*. Furthermore, counts of *Bacteroides* were lower in allergic children than in nonallergic children (Bjorksten et al., 1999). All together, this evidence strongly supports the notion that bacterial gut flora acquired in infancy plays a role in the immune responses that lead to allergies. Early colonization with lactobacilli and *Bacteroides* seem to protect against allergic illnesses, while colonization by clostridia, coliforms, and staphylococci favor allergies.

The full regulatory role played by specific strains of bacteria is far from clear. However, in the past few years, enormous strides have been made in our understanding. Experimental laboratory studies have found that live lactobacilli stimulate certain types of cytokines (interferon) better than inactive bacteria, indicating that certain structures on bacterial cell walls must bind to epithelial cells walls in order to trigger cytokine release. This direct interaction of normal gut flora with the intestinal wall is essential for maximum stimulation of the immune system to maintain homeostasis (Miettinen et al., 1996). Interactions of bacteria with epithelial cells stimulate cytokine secretion and these cytokines act as signals to either activate or suppress immune activities. However, bacterial strains don't all have the same effects. This is probably because different bacteria have different adhesive properties — that is, not all bacteria have the same ability to bind to epithelial cells.

This further explains why exposure to various microorganisms — at young ages — either primes the immune system for appropriate activity (lactobacilli, bifidobacteria) or inappropriate inflammatory and allergic dysfunction (clostridia, coliforms, staphylococci).

Healthy bacteria prevent allergies

Many studies have used probiotics, or "healthy bacteria" from yogurt cultures to investigate the roles of gut flora as they prime the immune system and sway it away from allergic responses. Lactobacilli and *Streptococcus thermophilus*, two bacterial genera found in yogurt and considered part of the "healthy" normal flora, stimulate secretion of certain cytokines, specifically IFN-α and IFN-γ (Pereyra et al., 1991). Lactobacilli and streptococci activate these cytokines by stimulating an enzyme required for their synthesis. In humans, this enzyme (called 2'-5'- A –synthetase) increases in abundance after eating yogurt that contains live and active bacterial cultures (Solis-Pereyra et al., 1997). IFN-α and IFN-γ prevent allergies in several ways. First, IFN-γ *inhibits* activities of IL-4, a pro-allergic cytokine. Second, IFN-α reduces pro-allergic IgE antibody levels; and third, IFN-α also promotes IFN-γ activities (Sareneva et al., 1998; Cross and Hill, 2001). Thus, probiotics nonspecifically stimulate immune functions through enhanced interferon activities, while simultaneously suppressing allergic functions by down-regulating the pro-allergic cytokine IL-4 and IgE (See figure 4-3).

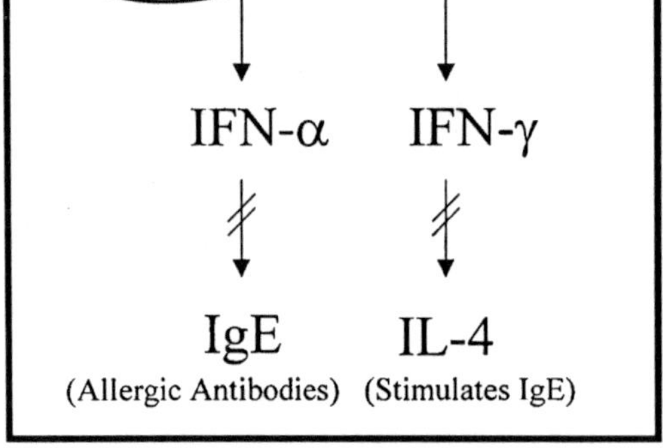

Figure 4-3. Probiotics stimulate secretion of interferons IFN-α and IFN-γ. These interferons turn off the allergic mediators, IgE and IL-4.

In laboratory experiments using immune cells from mice previously primed to be hyper-allergic, probiotic bacteria stimulate production of IFN-γ, while simultaneously reducing all the factors known to propagate allergic responses like cytokines IL-4, and IL-5 and IgE antibodies (Matsuzaki et al., 1998). Recent studies using human-gut-derived probiotics also suggest that these bacteria are potent inducers of cytokines IL-12 and IL-18 — interferons that nonspecifically trigger immune activities (Miettinin et al., 1998). Taken all together, these results indicate that bacteria modulate the immune system, preventing and alleviating symptoms of allergies by shifting immune responses away from secreting pro-allergic chemicals. Very simply, the bottom line is: *healthy gut bacteria redirect gut immune responses by decreasing production of the cytokines that cause allergies.*

It should be noted, however, that not all strains of bacteria produce the same responses. For example, some strains of *Lactobacillus* stimulate production of IL-5, a pro-allergic cytokine. As a result, not all strains of *Lactobacillus* are likely to be of benefit in allergy prevention.

Even bacterial strains known to be potent stimulators of IL-12 also stimulate production of IL-10, an inhibitor of cytokine synthesis (Hessle et al., 2000). This type of feedback at first seems contradictory, but it is both important and necessary. Although IL-12 is generally thought of as a good defense, stimulating immune activity against bacterial invaders, too much IL-12 promotes tissue inflammation. So you see, it is important that healthy bacteria not only "turn on" the immune system at the proper time, but the same microorganisms must also turn the immune system "off". Thus, gut bacteria and probiotics fine-tune the immune system in multiple ways to appropriately regulate host responses.

In addition to modulating cytokines, gut bacteria play other roles to suppress allergies. Normal gastrointestinal flora breaks down dietary proteins. If proteins do not get sufficiently degraded, they tend to be allergenic, stimulating the immune system to respond inappropriately. Inappropriate digestion, then, causes food allergies. The mere addition of healthy gut bacteria to the intestines improves break down of allergenic proteins into small non-allergic forms that are less capable of evoking harmful allergic responses (Apostolou et al., 2001). Additionally, "healthy" gut bacteria — especially commonly used probiotics like *Lactobacillus* GG — stabilize the mucosal barrier, preventing food particles from passing into direct contact with immune system mediators. This also prevents hypersensitivity to food components (Isolauri et al., 1993).

Regardless of the specific mechanisms by which "healthy" bacteria suppress development of allergies, numerous studies over the past two decades support the role of probiotic supplements in preventing allergic diseases. For example, in one study, *Lactobacillus* GG was administered prenatally to mothers who were at high risk for having a child with allergies. The probiotic supplement was also continued in the infants after birth. When the infants were 2 and 4 years of age, the incidence of allergies and eczema was evaluated. In the group of mothers and infants receiving probiotic supplements, the incidence of allergic eczema was half that of the group that did not receive any "healthy" bacteria (Kalliomaki et al., 2001; 2003).

Probiotics to treat allergies

Not only are healthy gut flora able to prevent allergies, but it is also possible to treat allergies by adding "healthy" gut bacteria back into the intestines. In fact, probiotics play dual immunomodulatory roles; probiotics stimulate the immune system of healthy individuals, while in folks with food allergies, probiotics suppress immune activities (Pelto et al., 1998). Take a look at how probiotics helped children with eczema.

> When children with eczema were given supplemental *Lactobacillus* GG, their symptoms reduced dramatically compared to children who were not given the bacterial supplement (Majamaa and Isolauri, 1997).
>
> An additional study examined the merits of probiotics in 27 infants, approximately 4 months in age, who had developed eczema. Results overwhelming showed that probiotic supplementation with either *Bifidobacterium lactis* or *Lactobacillus* GG reduced inflammatory, allergic eczema in these infants (Isolauri et al., 2000).

There are more studies, similar to the ones already described, covered in greater detail in chapter 7, which demonstrate the potent immunomodulatory properties of probiotics in prevention and treatment of allergic conditions. What these studies have in common is that they all support the notion that certain strains of "good" bacteria alleviate intestinal inflammation and skin sensitivities associated with food allergies.

Reasons for allergies in children

Newborns have many strikes against them when it comes to developing allergies. Many factors about a newborn's immune system favor development of allergies, rather than tolerance. (a) Until nearly one year of age, infants have a relative lack of IgA to fend off antigens via immune exclusion. (b) Additionally, there are major differences in the regulation of cytokine production in children versus adults, which make children more susceptible to infections (Lilic et al., 1997) and allergies. For example, a relative lack of IL-2 in infants increases their susceptibility to infections. Gut inflammation, associated with these infections, is accompanied by increased intestinal permeability, which *indirectly* leads to food allergies. Additionally, an abundance of the pro-allergic cytokine IL-4 in newborns *directly* makes them more susceptible to allergies. Alternatively, lack of the anti-inflammatory cytokine, TGF-β, prevents infants from acquiring oral tolerance and predisposes them to allergic diseases (Strober et al., 1998). (c) Young children often lack necessary gastric acids and pancreatic enzymes to sufficiently digest their foods. Food proteins that are not completely degraded by gastric acids and pancreatic enzymes can arouse the immune system, causing food allergies to develop. (d) Children are also more susceptible to certain intestinal infections of the gut. Often these infections, whether viral or bacterial in nature, can elicit secretion of pro-inflammatory cytokines like IFN-γ which disrupt tight junctions between epithelial cells and increase epithelial permeability (Heyman and Desjeux, 2000). The obvious symptom of these immune disturbances is diarrhea. Unfortunately, however, these alterations may do more than cause transient diarrhea. These alterations may do long term damage. Disrupted intestinal permeability prevents children from developing oral tolerance. As more and more antigens begin permeating across a compromised mucosal barrier, there is a greater likelihood that sensitization — food allergies and eczema — will occur as the local inflammation perpetuates itself.

To add insult to injury, during development of allergic conditions (the initial insult probably is worsened by IFN-γ secretion in response to viral or bacterial infections), children diagnosed with food allergies also seem to have abnormally high levels of TNF-α secretion (Heyman and Desjeux, 2000). Experiments have demonstrated that TNF-α and IFN-γ act together to increase gut permeability and perpetuate the vicious allergy cycle (Heyman and Desjeux, 2000).

Since abnormal gut flora is often the "inflammatory trigger" that initiates allergies, it is critical to ensure gut colonization by friendly bacteria from an early age. Infants who are formula-fed or who spend time in neonatal intensive care units are at a great disadvantage when it comes to acquiring a healthy repertoire of normal flora. As a result, there may be a tendency for these children to develop allergies later in life. Use of probiotics, in infancy, restores disrupted gut flora and reprograms the immune system to prevent allergic diseases. In European countries there has been much talk about incorporating probiotic bacteria into standard infant formulas.

Probiotics Modify the Immune System

As we have learned so far, the immune system can be negatively impacted by gastrointestinal dysbiosis. Strong inflammatory responses that ensue compromise normal barrier functions of the gut. Many infants don't acquire the right types of bacterial species immediately after birth, leading to a life-time of chronic inflammatory diseases and allergies. Can dietary supplementation with probiotics alter abnormal immune responses? This is what we will explore in the last section of this chapter.

It seems that probiotic bacteria *can* stabilize the gut's bacterial environment in several different ways — through improving gut IgA antibody responses and by more tightly controlling the balance between pro-inflammatory and anti-inflammatory cytokines.

Probiotics reinforce the various lines of gut defense that we talked about in chapter 3: immune exclusion, immune elimination, and immune regulation. Probiotics also stimulate non-specific host resistance to disease-causing invaders and aid in elimination of pathogens. Probiotics have been used successfully to treat various illnesses, reducing the risk of diseases associated with gut-barrier dysfunction.

Like "healthy" normal flora, probiotics participate nonspecifically in immune modulation in a variety of ways. Some probiotics alter the activities of macrophages (Perdigon et al., 1986; Perdigon et al., 1998; Schiffrin et al., 1994). These scavenger cells release toxic chemicals like peroxide, secrete enzymes that stimulate local inflammatory responses, and recruit more immune cells in response to disease-causing bacteria. Probiotics modulate these responses and prevent localized inflammation from getting out of control. Probiotics also alter production of cytokines (TNF-a, IL-6) and increase secretion of IgA antibodies to heighten immune responsiveness in the intestine. These activities prevent antigens from leaving the gut and keep them from causing a wide-spread allergic response throughout the entire body (Miettinen et al., 1996; Miettinen et al., 1998).

Recently, it was demonstrated that gram-positive bacteria — which is what most probiotics are — are more likely to stimulate the body's immune cells to release IL-12 and activate IFN-γ than gram-negative bacterial species (Hessle et al., 2000). In contrast, gram-negative species tend to secrete more IL-10, which inhibits or down-grades immune activities (Hessle et al., 2000). When IL-12, IFN-γ, and IL-10 are released in a controlled fashion in response to digestive flora or probiotics, intestinal awareness of antigens is heightened. These three cytokines permit effective communication between the immune system and the gut. It is clear that the gram-positive probiotic, *Lactobacillus* GG, a strain that has been widely studied for alleviating gastrointestinal inflammation and allergies, has dual immune properties. On the one hand, *Lactobacillus* GG generates pro-inflammatory mediators (IL-6, IL-12, IFN-γ, TNF-α) which heighten immune responses, but on the other hand, *Lactobacillus* GG stimulates release of anti-inflammatory mediators (IL-10), too. These dual effects keep inflammation and allergic reactions from getting out of control. The bottom line with probiotics, then, is that they fine tune the balance between immune suppression and immune stimulation. Probiotics definitely act as immune regulators, stabilizing dysregulated systems.

When we consider all that we currently know about the immunological merits of probiotics, it appears that probiotics reduce the synthesis of pro-inflammatory chemicals while simultaneously reinforcing production of chemicals that eliminate disease-causing invaders (Hessle et al., 2000).

IFN-α*	Antiviral activities
IFN-γ*	Activates macrophages
IL-2*	Activates a subset of T lymphocytes
IL-4**	IgE synthesis; promotes allergies
IL-5**	Eosinophil growth and differentiation; promotes allergies
IL-6**	T-lymphocyte and B-lymphocyte (antibody-producing cell) growth and activation
IL-10***	Suppresses macrophages; inhibits synthesis of IL-2, IL-4, IL-6, IL-12, IFN-γ, TNF-α, IgE
IL-12*	Activates a subset of T lymphocytes (Natural Killer cells) that kill tumors and intracellular bacteria
TNF-β*	Lyses or damages many types of cells

*Can nonspecifically activate the immune system, but can also perpetuate inflammation
** Usually considered to favor development of allergies
***Typically considered a suppressant of immune activity

Table 4-1. Actions of Selected Cytokines

Probably the most intriguing area of study within the field of probiotics at the present time is trying to understand the mechanisms by which bacteria modulate the immune system on a global, systemic level — not only in the gut. For example, several recent studies have documented that probiotics stimulate immune responses to vaccinations. Simultaneously taking a *Lactobacillus GG* supplement by mouth while being immunized with standard vaccinations somehow increases the body's immune response to the vaccination (Isolauri et al., 1995; Jung et al., 1999). Furthermore, we know that some probiotics activate immune-enhancing parts of the immune system while simultaneously suppressing allergic responses; however, we truly don't have any idea how these seemingly opposing effects occur. Clearly, we have much more to learn before we fully comprehend how the gut works as an amazing organ of the immune system and how dysbiosis imbalances this system.

Conclusion

In this chapter we have considered the "big picture" of inflammatory bowel diseases and allergic disorders. Both of these ailments can originate from abnormal gut flora. Abnormal gut bacteria trigger release of certain cytokines which "communicate" with our immune systems. Inflammation and allergies are widely dependent upon which cytokines are released in response to gut bacteria, since cytokines can perpetuate inflammatory or allergic responses. Just how the immune surveillance system in the gut distinguishes between friendly microorganisms and potential disease-causing bacteria in the first place is not entirely clear. However, it is clear that when the immune system is not appropriately "primed," early in life, a life-time of hyper-allergic and hyper-inflammatory disease states can ensue. However, as bleak as this sounds, it is possible to "re-program" and modify the activities of the immune system by introducing healthy probiotic bacteria. This will be discussed in much more detail in subsequent chapters when we discuss the role of probiotics as treatments for allergies (chapter 7) and inflammatory bowel diseases (chapter 6).

Notes

Notes

References

Apostolou E, Pelto L, Kirjavainen PV et al. Differences in the gut bacterial flora of healthy and milk-hypersensitive adults, as measured by fluorescence *in situ* hybridization. FEMS Immunol Med Microbiol. 2001;30:217-221.

Bjorksten B, Naaber P, Sepp E, et al. The intestinal microflora in allergic Estonian and Swedish 2-year-old children. Clin Exp Allergy. 1999;29:342-346.

Chapman MAS. The role of colonic flora in maintaining a healthy large bowel mucosa. Ann R Coll Surg Engl. 2001;83:75-80.

Cross ML and Hill HS. Can immunoregulatory lactic acid bacteria be used as dietary supplements to limit allergies? Int Arch Allergy Immunol 2001;125:112-119.

Duchmann R, Kaiser I, Hermann E, et al. Tolerance exists towards resident intestinal flora but is broken in active inflammatory bowel disease (IBD). Clin Exp Immunol. 1995;102:448-455.

Fabia R, Ar'rajab A, Johansson M-L. The effect of exogenous administration of *Lactobacillus reuteri* R2LC and oat fiber on acetic acid-induced colitis in the rat. Scan J Gastroenterol. 1993;28:155-162.

Gionchetti P, Rizzello F, Venturi A, et al. Oral bacteriotherapy as maintenance treatment in patients with chronic pouchitis: A double-blind, placebo-controlled trial. Gastroenterol. 2000;119:305-309.

Gronlund MM, Arvilommi H, Kero P, et al. Importance of intestinal colonization in the maturation of humoral immunity in early infancy: A prospective follow up study of healthy infants aged 0-6 months. Arch Dis Child Fetal Neonatal Ed. 2000; 83:F186-F192.

Gupta P, Andrew H, Kirschner BS, et al. Is *Lactobacillus* GG helpful in children with Crohn's disease? Results of a preliminary, open-label study. J Pediatr Gastroenterol. Nutr. 2000;31:453-457.

Harper PH, Truelove SC, Lee ECG, et al., Split ileostomy and ileocolostomy for Crohn's disease of the colon and ulcerative colitis: A twenty year survey. Gut. 1983;23:106-113.

Hessle C, Andersson B, Wold AE. Gram-positive bacteria are potent inducers of monocytic interleukin-12 (IL-12) while gram negative bacteria preferentially stimulate IL-10 production. Infect. Immunol. 2000;68;3581-3586.

Heyman M and Desjeux JF. Cytokine-induced alteration of the epithelial barrier to food antigens in disease. Ann NYAS. 2000;915:304-311.

Isolauri E, Arvola R, Moilanen E, et al. Probiotics in the management of atopic eczema. Clin Exp Allergy. 2000;30:1604-1610.

Isolauri E, Joensuu J, Suomalainen H, et al. Improved immunogenicity of oral D x RRV reassortant rotavirus vaccine by *Lactobacillus casei* GG. Vaccine. 1995;13:310-312.

Isolauri E, Kirjavainen PV, and Slaminen S. Probiotics: A role in the treatment of intestinal infection and inflammation? Gut. 2002;50:iii54-iii59.

Isolauri E, Majamaa H, Arvola T, et al. *Lactobacillus casei* strain GG reverses increased intestinal permeability induced by cow milk in suckling rats. Gastroenterology. 1993;105:1643-1650.

Isolauri E, Sutas Y, Kankaanpaa P, et al. Probiotics: Effects on immunity. Am J Clin Nutr. 2001;73:444S-450S.

Jung LKL. *Lactobacillus* GG augments the immune response to typhoid vaccination: A double-blind, placebo-controlled study. *Faseb J.*1999;13:A872.

Kalliomaki M, Salminen S, Arvilommi H, et al. Probiotics in primary prevention of atopic disease: A randomised placebo-controlled trial. Lancet. 2001;357:1076-9.

Kalliomaki M, Salminen S, Poussa T, et al. Probiotics and prevention of atopic disease: 4-year follow-up of a randomised placebo-controlled trial. Lancet. 2003;361:186-1871..

Kennedy RJ, Kirk SJ, Gardiner KR. Promotion of a favorable gut flora in inflammatory bowel disease. JPEN. 2000;24:189-195.

Kruis W, Schultz E, Fric P, et al. Double-blind comparison of an oral *Escherichia coli* preparation and mesalamine in maintaining remission of ulcerative colitis. Aliment Pharmacol Ther. 1997;11:853-858.

Kuhn R, Lohler J, Rennick D, et al. Interleukin-10-deficient mice develop chronic enterocolitis. Cell. 1993;75:263-274.

Lilic D, Cant AJ, Abinum M, et al. Cytokine production differs in children and adults. Pediatric Res. 1997; 42:237-240.

Linskens RK, Huijsdens XW, Savelkoul PHM, et al. The bacterial flora in inflammatory bowel disease: Current insights in pathogenesis and the influence of antibiotics and probiotics. Scand J Gastroenterol. 2001;Suppl 234:29-40.

MacDonald TT. Breakdown of tolerance to the intestinal bacterial flora in inflammatory bowel disease (IBD). Clin Exp Immunol. 1995;102:445-447.

Macpherson A, Khoo UY, Forgacs I, et al. Mucosal antibodies in inflammatory bowel disease are directed against intestinal bacteria. Gut. 1996;38:365-375.

Madsen KL, Doyle JSG, Jewell JD, et al. Lactobacillus species prevents colitis in interleukin 10 gene-deficient mice. Gastroenterol. 1999;116:1107-1114.

Majamaa H, Isolauri E. Probiotics: A novel approach in the management of food allergy. J Allergy Clin Immunol 1997;99:179-185.

Malin M, Verronen P, Mykkanen H, et al. Increased bacterial urease activity in faeces in juvenile chronic arthritis: Evidence of altered intestinal microflora? Br J Rheumatol. 1996;35:689-694.

Matsuzaki T, Yamazaki R, Hashimoto S, et al. The effect of oral feeding of *Lactobacillus casei* strain Shirota on immunoglobulin E production in mice. J Dairy Sci. 1998;81:48-53.

Miettinen M, Matikainen S, Vuopio-Varkila J, et al. Lactobacilli and streptococci induce interleukin-12 (IL-12), IL-18, and gamma interferon production in human peripheral blood mononuclear cells. Infect Immun. 1998;66:6058-6062.

Meittinen M, Vuopoi-Varikila J, Varkila K. Production of tumor necrosis factor alpha, interleukin-6, and interleukin-10 is induced by lactic acid bacteria. Infect Immunol. 1996;64:5403-5405.

Monteleone I, Vavassori P, Biancone L, et al. Immunoregulation in the gut: Success and failures in human disease. Gut. 2002;50:iii60-iii64.

Okamoto T, Sasaki M, Tsujikawa T, et al. Preventive efficacy of butyrate enema and oral administration of *Clostridium butyricum* M588 in dextran sodium sulfate-induced colitis in rats. Gastrolenterol. 2000;35:341-346.

Pelto L, Isolauri E, Lilius EM, et al. Probiotic bacteria down-regulate the milk-induced inflammatory response in milk-hypersensitive subjects but have an immunostimulatory effect in healthy subjects. Clin Exp Allergy. 1998;28:1474-1479.

Perdigon G, deMacfas ME, Alvarez S, et al. Effect of perorally administered lactobacilli on macrophage activation in mice. Infect Immunol. 1986;53:404-410.

Perdigon G, de Macfas ME, Alvarez S, et al. Systemic augmentation of the immune response in mice by feeding fermented milks with *Lactobacillus casei* and *Lactobacillus* GG-derived enzymes. Immunol. 1998;63:17-23.

Pereyra BS, Falcoff R, Falcoff E, et al. Interferon induction by *Lactobacillus bulgaricus* and *Streptococcus thermophilus* in mice. Eur Cytokine Netw. 1991;2:299-303.

Rembacken BJ, Snelling AM, Hawkey PM, et al. Non-pathogenic *Escherichia coli* versus mesalamine for the treatment of ulcerative colitis: A randomised trial. Lancet. 1999;354:635-639.

Sadlack B, Merz H, Schorle H, et al. Ulcerative colitis-like disease in mice with a disrupted interleukin-2 gene. Cell. 1993;75:253-261.

Sareneva T, Matikainen S, Kurimoto M, et al. Influenza A virus-induced IFN-alpha/beta and IL-18 synergistically enhance IFN-gamma gene expression in human T cells. J Immunol. 1998; 160:6032-6038.

Schiffrin EJ, Rochat F, Link-Amster H, et al. Immunomodulation of human blood cells following the ingestion of lactic acid bacteria. J Dairy Sci. 1994;78:491-497.

Sepp E, Julge K, Vasar M, et al. Intestinal microflora of Estonian and Swedish infants. Acta Paediatr. 1997;86:956-961.

Solis-Pereyra B, Aattouri N, Lemonnier D. Role of food in the stimulation of cytokine production. Am J Clin Nutr. 1997;66:521S-525S.

Steinhart AH, Feagan BG, Wong CJ, et al. Combined budesonide and antibiotic therapy for active Crohn's disease: A randomized controlled trial. Gastroenterol. 2002; 123:33-40.

Strober W, Kelsaa B, Marth T. Oral tolerance. J Clin Immunol. 1998;18:1-30.

Sudo N, Sawamura S, Tanaka K, et al. The requirement of intestinal bacterial flora for the development of an IgE production system fully susceptible to oral tolerance induction. J Immunol. 1997;159:17391745.

Taurog JD, Richardson JA, Croft JP, et al. The germ free state prevents development of gut and joint inflammatory disease of HLA-B27 transgenic rats. J Exp Med. 1994;180:2359-2364.

Chapter 5

A Gut Wrenching Experience Probiotics and Diarrhea

Probiotics have been effective time and time again for treating and preventing diarrhea. Most studies have been small; however, the majority of data overwhelmingly supports the use of probiotics for treating diarrhea, regardless of its cause.

This chapter focuses initially on the use of probiotics as a treatment for diarrhea caused by a bacterium known as *Clostridium difficile* (*C. difficile*). Although not widely known outside of the medical community, *C. difficile* can cause severe, persistent, and even life-threatening diarrhea. Diarrhea caused by *C. difficile* is sometimes referred to as "antibiotic-associated diarrhea" because it commonly occurs during or shortly after antibiotic use. Unfortunately, when we take antibiotics, the drugs not only kill bacteria causing our infection, but also wipe out our normal flora. As a result, it is not uncommon for antibiotics to cause an imbalance in normal gastrointestinal flora, leading to overgrowth of disease-causing bacteria like *C. difficile*. (Occasionally, there have been instances where *C. difficile* overgrows in the absence of antibiotic use.) Although the majority of folks who end up with *C. difficile* diarrhea recover quite nicely with antibiotic therapy, it has become increasingly apparent during the last decade that there is a subset of individuals who have extreme difficulty overcoming *C. difficile* diarrhea, probably due to a focal — or very specific — immune deficiency. For these individuals, *C. difficile* can cause chronic, persistent, life-threatening diarrhea for the rest of their lives unless they are fortunate enough to find an expert who knows how to deal with this microorganism. It is primarily for these folks that I began to investigate probiotics and it is these individuals that, I hope, will find probiotic therapy to be the answer to gaining control over their lives again.

For those who suffer from chronic, persistent *C. difficile* diarrhea, probiotics can be a remarkably successful, life-saving therapy. Since I feel so passionately about helping those who suffer from *C. difficile* diarrhea, I have devoted part of this chapter to describing what makes this microorganism tick and what therapies may eradicate it.

The last sections of this chapter also describe benefits of probiotics for diarrhea caused by other things, like rotavirus infection and traveler's diarrhea, for example. Diarrhea associated with inflammatory bowel diseases like Crohn's disease and ulcerative colitis will be dealt with in detail in chapter 6.

C. difficile Diarrhea

We are going to begin this section with a true story of one child who suffered from a chronic, persistent infection with *C. difficile.* After nearly a year of battling the illness, this little boy was cured with probiotics after all other medical interventions had failed. Probiotics literally saved this child's life! Although this story is included here first and foremost to describe the role of probiotics in treating diarrhea, as you read this child's history, consider everything you have learned so far about normal gastrointestinal flora. Keep in mind, healthy flora is essential from birth to prevent a life-time of food allergies, asthma, eczema, and inflammatory disorders. Due to complications at birth, this child started life with antibiotics that disrupted his gut normal flora and he will probably suffer with the ramifications for the rest of his life.

K.K. had numerous complications during the birthing process. During delivery, K.K.'s mother developed an infection in her uterine membranes when her waters broke prematurely. As a result, K.K. received intravenous antibiotics in the neonatal intensive care unit for the first three days of life to prevent meningitis. K.K. was discharged from the hospital when he was 5 days old. However, at 10 days of age, K.K. was readmitted to the hospital when he stopped feeding, stopped awakening, and was completely unresponsive. K.K. was again given intravenous antibiotics to treat what was thought to be late-onset meningitis due to complications associated with his birth. However, cultures failed to grow any viruses or bacteria and 72 hours after re-admission, K.K. was feeding and awakening every few hours as expected for an infant his age.

At 9 months of age, K.K. was diagnosed with asthma. The asthma was mild and intermittent in nature and was well-controlled with maintenance breathing treatments using anti-inflammatory drugs. Acute flare-ups of asthma were infrequent, usually associated with respiratory tract infections, and treated successfully with the bronchodilator, levalbuterol (Xopenex®). K.K.'s next 9 months were medically insignificant. However, at 18 months of age, K.K. developed an anaphylactic allergic reaction to eggs. All egg-containing products were removed from his diet and no other food allergies were noted.

At age 2 years and 3 months, K.K. developed a yeast infection in his diaper area which resolved with antifungal creams, and at age 2 years and 4 months, K.K. developed diarrhea. Stools were green, foul-smelling, and accompanied by large amounts of mucus. Frequently, mucus was passed even in the absence of stools. Bowel movements occurred as often as fifteen times a day. Blood was also detected in the stools at times. K.K.'s stools were tested for numerous bacteria and viruses. *Clostridium difficile* toxins were present in stool specimens. All other bacteria, bacterial toxins, and parasites were absent from his stools.

Initially, a ten day course of the antibiotic, metronidazole (Flagyl®) was prescribed. K.K.'s symptoms initially responded to this treatment, however, five days after stopping metronidazole, K.K.'s diarrhea returned. K.K. was again given metronidazole and this time the drug was not stopped abruptly, but was slowly tapered off over a period of 35 days. At this point, a probiotic containing *Lactobacillus* GG was added to his therapy and was continued for nine months. Again, symptoms of the intestinal infection improved while taking metronidazole, but returned five days after the antibiotic was stopped. Another antibiotic, vancomycin was then tried. Once again, during a ten day course of vancomycin, K.K.'s diarrhea responded to the antibiotic, but within 72 hours of stopping the drug, his diarrhea returned. A long-term slow tapering regimen of vancomycin was then used, slowly withdrawing the drug over a period of five months; however, as the dosage of the drug was tapered off, diarrhea returned.

While using vancomycin, K.K.'s intestines were flushed with Colyte® — a potent bowel cleansing agent often used prior to surgical procedures of the gut. This was attempted in the hopes that the bacteria and their toxins would be removed from his intestines. But, alas, symptoms of diarrhea returned within days.

After 10 months of antibiotic therapy, K.K. had not gained any weight and could not stop taking antibiotics without symptoms of *Clostridium difficile* returning within 3-5 days. Ten months after diarrhea began, K.K. was started on a relatively high dose of a probiotic that contained a total of 450 billion bacteria in each dose. The probiotic was called VSL#3® and each dose contained eight different strains of bacteria. Within days of starting the probiotic, K.K.'s symptoms improved. Ten days after VSL#3® was started, vancomycin was stopped, and VSL#3® was continued. VSL#3® was given in a dose of 1/2 packet in the morning and 1/2 packet in the afternoon, one hour prior to meals. Within one month of beginning therapy with VSL#3®, K.K. gained three pounds. Additionally, for the first time since his symptoms began, the foul smell and mucus associated with *C. difficile* in his stools disappeared. After taking VSL#3® for four months, no traces of *C. difficile* bacteria or *C. difficile* toxins could be found in his stools.

About *Clostridium difficile*

Clostridium difficile is a gram-positive rod shaped bacteria that produces at least two toxins, toxin A and toxin B. These toxins work together to cause a serious and potentially life-threatening disease. *C. difficile* is found in the stools of many infants and about 5% of healthy adults. While it is possible to carry *C. difficile* in the intestines without experiencing any problems, a serious infection may occur when a toxin-secreting strain of *C. difficile* overgrows in the bowel. As mentioned earlier, most individuals with *C. difficile* diarrhea develop symptoms after taking a course of antibiotic therapy (symptoms may be delayed until 6-8 weeks after antibiotic use). But it is also not uncommon to have difficulties with *C. difficile* after chemotherapy treatments or during hospitalization.

Nearly all antibiotics can cause *C. difficile* overgrowth. However, penicillins, cephalosporins, and clindamycin are the most common culprits. Although *C. difficile* is implicated in only 10-20% of cases of antibiotic-associated diarrhea, it accounts for most incidences of colitis (inflammation of the colon) associated with antibiotic therapy (Bartlett, 2002). Studies have determined that hospitalized adults have a much greater likelihood of having *C. difficile* in their stools — at a rate of 20-35% — compared to only 3% of adults treated as outpatients. In addition to antibiotic use, chemotherapy, and hospitalization, another risk factor for developing *C. difficile* diarrhea is simply advancing age. Older individuals are more likely to be colonized with *C. difficile*. One study conducted in Sweden found that individuals older than 60 years of age are 20 to 100 times more likely to have *C. difficile* in their stools compared to 10-20 year olds (Bartlett, 2002). Sometimes, outbreaks of *C. difficile* diarrhea occur in hospitals, nursing homes, or daycare centers.

Symptoms of *C. difficile* diarrhea vary widely in severity. Some individuals experience recurrent mild-to-moderate diarrhea, while others suffer from recurrent bouts of severe abdominal and back cramping, frequent loose and watery, greenish, foul-smelling stools, flatulence, fever, as well as variable amounts of mucus and blood in the stool. *C. difficile* diarrhea with accompanying inflammation of the colon can lead to toxic dilation of the colon, perforation of the colon, dehydration, loss of water volume, shock, and death. Interestingly, the toxins produced by *C. difficile* can also trigger a whole host of extra-intestinal complications, too, including joint pain and sleep disorders.

C. difficile diarrhea is most often diagnosed by the presence of *C. difficile* toxins in the stools. However, other signs of infection include high levels of white blood cells in the blood stream, white blood cells in the stools, and characteristic changes of the colon seen by endoscopic visual inspection or biopsies. The term **pseudomembranous colitis** is used to describe the toxin-induced inflammation and nodules — or loose plaques — that are evident during colonoscopic examination. These pseudomembranes — or plaques — contain white blood cells, mucus, and epithelial cells that are loosely adherent to the inflamed and dying mucosal lining of the intestine.

C. difficile is an **anaerobic**, **sporulating** organism. Anaerobic means the bacteria cannot grow and multiply in the presence of oxygen and sporulating refers to that fact that these bacteria have the ability to form spores and lie in a dormant state. When the environment is unfavorable, *C. difficile* stops growing and lies dormant, until more favorable conditions are encountered. As a result, *C. difficile* is difficult to eliminate because it can persist in the intestines and in the outside environment for long periods of time, easily spreading from one individual to another. Antibiotics and chemotherapy treatments are viewed by *C. difficile* as "unfavorable environments." Thus, during antibiotic therapy, antibiotics disrupt normal gastrointestinal flora by killing many bacterial species; however, *C. difficile* persists in the intestines in a dormant state to avoid being killed. After a course of antibiotics is completed, there is often an insufficient number of "good" flora left to suppress the growth of *C. difficile* and *C. difficile* grows uninhibited.

The story presented earlier that described *C. difficile* diarrhea experienced by K.K. is somewhat unusual because K.K. had not taken antibiotics immediately prior to the onset of his symptoms. However, given his case history, it is possible that he initially picked up the bacteria while in the neonatal intensive care unit at birth. In fact, from personal communication with mothers who have had newborn infant children test positive for *C. difficile* toxins, I learned that it is not unusual for symptoms of *C. difficile* infections to mimic symptoms of meningitis in infants less than 2 weeks of age.

It is likely that K.K. was originally exposed to *C. difficile* in the neonatal intensive care unit and that the earliest symptoms he experienced occurred several days later — in the form of meningitis-like symptoms. Typically children under the age of two years do not exhibit gastrointestinal symptoms even when colonized by *C. difficile*, because immaturely-developed intestines do not make the protein that *C. difficile* toxins bind to in the gut. This could explain why K.K. did not experience gastrointestinal symptoms earlier in life. If *C. difficile* was present from birth, inappropriate oral tolerance may have developed in this child such that the immune system did not recognize *C. difficile* as "foreign." This inappropriate oral tolerance explains why K.K.'s immune system failed to mount typical immune responses against the bacterium. The fact that this child experienced food allergies (egg) and asthma is also consistent with long-standing gastrointestinal inflammation caused by an imbalance in normal bacterial flora due to the persistence of *C. difficile* microorganisms. The yeast infection that immediately preceded this child's onset of *C. difficile* diarrhea also is indicative of disturbances within normal gut flora.

C. difficile diarrhea is typically diagnosed by testing for the presence of *C. difficile* toxins — either looking for toxin A or toxin B. These tests typically take less than 24 hours. However, most commercial testing laboratories using toxin-detecting tests have a false negative rate of 10 to 20% (Bartlett, 2002). This means that up to 20% of the time, *C. difficile* toxins may be present in the stools and be the underlying cause of the diarrhea, but the laboratory tests are not *sensitive* enough to detect toxins in the specimen. In fact, some folks with symptoms of *C. difficile* diarrhea have repeatedly had their stools test "negative" for this toxin for several years, only to find out, once they switched to a different laboratory with more sensitive detection methods, that their diarrhea was, in fact, caused by this microorganism. For this reason, it is often recommended that more than one stool specimen be tested for *C. difficile* toxins to increase the likelihood of accurate detection. Another method for detecting *C. difficile* is to place stool samples on selective petri dishes. This method, when performed correctly, can identify and isolate the *C. difficile* microorganism itself rather than relying upon detection of toxins, but this method takes 3-4 days for bacteria to grow and few laboratories offer this test. Other less specific signs that *suggest C. difficile* infection, but that are not definitively diagnostic are elevated white blood cells counts in the blood stream, white blood cells in feces, and low levels of protein in the blood (hypoalbuminemia) (Bartlett, 2002). In rare situations, when *C. difficile* is suspected, but has not been able to be confirmed by standard laboratory methods, a colonoscopy may be necessary. A colonoscopy is a test that allows visual inspection of the inside of the intestines by inserting a long, flexible fiberoptic tube. Findings in the colon may range from normal-to-mild inflammation all the way to severe pseudomembranous colitis. Pseudomembranous colitis, although rare, is nearly always caused by *C. difficile*.

Standard Medical Treatments for *C. difficile*

Initial treatment of *C. difficile* diarrhea begins with discontinuing use of any antibiotics that may have contributed to the infection. Many times, just stopping the offending antibiotic is sufficient for normal gut flora to re-populate the intestines. However, if diarrhea persists or is severe and *C. difficile* is implicated, one of two oral antibiotics is typically recommended. Metronidazole (Flagyl®) or vancomycin (Vancocin®) are typically taken by mouth three or four times per day. Roughly 90-97% of people with *C. difficile* diarrhea respond to these antibiotics. Fevers usually resolve within 24 hours and diarrhea typically stops within 3-4 days. Most often, a 10 day course of antibiotic is used initially, although some studies have found it more beneficial to use longer treatment regimens.

Metronidazole is usually the initial drug of choice because it is less expensive than vancomycin. Additionally, there is less chance that metronidazole will cause antibiotic-resistant strains of bacteria to emerge, which can, of course, lead to other complications. However, a common unpleasant side effect associated with metronidazole is a metallic taste in the mouth, and many individuals have difficulty tolerating this. Additionally, when taking metronidazole, abstinence from alcohol is absolutely necessary. Severe reactions have occurred in individuals taking metronidazole when alcohol was consumed. Oral vancomycin is usually reserved for patients who do not respond to metronidazole or who continuously relapse each time metronidazole is discontinued. In patients who fail to respond to either of these antibiotics, an evaluation should be performed to make certain that there is no bowel obstruction, preventing antibiotics from reaching the colon. Severely ill patients who do not respond to metronidazole or vancomycin may require surgical removal of the colon to completely eliminate the bacterium from their intestines.

Although symptoms of *C. difficile* diarrhea clear up in most people once a complete course of metronidazole or vancomycin has been used, symptoms of diarrhea return in 20-25% of individuals within three weeks of stopping these antibiotics. These relapses often resolve after another course of antibiotic therapy. However, 3-5% of patients have continual relapses and are diagnosed with chronic, persistent *C. difficile* diarrhea (Bartlett, 2002). In fact, according to a personal communication with Dr. Thoerig, medical director for Mucovax©, a pharmaceutical company located in the Netherlands that is investigating new treatment approaches for *C. difficile* diarrhea, it is estimated that as many as 3 million people in the United States suffer from *Clostridium difficile*-associated diarrhea.

Recent evidence suggests that chronic, persistent *C. difficile* disease may be associated with a focal immune deficiency. It appears that individuals who have difficulty recovering from *C. difficile* diarrhea fail to make antibodies against *C. difficile* toxin A. The ability to make antibodies against this toxin protects against reoccurring infections (Kyne et al., 2001).

Treatment of persistent *C. difficile* diarrhea tends to become quite expensive. Estimated costs average $10,970 per person according to one report (McFarland et al., 1999). Unfortunately, there is no clear answer for appropriate treatment in cases of chronic relapsing *C. difficile* diarrhea. Some treatment approaches prove to be curative in some individuals, yet these same regimens do not benefit others. Numerous antibiotic regimens have been tried, sometimes successfully and sometimes not. For example, extended tapering regimens of vancomycin including pulse dosing (several days of drug, followed by several days without drug) (Tedesco et al., 1985) or long periods of very low doses of vancomycin (either once daily or once every other day) have been used with success in some patients. However, these same regimens have not benefited others. Part of the problem with persistent *C. difficile* infection is that: (1) as long as antibiotics (metronidazole/vancomycin) are used, the drugs not only prevent growth of *C. difficile*, but also continue to disrupt normal gastrointestinal flora and (2) antibiotics don't eliminate *C. difficile* spores, since these bacteria simply lie dormant until antibiotics are stopped.

Some individuals have been successfully treated for *C. difficile* diarrhea using approaches other than antibiotics. For example, bismuth-containing drugs such as Pepto Bismal® seem to be selectively toxic to *C. difficile* when used in high doses (Mahony et al, 1999). However, because Pepto Bismal® contains salicylates, this approach is not suitable for children (due to the risk of Reye's syndrome), for those with a history of peptic ulcer disease, or for people taking anticoagulants ("blood thinners").

Others have had success eliminating *C. difficile* with a cholesterol-lowering drug called cholestyramine (Questran®). Cholestyramine is a resin and binds to nearly everything it comes in contact with, including *C. difficile* toxins. By binding to bacterial toxins, cholestyramine may prevent the toxins from irritating the colon, thereby preventing diarrhea and allowing normal gastrointestinal flora to regrow.

Another approach that has been used with some success involves flushing the intestines with a potent bowel cleansing agent such as Colyte®. Colyte® is a drug normally used to clean out the bowel prior to gastrointestinal surgeries or colonoscopies. It typically causes severe diarrheal symptoms which continue for several hours after ingestion. This method, sometimes, successfully removes both *C. dif-*

ficile bacteria and their toxins from the digestive tract.

Other management regimens have used intravenous immunoglobulins (IVIG) — essentially antibodies pooled together from the blood or plasma of healthy individuals. Since, for some reason, those with chronic, persistent *C. difficile* diarrhea don't make their own antibodies to ward off this bacterium, intravenous infusions of IVIG provide the lacking antibodies (Leung et al., 1991). This approach is effective for some individuals — especially those folks whose diarrhea initially improves while taking either metronidazole or vancomycin — but it does not work for everyone. It is usually necessary to repeat IVIG intravenous infusions every four weeks for a total of three treatments to completely eliminate *C. difficile* infection (Dr. Ciaran Kelly, Beth Israel Deaconess Medical Center, Harvard Medical School, personal communication). IVIG is expensive and is associated with risks including anaphylactic allergies, kidney damage, and the theoretical risk of contracting a blood-borne infection.

Other experimental approaches for treating *C. difficile* diarrhea — in individuals whose immune systems simply don't recognize the bacterium as a foreign, disease-causing invader — are currently being investigated. One approach undergoing clinical trials involves immunizing affected individuals with *C. difficile* toxins, with the intention of stimulating immune responses (Aboudola et al., 2003). Another approach involves "immune milks." Cow's milk, collected soon after delivery of calves — called colostrum — is rich in antibodies. Pharmaceutical companies have investigated the possibility of immunizing female cows with *C. difficile* toxins; in this way, colostrum will become rich in antibodies directed against *C. difficile* organisms. Purification and subsequent ingestion of milk containing these antibodies by affected individuals may eradicate *C. difficile* infection (Louis Thoerig, Mucovax©, personal communication.)

A big advantage for using one of the non-antibiotic treatments (like Pepto Bismal®, cholestyramine, IVIG, or colostrum), as opposed to using antibiotics (metronidazole or vancomycin) to eliminate *C. difficile* is that the non-antibiotics greatly facilitate growth of normal flora. When antibiotics are used to eradicate this type of infection, the antibiotics kill many of the "good" gastrointestinal floral species, but only kill non-spore forms of *C. difficile*. The *C. difficile* spores are still present. In order to eradicate *C. difficile* spores, you **need** to have some "good" normal flora present. It is the toxins produced by various normal floral species that kill *C. difficile* spores. However, if antibiotics wipe out all the "good" flora, there's nothing left to eliminate the spores and the infection just keeps coming back, over and over again.

Probiotics in *C. difficile* Diarrhea

Saccharomyces boulardii

In the past two decades, numerous probiotic approaches have been tried as treatments for persistent *C. difficile* diarrhea. Many of these approaches have worked for large numbers of people; but, keep in mind, not every treatment works for everyone.

In the late 1980s, a well-designed clinical trial used a non-disease-causing yeast called *Saccharomyces boulardii* to prevent diarrhea in hospitalized patients receiving antibiotics. *Saccharomyces boulardii* has many properties that make it an ideal probiotic agent. Although the normal environment where *Saccharomyces boulardii* grows is on lychee fruit, it also grows well at body temperature in the intestines. This yeast survives passage through the intestinal tract, but it is rapidly eliminated from the body when therapy is stopped. A big advantage of *Saccharomyces boulardii* over many other probiotics is that, since it is a yeast, it is unaffected by antibiotics (although, it will be killed by antifungal drugs). Therefore, it can be used simultaneously with antibiotics, if desired.

> When *Saccharomyces boulardii* was given as a supplement to prevent diarrhea, only 9.5% of hospitalized patients taking antibiotics experienced antibiotic-associated diarrhea compared to 22% of patients that received antibiotics without *Saccharomyces boulardii* supplements (Surawicz et al., 1989b). These results indicate that *Saccharomyces boulardii* reduces the risk of acquiring antibiotic-associated diarrhea in patents who are hospitalized.

Based on encouraging preliminary data indicating that this yeast could *prevent* antibiotic-associated diarrhea, numerous studies, both in humans and experimental animals, have gone on to evaluate *Saccharomyces boulardii*, as a *treatment* for active *C. difficile* diarrhea. Early in the 1990s, a well designed randomized, placebo-controlled clinical trial demonstrated that addition of *Saccharomyces boulardii* to traditional antibiotic therapies (metronidazole or vancomycin) for treatment of recurrent *C. difficile* diarrhea, resulted in a lower reoccurrence rate of diarrhea for those suffering from chronic, persistent diarrhea (McFarland, 1994).

> To be precise, either **placebo** or 1 gram of *S. boulardii* per day was administered to 124 patients. The risk of recurring *C. difficile* diarrhea was substantially reduced for those who had been suffering from recurrent *C. difficile* infection (reoccurrence rates were 35% with *S. boulardii* versus 64% with placebo).

Numerous other small studies indicate *Saccharomyces boulardii* is beneficial in treating *Clostridium difficile* infections, but I won't describe every study in detail. However, I have included references for those who are interested in learning more. (Kimmey et al., 1990; Buts et al., 1993; Surawicz et al., 1989a; Surawicz et al., 2000).

> For example, 13 patients with recurring *C. difficile* diarrhea were treated simultaneously with a 10 day course of vancomycin and a 30 day course of *Saccharomyces boulardii.* Although prior to the addition of *Saccharomyces boulardii,* the patients in this study had experienced multiple recurrences of *C. difficile* diarrhea, after treatment with *Saccharomyces boulardii,* eleven of the patients (85%) had no further recurrences of *C. difficile* diarrhea (Surawicz et al., 1989a).

It is interesting to note that the combination of vancomycin with *Saccharomyces boulardii* achieves a higher cure rate in cases of persistent *C. difficile* diarrhea than vancomycin alone. Thus, here is an example where combining conventional medicine with an "alternative" medicine achieves a higher success rate in eliminating harmful bacteria than conventional medicine alone (Surawicz et al., 2000). Since *Saccharomyces boulardii* is a yeast, this probiotic is not destroyed if used simultaneously with antibiotics, although *Saccharomyces* supplements would be killed if used with anti-fungal drugs.

> In another study, 19 infants and children with persistent intestinal symptoms related to *C. difficile* overgrowth were administered *Saccharomyces boulardii* for 15 days. Within one week of treatment, gastrointestinal symptoms cleared up in 18 patients (95%). Furthermore, *C. difficile* toxin B was no longer detectable in the stools of 85% of these patients and complete elimination of the *C. difficile* microorganism from stools occurred within one month in 73% of individu-

> als. Although two patients experienced a relapse of symptoms, a second 15-day course of *Saccharomyces boulardii* eliminated adverse gastrointestinal effects in these study participants also (Buts et al., 1993).

Another case study described the experience of one patient with *C. difficile* diarrhea who relapsed six times over an eight month period, despite treatment with vancomycin, metronidazole, bacitracin (another antibiotic rarely used due to side effects), and cholestyramine. *Saccharomyces boulardii* was initiated simultaneously with vancomycin during the last course of treatment, and the yeast was continued for three months. No further reoccurrence of diarrhea occurred during the three months that the patient received *Saccharomyces boulardii* or during the 18 months that the patient was followed after discontinuing the yeast supplement (Kimmey et al., 1990). Thus, for patients dealing with chronically, recurring *C. difficile* diarrhea, probiotics can offer some pretty amazing advantages over traditional antibiotic therapies alone.

The exact mechanism by which *Saccharomyces boulardii* is effective in treating *C. difficile* is not known, but some studies indicate that *Saccharomyces* interferes with *C. difficile* toxin A. This probiotic produces a protease (an enzyme that breaks down proteins) that destroys either the intestinal wall site to which toxin A binds (Pothoulakis et al., 1993) or destroys *C. difficile* toxin A directly (Castagliuolo et al., 1996). In addition, *Saccharomyces boulardii* stimulates the intestinal immune system to secrete *C. difficile* toxin A-specific antibodies (IgA) in the gut (Qamar et al., 2001). Regardless of its precise mechanism, it is clear that *Saccharomyces boulardii* disrupts toxins that would normally irritate the intestines and by doing so has cured many people when conventional medicine has failed.

Dr. Christina Surawicz, a gastroenterologist with the University of Seattle at the Harborview Medical Center, is one of the world's leading experts in this area. Surawicz has 15 years of experience under her belt researching and prescribing *Saccharomyces boulardii* as a treatment for *Clostridium difficile* diarrhea. According the Surawicz, she became interested in studying the clinical effects of *Saccharomyces boulardii* in humans through a collaboration she had with the university's pharmacology department. While studying a completely unrelated topic — drug metabolism in guinea pigs — investigators noted that

Saccharomyces boulardii cleared up colitis in these animals.

According to Surawicz, "This yeast has been marketed in Europe and Africa for 40 years, but there was really nothing known about it, no studies done other than for use in traveler's diarrhea." Surawicz summarized our current understanding, "*Saccharomyces* decreases the incidence of antibiotic-associated diarrhea when compared to placebo. It doesn't appear effective for primary *Clostridium difficile* diarrhea, but it is effective in recurrent disease models [those with chronic, persistent *C. difficile* diarrhea]." Surawicz indicated that the best research to date suggests, "The yeast secretes a protease that inactivates *C. difficile* toxin A, although we can't rule out other mechanisms. Since yeast is thousands of times bigger than bacteria, it is possible that this yeast elbows out the bad bacteria. There are also effects on the immune system, like increased IgA levels. There are multiple levels by which it works." For those who are interested, at least one form of *Saccharomyces boulardii* is commercially available as a product called Florastor®.

Probiotic bacteria

Over the years, numerous studies have also examined the effects of lactic acid-producing bacteria as a treatment for *C. difficile*. Time and time again, *Lactobacillus* GG given at ***high*** doses (10 billion live bacteria daily) for as little as 7-10 days following traditional antibiotic therapy (metronidazole or vancomycin) has cured patients with relapsing *C. difficile* diarrhea (Gorbach et al., 1987). Several reasons have been proposed to explain the effectiveness of *Lactobacillus* GG, including its resistance to gastric and bile acids, its ability to adhere to and colonize the gastrointestinal tract, and its production of an antimicrobial substance that inhibits growth of other anaerobic bacteria in the gut.

Since initial positive studies published in the late 1980s, numerous smaller studies have been conducted using various probiotic regimens. Results from these studies indicate *Lactobacillus* GG and *Lactobacillus plantarum* may be effective treatments for recurrent, relapsing *C. difficile* diarrhea (Biller et al., 1995; Levy et al., 1997).

> For example, *Lactobacillus* GG was used to cure 4 children of *Clostridium difficile*-associated diarrhea. Prior to using *Lactobacillus* therapy, each of the children had been treated previously with vancomycin or metronidazole, had suffered from severe diarrhea for 3-5 months, and had previously experienced multiple (3-5) relapses. (Biller et al., 1995).

In the patient example mentioned earlier, K.K. had been using *Lactobacillus* GG supplements for 10 months while simultaneously taking antibiotics, yet in this child *Lactobacillus* GG was not effective. It is likely that the dose of probiotic recommended to this child was not large enough to overcome the influence of *C. difficile*, especially since he was taking the *Lactobacillus* supplement concurrently with vancomycin. Since vancomycin is an antibiotic, it is likely that each time a dosage of *Lactobacillus* GG was given to the child, the next dose of vancomycin eliminated the majority of "healthy" bacteria. The probiotic preparation that cured K.K. contained 450 billion live and active microorganisms in each dose, and each dose contained 8 different bacterial species rather than just one. When it comes to probiotics in the gastrointestinal tract, experts now agree on two things: a critical **number** of microorganisms must be consumed in order to alter the bacterial populations in the gut, and **several different species** of bacteria given simultaneously are preferable to using just one species, in order to exert positive effects in an environment where at least 500 different bacterial populations flourish.

Other probiotic approaches have been used with success both to prevent and to treat *C. difficile* diarrhea, but larger studies are needed before conclusions can be drawn. One example of a therapeutic regimen that uses probiotics to *prevent* infections caused by *C. difficile* is the use of *Clostridium butyricum* (Miyairi 588 strain) in eastern countries. In Japan, China, and Korea, for instance, all hospitalized patients are automatically prescribed *Clostridium butyricum* as a preventative measure — to prevent *C. difficile* acquisition during hospitalizations (Borody, 2002). It is believed that this is a friendly clostridium species that can live normally in the human intestines. *C. butyricum* is assumed to interfere with the growth of *C. difficile* by competing for binding sites on the intestinal wall or competing for essential nutrients.

> One hundred ten Japanese children receiving antibiotics were divided into three groups. One group received antibiotics alone, another group received antibiotics and *C. butyricum* simultaneously from the beginning of antibiotic treatment, and the third group received the probiotic only mid-way through antibiotic treatment. During treatment, 59% of those who received just antibiotics had diarrhea, compared to only 5% and 9% of those who received probiotics simultaneously with antibiotics from the middle or beginning of therapy,

> respectively. Additionally, only patients who did not take the probiotic had significantly reduced numbers of bifidobacteria in their intestines.
>
> Thus, it can be concluded from this study that simultaneous administration of *C. butyricum* with antibiotics prevents decreases in intestinal bifidobacteria by normalizing disturbed normal flora. Furthermore, this probiotic was effective for both treatment and prevention of antibiotic-associated diarrhea in children (Seki et al., 2003).

Although *C. butyricum* is widely used in the Far East, there is little information about this probiotic in the Western literature.

Another example of a novel probiotic approach that has worked successfully to *treat* continual relapses of *C. difficile* diarrhea involves administration of a strain of *C. difficile* that does not produce toxins (Seal et al., 1987). Patients in whom this therapy was tried responded favorably without side effects. It appears that a non-toxin-producing *C. difficile* strain, "crowds out" toxic strains of *C. difficile.* Administration of non-toxin-producing *C. difficile* strains successfully cured two patients of *C. difficile* diarrhea after they had each suffered from multiple relapses of continual diarrhea every time metronidazole and vancomycin therapy were discontinued.

Less aesthetically pleasing probiotic alternatives

Other more invasive probiotic approaches have been used with great success in some individuals with chronic *C. difficile* diarrhea. Although these procedures are not routinely needed, they have great potential to be curative in patients who have been severely ill with *C. difficile.* I am including these treatments here for completeness sake, since patients who have been severely ill — after having failed all other treatments — are sometimes willing to try anything to get well again.

One of these approaches is referred to as the "broth" method. Dr. Mark Allen, at St. Luke's Hospital in Kansas City, MO, uses laboratory-grown *Escherichia coli* and Bacteroides species of bacteria to treat patients with persistent *C. difficile* gastrointestinal symptoms. At first glance, some of you are, no doubt, skeptical saying to yourself, "Isn't *Escherichia coli* the bacteria that causes disease?" You would be partially correct. A specific toxin-secreting strain, *Escherichia coli*

0157:H7 can be deadly. It is this strain that you sometimes hear about from the media when it causes sickness after people eat contaminated meats. But, the truth of the matter is, we need *Escherichia coli* in our bodies, and Dr. Allen does not use the harmful strain in his practice. In fact, around the world, different strains of *Escherichia coli* are commercially available as probiotics. Some of the trade names by which these products are sold include Mutaflor® and Probactrix®.

Using an endoscopic procedure in which a naso-jejunal tube is inserted via the nose down into the small intestines, Dr. Allen delivers live bacteria into the upper bowel region of the gastrointestinal tract. According to Dr. Allen, delivery of the bacteria to the small intestines allows the microorganisms to slowly "percolate through the lower portions of the colon." According to Allen, "This procedure is approximately 60% effective in curing *C. difficile* diarrhea." Failure to beat *C. difficile* after one "broth" treatment does not predict future failures. Some of Dr. Allen's patients have failed to get better with the first broth infusion, but have beaten *C. difficile* diarrhea with subsequent treatments.

Perhaps the ultimate in "distasteful" probiotic approaches is using fecal matter from healthy people as a source of probiotics to replace the normal gastrointestinal flora in individuals who have failed other *C. difficile* treatments. Yes, this approach is aesthetically unattractive and distasteful to think about, but it has a very high rate of success! When I first read about this in the literature, my reaction was, "Ugh! You've got to be kidding!" However, on thinking about it further, it makes perfect sense. Quite frankly, 100 years ago, the idea of blood transfusions — giving blood from one individual to another — was just as distasteful to people. In this case, "swapping poop" from a healthy person to a sick person is less invasive than a blood transfusion. Where do you think most commercially-available probiotics came from initially? Most, if not all, probiotic bacteria were originally isolated from human feces! There are definite advantages of "fecal transplants" since the procedure replaces *all strains* of healthy normal flora in *large quantities* and does so all at one time, without a need for continuous daily probiotic therapy.

Although this procedure is neither routine nor widely accepted, individuals with incurable symptomatic *C. difficile* are often willing to seek out any form of therapy rather than continue suffering. Of course, the biggest concern with this approach is that another communicable disease may be transmitted from the "healthy" person to the "sick" person. For this reason, it is necessary that the fecal donor undergo extensive laboratory and physical evaluation to rule out as many infectious diseases as possible, including HIV and hepatitis. I don't necessarily recommend this method. However, it has been highly curative for those with chronic, persistent *C. difficile* diarrhea for whom all other treatments have failed.

Using "healthy" feces as a probiotic, some physicians have deposited the stools (and associated probiotic bacteria) directly into the intestines of patients during colonoscopies so that the beneficial bacteria could be uniformly distributed along the entire wall of the colon (Persky and Brandt, 2000). Other physicians have replaced the normal gastrointestinal flora using fecal enemas (Eiseman et al., 1958; Bowden et al., 1981; Schwan et al., 1983; Schwan et al., 1984; Tvede and Rask-Madsen, 1989; Flotterod et al., 1991; Paterson et al., 1994; Lund-Tonnesen et al., 1998), have delivered feces via a naso-intestinal tube (Flotterod et al., 1991), or have suspended feces in milk (Gustafsson et al., 1998) to treat *C. difficile* diarrhea or other gastrointestinal ailments.

The earliest report using total human fecal flora to treat pseudomembranous colitis was in 1958. At that time, *C. difficile* hadn't even been identified so the doctors in charge of the study didn't even know what "bug" they were fighting. Four patients who were literally at death's door, were given fecal enemas to replace their entire gut flora, and amazingly these patients recovered in a matter of hours (Eiseman et al., 1958). Other success stories follow:

> Over an eighteen year period, 16 patients with refractory pseudomembranous colitis were treated with fecal enemas to restore intestinal flora when standard accepted forms of therapy had failed to resolve the disease. Thirteen of the patients responded dramatically with decreases in diarrhea, lowered temperature, and improved white blood cell counts. No adverse effects from fecal enemas were observed (Bowden et al., 1981).

> In a similar study, six patients with chronic relapsing diarrhea caused by *Clostridium difficile* were treated by rectal instillation of feces or a mixture of ten different bacteria. It is interesting to note that prior to successful treatment with probiotic enemas, there was a lack of bacteroides species present in the stools of these individuals. However after treatment, growth of *Clostridium difficile* was inhibited, presumably by *Bacteroides* that re-colonized the colon. These findings suggest that absence of bacteroides species contributes to chronic relapsing *Clostridium difficile* diarrhea and that the presence of *Bacteroides* prevents colonization by *Clostridium difficile* (Tvede and Rask-Madsen, 1989).

> Most recently, in a **retrospective** report, 18 patients with refractory *C. difficile* diarrhea were treated with stools donated by healthy individuals. Fecal flora infusions were delivered to patients via a nasogastric tube. Although two patients died due to other illnesses, of the remaining 16 patients, only a single patient experienced a recurrence of *C. difficile* diarrhea (94% cure rate). This one patient was re-treated with vancomycin without any further problems (Aas et al., 2003). By the way, this study was published just this year and was carried out at a major U.S. medical center.

According to Dr. Borody, a gastroenterologist in Sydney, Australia, who has used fecal enemas in hundreds of patients (including many who have traveled to him from the United States), the clinical improvement following fecal enemas is usually quite dramatic. Typically within 1-4 days diarrhea stops, pseudomembranes resolve, and other adverse gastrointestinal effects subside. Dr. Borody has unparalleled experience and expertise in the delivery of healthy fecal flora, which he refers to as "human probiotic infusions". Dr. Borody currently serves as director of the Centre for Digestive Diseases and the director of the world's only Probiotic Therapy Research Centre (PTRC). The goal of the PTRC is to diagnose and treat disorders caused by abnormal bowel flora by preparing and developing probiotics to treat various disease states.

According to the PTRC's website, the reason that patients with *C. difficile* relapse after seeming to get better initially with antibiotic therapy is because *C. difficile* spores persist and grow again after conventional pharmacological therapies are stopped. At the present time, we don't have any medicines that kill *C. difficile* spores. On the other hand, human probiotic infusions *can* permanently eradicate *C. difficile* spores, since normal gut flora secrete bacteriocins that are toxic to *C. difficile* spores. Using fresh fecal matter from healthy donors as the source of probiotics, human fecal infusions have a *C. difficile*-cure rate of 90-95%.

The problem with *C. difficile* isn't the *presence* of the pathogen, but the *absence* of healthy flora to keep the growth of the microorganism suppressed. According to Dr. Borody, "People with *C. difficile* don't have *Bacteroides*. *Bacteroides* can kill *C. difficile*." Borody also said, "Human probiotic infusions are comprised almost entirely of *Bacteroides*; *Bacteroides fragilis* makes up 90%."

Although some physicians argue that it is impossible to permanently alter the gut's flora with a simple fecal infusion, Dr. Borody's research center has "compared the genetic cross section of bugs" in sick people prior to fecal transplant, in the healthy fecal donor, and in the "former patient" six months after fecal flora infusion. With human probiotic infusions, there is between a 40% to 60% long-term gut colonization rate with the new flora six months after the procedure. In his experience, Dr. Borody finds that children with chronic, persistent *C. difficile* can be cured with commercially available probiotics more often than adults; adults commonly require human probiotic infusions to cure *C. difficile* diarrhea.

Dr. Borody indicated that patients who fail to be cured using fecal infusions are usually those who have been treated late in the course of their illness and die of overwhelming pseudomembranous colitis (Borody, 2000). See below for one patient's story of how fecal enemas cured her of the *C. difficile* nightmare.

> Although generally healthy as a child, C.P. suffered from mild asthma symptoms especially during her junior high years. At 13 years of age, IVIG was administered to "boost her immune system". Eight years later, at 22 years of age, C.P. was hospitalized for severe diarrhea after taking cephalexin (Keflex®) for tonsillitis. A sigmoidoscopy revealed pseudomembranous colitis caused by *C. difficile.* A standard dosing regimen of metronidazole was given and a strict diet was followed for one year. Although *C. difficile*-associated diarrhea improved, C.P. was left with what doctors termed "irritable bowel syndrome."
>
> During the next 18 years, C.P. had no further recurrences of *C. difficile* diarrhea. However, at 39 years of age, C.P. was prescribed cefixime (Suprax®) to treat a chronic sinus infection and *C. difficile*-associated diarrhea reoccurred, necessitating hospitalization. This second episode of *C. difficile* diarrhea resolved after treatment with a standard course of vancomycin.
>
> However, the third time *C. difficile* diarrhea flared up — following antibiotic treatment for tonsillitis — hospitalization was required for pseudomembranous colitis. Although given the standard 10 day course of vancomycin, C.P. failed to recover from this episode of *C. difficile* diarrhea, despite her stools repeatedly testing negative for *C. difficile* toxins (an example of the false negative results that sometimes occur with some standard laboratory testing procedures). For three years, C.P. spent 3-4 hours on the toilet every day. C.P. took codeine pills (to intentionally make herself constipated) whenever she had to leave the house. According to C.P., "When I drank water, it poured right through me. Sometimes I sat on the toilet just to get something to drink."

> After being quite ill for nearly three years, C.P. sent a stool sample to another medical center with different laboratory testing capabilities. At this institution, C.P.'s stools tested positive for the *C. difficile* microorganism and its toxins. C.P. was prescribed vancomycin. However, despite various antibiotic dosing regimens, supplementation with commercially-available probiotics like *Saccharomyces boulardii* and *Lactobacillus GG*, and dietary changes in which she ate only white rice and fish or only brown rice, C.P.'s diarrhea continued for months.
>
> At this point, C.P. felt she had no other options. C.P. opted to use fecal enemas from a healthy, extensively screened donor (in this case, her husband) to cure *C. difficile* diarrhea. Enemas were administered once daily for 10 days, with each enema retained rectally for a minimum of 5-6 hours. While receiving fecal enemas, C.P. began feeling better within the first week and within 2-3 weeks she was having diarrhea only once or twice a week. It has been several months since C.P.'s fecal enemas, and she is *C. difficile* symptom-free. For the first time in 25 years (since her first episode with *C. difficile* diarrhea), C.P. can eat whatever she wants without suffering adverse gastrointestinal effects.

While fecal enemas are not a treatment-of-first-choice and should be performed only with medical supervision, C.P.'s story indicates the dramatic improvements that this type of therapy has been associated with in nearly 1000 patients to date (personal communication with Dr. Borody). It is my personal belief that commercially available supplements of probiotic bacteria should be utilized whenever possible since many of these strains have documented efficacy and a safe track record. However, for some individuals, commercially-available supplements that replace only one (or several) strain(s) of bacteria, may simply not be sufficient to re-establish normal gastrointestinal flora in some severely ill patients. Perhaps the only way to restore homeostasis in these patients is to re-introduce *all* strains of normal digestive tract flora (possibly 500 or more strains) simultaneously.

To further illustrate the amazing capability of human bacterial flora to fight *C. difficile*, I've included an e-mail communication sent from a Canadian physician to a gastroenterologist who had recommended human probiotic infusions to combat resistant and persistent *C. difficile* in a Canadian patient.

> I thought I'd keep you up to date. A week ago my patient was literally at death's door. She was having 15 bowel movements per day. She was mentally and physically exhausted. She was anorexic, had continuous nausea and vomiting. She

> wanted to die. She was chronically ill, wasting, and bed-ridden. I insisted she have a colonoscopy and fecal infusions since there were no other options except surgical removal of her intestines!
>
> ...The patient's daughter donated stool and improvements were noted within 24 hours. After 5 infusions, there is no more diarrhea, pain, nausea, or vomiting. Her appetite is returning and she is tolerating foods. She smiles and is talkative. She has gone from wanting to die to looking forward to getting out of the hospital for the first time in a month. She has regained her sense of humor.
>
> This is a lady who walked 10 km daily until she received clindamycin [an antibiotic] for a dental infection. Personally, I thought she was going to die, but now it looks like she has turned the corner. The nursing staff is incredulous.

Other Types of Diarrhea

Antibiotic-associated diarrhea

Although roughly 20% of patients taking antibiotics experience diarrhea, *C. difficile* is not always identified as the cause. In fact, the precise cause of antibiotic-associated diarrhea is often not identified, but a gastrointestinal imbalance between "good" and "bad" bacteria is suspected. Antibiotic-associated diarrhea not caused by *C. difficile* is relatively mild, self-limiting, and not associated with intestinal lesions such as pseudomembranous colitis. Numerous studies have successfully used probiotics to *prevent* development of gastrointestinal symptoms — mainly diarrhea — during antibiotic therapy. Supplements of *Lactobacillus acidophilus*, *Lactobacillus bulgaricus*, *Lactobacillus rhamnosus* GG, *Bifidobacterium longum*, *Enterococcus faecium*, and *Sacchromyces boulardii* have *prevented* diarrhea during antibiotic therapies in numerous studies (Gotz et al., 1979; Clements et al., 1983; Witsell et al., 1995; Borgia et al., 1982; Wunderlich et al., 1989; Siitonen et al., 1990; Surawicz et al., 1989b; McFarland et al., 1995; Vanderhoof et al., 1999).

Perhaps the earliest study of probiotics as a preventative for antibiotic-associated diarrhea was conducted in 1979 when it was noted that simultaneous administration of a product called Lactinex® (which contains both *Lactobacillus acidophilus* and *Lactobacillus bulgaricus)* was effective in preventing diarrhea in hospitalized patients receiving ampicillin. In this study, none of the patients taking probiotics developed diarrhea compared to 14% in the placebo group (Gotz et al., 1979).

Other examples of positive studies follow.

> Administration of *Saccharomyces boulardii* — given within 72 hours of initiating beta-lactam antibiotics (penicillins and cephalosporins are some examples of beta-lactam antibiotics), causes significantly fewer patients to develop diarrhea (7 of 97) compared to those receiving placebo (14 of 96). These results indicate that prophylactic use of *Saccharomyces boulardii* results in significantly fewer cases of antibiotic-associated diarrhea. (McFarland et al., 1995).
>
> In another study it was shown that *Lactobacillus* GG reduced diarrhea, abdominal distress, stomach pain, and flatulence associated with erythromycin therapy. Despite simultaneous use of an antibiotic, the intestines of those receiving *Lactobacillus* GG were still colonized by the probiotic bacteria as measured by total fecal counts of *Lactobacillus* GG (Siitonen et al., 1990).
>
> Still another study demonstrated that yogurt supplemented with *Bifidobacterium longum* reduced gastrointestinal side effects associated with use of the antibiotic erythromycin. In this study, 60% of those who received placebo experienced antibiotic-associated diarrhea, while only 10% of individuals who took the probiotic ended up with diarrhea (Colombel et al., 1987).
>
> Additionally, simultaneous administration of *Lactobacillus acidophilus* with the antibiotic amoxicillin/clavulanic acid (Augmentin®) resulted in significantly fewer gastrointestinal side effects and yeast superinfections (Witsell et al., 1995) than when no probiotics were administered.
>
> Recently, 202 children taking antibiotics were simultaneously administered either *Lactobacillus* GG or placebo. Only 7 probiotic-treated children, compared to 25 children taking placebo, experienced diarrhea — indicating that *Lactobacillus* GG reduced the incidence of antibiotic-associated diarrhea in these children (Vanderhoof et al., 1999).

Another study also found a lower incidence of diarrhea in children taking *Lactobacillus* GG during antibiotic therapy when compared to placebo (5% versus 16%) (Arvola et al., 1999). In contrast, there are a few studies that failed to find any substantial benefits of probiotics when used to prevent antibiotic-associated diarrhea. (Thomas et al., 2001; Tankanow et al., 1990). The discrepancy between the results from these studies and all the other studies is unclear. However, it is possible that the lack of effect may be related to the relatively low dose of probiotics used in these investigations. Alternatively, for unknown reasons, we know that everyone does not respond in the same way to a given probiotic, probably due to individual differences in normal gut flora. With the exception of two negative results, most studies overwhelmingly indicate that probiotics are warranted in patients taking broad-spectrum antibiotics to prevent gastrointestinal side effects.

Although lactobacilli are probably the most widely studied probiotic, other bacterial microorganisms have also been investigated as probiotics to prevent antibiotic-associated diarrhea.

> A multi-center study evaluated the use of another bacterium, *Enterococcus* SF68, to prevent antibiotic-associated diarrhea. *Enterococcus* SF68 reduced the incidence of antibiotic-associated diarrhea (8.7%) compared to placebo (27.2%) (Wunderlich et al., 1989).
>
> In another trial, *Streptococcus faecium* significantly reduced the number of hospitalized patients who experienced diarrhea while taking multiple antibiotics. It is believed that enterococci, like other probiotics, may suppress growth of disease-causing bacteria either by competing for essential nutrients or by producing antimicrobial substances (Borgia et al., 1982).

Gastroenteritis

Gastroenteritis is defined as inflammation of the stomach and intestines. It may be caused by infection with viruses or bacteria, or by the presence of bacterial toxins. Gastroenteritis may cause severe vomiting and diarrhea, but it is usually short-lived and resolves spontaneously in 3-5 days. In infants and children, gastroenteritis is most often due to a specific virus called rotavirus.

Several human studies indicate that probiotics may help to *prevent* and *treat* diarrhea in infants and adults with gastroenteritis. Beneficial effects have been explained by stabilization of normal gut flora, reduced gastrointestinal permeability, and increased IgA antibody responses to infection (Isolauri et al., 2002). For example, recently *Lactobacillus* GG was shown to be significantly effective in *preventing* hospitalized infants from acquiring diarrhea — especially rotavirus enteritis (Szajewska et al., 2001).

> Eighty-one children hospitalized for reasons other than diarrhea, ages one month to 3 years, were enrolled in a randomized, **double-blind** trial. Children received either probiotics or placebo during their hospitalization. *Lactobacillus* GG substantially reduced the incidence of hospital-acquired diarrhea (6.7% for probiotics versus 33.3% for placebo).

Numerous studies have found that probiotic bacteria effectively *treat* rotaviral diarrhea, as well.

> In a double blind **placebo-controlled** study, *Bifidobacterium bifidum* and *Streptococcus thermophilus* were given to hospitalized infants. The combination of these probiotics reduced diarrhea and shedding of the virus (Saavedra et al., 1994).

Most probiotic studies in infants with rotavirus-associated diarrhea have used various strains of lactobacilli (Isolauri et al., 1991; Kaila et al, 1992; Majamaa et al., 1995; Isolauri et al., 1994).

> In one study of children ages 4-45 months with acute diarrhea (82% of the children had rotavirus), *Lactobacillus* GG significantly shortened the duration of diarrhea (Isolauri et al., 1991). Another study found similar results in 42 children with rotavirus diarrhea ages 5-28 months (Isolauri et al., 1994).

> Another probiotic strain, *Lactobacillus reuteri,* effectively colonized the gastrointestinal tract of children ages 6-36 months and significantly shortened the duration of watery diarrhea caused by rotavirus. In this study, there was also a correlation between dosage of probiotic and clinical effect (Shornikova et al., 1997b) — the higher the probiotic dosage, the more dramatic the clinical response.

These results indicate that oral bacterial therapy counteracts the disturbed microbial balance following rotavirus infections, shortens the duration of diarrhea, and speeds gastrointestinal healing. Furthermore, this last study supports the theory that there is a critical **number** of probiotics needed to make a difference when using probiotics to treat gastrointestinal infections.

Several other studies attempted to identify the mechanism by which lactobacilli fight gastroenteritis. These studies noted an increase in IgA antibodies against rotavirus in patients treated with *Lactobacillus casei* strain GG. These results indicate that probiotics stimulate the immune system by enhancing local defense mechanisms in the gastrointestinal tract in order to eliminate the infection. In theory, by stimulating antibody production, lactobacilli may also *prevent re-infections* with the same virus (Kaila et al., 1992; Kaila et al., 1995; Majamaa et al., 1995).

> Forty-four children between the ages of 7 and 37 months of age were admitted to the hospital for gastroenteritis during a rotavirus epidem-

> ic. The children were randomized to receive either *Lactobacillus* GG or placebo. The duration of diarrhea was significantly shorter in the group that received the probiotic. Additionally, there was a substantially greater IgA antibody response in children who received *Lactobacillus* GG. These results indicate *Lactobacillus* GG promotes recovery from rotaviral diarrhea by stimulating immune defenses, an action that may protect against subsequent reinfections in the future (Kaila et al., 1992).
>
> Similarly, during another rotavirus epidemic, 60 children between the ages of 4 and 35 months were hospitalized for acute gastroenteritis. These children were randomly and double-blindly assigned to receive either *Lactobacillus* GG, *Lactobacillus* casei, or a combination of *Streptococcus thermophilus*, *Lactobacillus delbrucki*, and *Lactobacillus casei*. The children that received *Lactobacillus* GG had a shorter duration of diarrhea than children who received other probiotic preparations. Again, in this study, *Lactobacillus* GG was associated with enhanced activity of IgA antibodies.

These results demonstrate that *Lactobacillus* GG promotes clinical recovery from acute gastroenteritis and increases gut immune responses to rotavirus. This last study is significant because it suggests that *Lactobacillus* GG differs from some other commonly used strains of probiotic bacteria. This is important to understand because this result implies that probiotics are not all created equally for treating disease and modifying the immune system (Majamaa et al., 1995).

Although I won't describe the details, *Lactobacillus* has also been effective in numerous other studies when used as a treatment for acute gastroenteritis that was not necessarily caused by rotavirus (Raza et al., 1995; Pant et al., 1996; Guarino et al., 1997; Shornikova et a., 1997a, 1997c; Rautanen et al., 1998; Guandalini et al., 2000; Kaila et al., 1995).

Since childhood diarrhea is a significant health problem all around the world, a recent study set out to analyze the *outcome data* of all medical literature that used probiotics to treat children with gastroenteritis. All literature published from 1966 to 2000 was reviewed. After analyzing the data, it was concluded by numerous health care professionals that *Lactobacillus* is a safe, effective, and useful treatment for children with acute infectious diarrhea (Van Niel et al., 2002). (For a comprehensive review of clinical trials using probiotics to prevent or treat gastroenteritis, clinicians are directed to Marteau et al., 2002).

Other probiotics have been used successfully to treat gastroenteritis. For example, *Saccharomyces boulardii* has been associated with significant therapeutic benefits in infants with gastroenteritis. Another probiotic bacterium, *Enterococcus faecium,* has produced beneficial effects in both infants (Bellomo et al., 1980) and adults with diarrhea (Wunderlich et al., 1989; Camarri et al., 1981; Buydens and Debeuckelaere, 1996).

> The beneficial effects of a preparation containing *Enterococcus* SF68 were evaluated in 211 adult patients with diarrhea. Compared to patients receiving placebo, on the second day of therapy only 61% of patients receiving *Enterococcus* SF68 continued to have diarrhea compared to 96% of those receiving placebo. By the third day of treatment, diarrhea was present in only 8% of individuals administered *Enterococcus* compared to 66% of those taking placebo.

These results indicate that *Enterococcus* SF68 shortens the duration and severity of diarrhea (Buydens and Debeuckelaere, 1996).

Streptococcus faecium was also compared directly to a combination regimen of neomycin and bacitracin (two antibiotics) for treatment of acute enteritis in adults.

> Elimination of diarrhea and related gastrointestinal disturbances was significantly more rapid and complete in individuals receiving *Streptococcus faecium* than those who received the antibiotic combination (56% cured at 48 hours compared to 31%).

This study indicates that *Streptococcus faecium* may be a useful adjunct in the treatment of acute enteritis (Camarri et al., 1981).

Necrotizing enterocolitis (NEC)

Necrotizing enterocolitis affects premature babies and is characterized by intestinal inflammation that can cause illness and death. Most times we don't have any idea what causes NEC, but we do know that infants have fragile bowels that are very sensitive to infection. NEC is quite a serious problem. As many as 25% of pre-term, low birth-weight infants are affected by NEC. Of these, half require surgery to remove a portion of their intestines, 25% have long-term complications, and as many as 30% die.

Since a wide variety of bacteria and toxins have been associated with NEC, a recent study examined whether oral administration of the probiotics *Lactobacillus acidophilus* and *Bifidobacterium infantis* decreased the incidence of NEC in a neonatal intensive care unit (NICU).

For one year, all 1237 newborns infants admitted to the NICU of a hospital in Bogota, Columbia, were given *Lactobacillus acidophilus* and

Bifidobacterium infantis daily until the infants were sent home from the hospital. During the year long study, 34 infants developed NEC and 14 of these babies died. These results were compared to data from the previous year in which 1282 infants were admitted to the NICU, but did not receive probiotics. In infants not treated with probiotics, 85 babies developed NEC and 35 of these infants died. The dramatically reduced incidence of NEC and substantially fewer deaths when probiotics were added in this NICU clearly demonstrate that further investigation into the association between bacterial colonization and its role in NEC is needed (Hoyos, 1999).

As you will recall from chapter 1, a variety of factors disrupt acquisition of healthy normal flora in infants. One factor is antibiotics, another is lack of breast milk. Unfortunately, infants requiring NICU attention are placed at a tremendous disadvantage compared to their peers in the regular hospital nursery, since they are typically given antibiotics, and breast milk feedings are often not an option. Both of these things set the stage for a variety of "bad" bacteria to become established in their intestines, in preference to "healthy" bacteria.

Since we don't know exactly which infectious microorganisms cause NEC, it would be nice if we could simultaneously suppress growth of all "harmful" bacteria in preemies, to give them an additional advantage as they begin their lives. To investigate the feasibility of suppressing pathogenic bacteria with probiotics, a randomized, double-blind study was conducted using 54 healthy newborns. *Escherichia coli* strain Nissle 1917 was given to half the infants for the first 5 days of life, to see if this non-disease-causing probiotic strain decreased the likelihood that these children would pick up disease-causing bacteria in their intestines. By the third day of life, potential disease-causing bacteria were identified in 15% of probiotic-treated children versus 57% of placebo-treated children. These differences were even more striking five days after birth (15% versus 62%).

Although children were supplemented with the probiotic for only five days after birth, infants who received the probiotic were still less likely to have disease-causing bacteria in their stools (28% versus 85%) six months later. Remarkably, and unlike most probiotics, *Escherichia coli* strain Nissle 1917 was still detected in stools of probiotic-treated infants 6 months after their last dose of the probiotic, indicating that this microorganism is able to colonize and persist in the intestines for extended periods of time (Lodinova-Zadnikova and Sonnenborn, 1997)!

Traveler's diarrhea

Acute diarrhea occurs in about half of travelers visiting high-risk areas. Although not all studies have found probiotics to offer significant protection against diarrhea when traveling to foreign locations (Pozo-Olano et al., 1978; Katelaris et al., 1995), some studies have found a significantly lower incidence of diarrhea when probiotics such as lactobacilli, bifidobacteria, streptococci, and *Saccharomyces boulardii* (Black et al., 1989; Oksanen et al., 1990; Hilton et al., 1996) are used.

> For example, a mixture of *Lactobacillus acidophilus*, *Lactobacillus bulgaricus*, bifidobacteria, and *Streptococcus thermophilus* reduced the frequency of diarrhea from 71% to 43% in Danish travelers touring Egypt (Black et al., 1989).
>
> Similarly, taking *Lactobacillus* GG when traveling in Turkey reduced the risk of contracting traveler's diarrhea by 39.5% (Oksanen et al., 1990).
>
> There may also be a role for *Saccharomyces boulardii* in preventing traveler's diarrhea, for those visiting northern Africa and Turkey (Kollaritsch et al., 1993).

A few other studies have also demonstrated the merits of probiotics in preventing traveler's diarrhea, but it is difficult to draw conclusions from these studies since the travelers did not take the probiotics regularly as prescribed (Marteau et al., 2002).

Other conditions associated with diarrhea

Irritable bowel syndrome is a common disorder of the intestines that leads to cramping abdominal pain, bloating, flatulence, and either constipation or diarrhea (or sometimes both). Some studies have suggested that probiotics may be beneficial. For example, in one study, the use of probiotics alleviated constipation in individuals with irritable bowel syndrome (Andrews and Borody, 1993). Other studies indicate probiotics reduce many bothersome gastrointestinal symptoms of this illness.

> In one small clinical trial, investigators evaluated *Lactobacillus* in 29 patients with irritable bowel syndrome. The following signs and symptoms of irritable bowel syndrome were recorded: abdominal pain, bloating or gas, number of daily stools, consistency of stools, mucus content of stools, and general physical state. The trial lasted for a total of 14 weeks. During the first six weeks either *Lactobacillus acidophilus* or placebo was administered. This was followed by 2 weeks without receiving any supplements. Then, whichever treatment — probiotic or placebo — had not been used during the first six weeks, was administered during the next six week period. During the

> trial, patients were asked to keep track of their symptoms on a daily basis. Neither doctors nor patients knew whether placebo or probiotic was administered at any given time. When the data was analyzed, there was a significant therapeutic benefit — assessed by reduction of gastrointestinal symptoms — for 50% of patients while they received *Lactobacillus* compared to placebo (Halpern et al., 1996).

Critically ill patients often experience diarrhea due to overgrowth of bacteria in their small intestines. From clinical trials, it has been suggested that lactobacilli (Vanderhoof et al., 1998) reduce small bowel bacterial overgrowth in patients with short bowel syndrome. Additionally, *Saccharomyces boulardii* may offer benefits to these patients by reducing the number of days that patients experience diarrhea (Bleichner et al., 1997).

> In one double-blind, placebo-controlled clinical trial involving 128 patients hospitalized in an intensive care unit and requiring tube feedings for more than six days, some received supplements with *Saccharomyces boulardii* while others received placebo. (Tube feedings are frequently associated with diarrhea due to small intestinal bacterial overgrowth.) In this trial, *Saccharomyces boulardii* reduced the percentage of days with diarrhea per tube feeding from 18.9 to 14.2%. In fact, when the study was evaluated in terms of other risk factors associated with development of diarrhea — such as fever, malnutrition, low levels of albumin in the blood, or infection — the protective effect of *Saccharomyces boulardii* was even more significant. The investigators concluded that *Saccharomyces boulardii* prevents diarrhea in critically ill tube-fed patients, especially in patients with other risk factors for diarrhea (Bleichner et al., 1997).

Small bowel overgrowth is a well-known complication of end-stage kidney failure. Oral administration of *Lactobacillus acidophilus* reduces production of toxins and carcinogens and improves the nutritional status of patients undergoing hemodialysis (Simenhoff et al., 1996).

Radiation to the pelvis almost always causes diarrhea. *Lactobacillus acidophilus* significantly decreases diarrhea in such patients (Salminen et al., 1988).

> In women receiving pelvic radiation therapy for gynecological malignancies, *Lactobacillus acidophilus* in combination with lactulose (a food substrate for the bacteria) prevented radiation-associated diarrhea. However, the women receiving the probiotic had a much higher incidence of flatulence — presumably, due to the lactulose supplement.

Additionally, there is a small amount of evidence suggesting that probiotics such as *Lactobacillus plantarum* 299v may also help to reduce HIV-associated chronic diarrhea by colonizing the gut and helping to reestablish normal gastrointestinal flora (Cunningham-Rundles et al., 2000).

In third world countries, diarrhea is a major cause of death in children. Two studies, one based in Thailand and another conducted in Peru, found that probiotic supplementation in children significantly reduces the risk of diarrhea.

> In the first study, Thai children aged 3-24 months with acute diarrhea and dehydration were enrolled into a study in which 37 children were rehydrated and received *Lactobacillus acidophilus* while 36 children were rehydrated and received placebo. The length of time that diarrhea persisted was significantly less in children that received the probiotic (Simakachorn et al., 2000).
>
> In the other study, 204 undernourished children aged 6-24 months from a poor Peruvian town participated in a clinical trial in which they received either placebo or *Lactobacillus* once daily for 15 months. The children that received the probiotic had significantly fewer diarrheal episodes than the children that got placebo, especially non-breastfed toddlers (Oberhelm et al., 1999).

When all of these studies are combined and evaluated simultaneously, there is overwhelming support for use the of probiotics to prevent and treat numerous types of diarrhea. Probiotics are not only remarkably effective treatments for diarrhea, but they are also incredibly safe — with no adverse effects more severe than flatulence reported in any clinical trial.

Conclusion

An overwhelming number of studies demonstrate the benefits of probiotics in treating diarrhea. Probiotic supplements may cure chronic, relapsing *C. difficile* diarrhea even in extremely ill patients. Probiotics may reduce the duration and severity of rotaviral diarrhea. Additionally, probiotics may prevent antibiotic-associated diarrhea, traveler's diarrhea, and episodes of acute gastroenteritis. In the future, perhaps specific strains of probiotic bacterial supplements and clear dosage regimens will be identified as therapies-of-choice for each of the many causes of diarrhea.

Notes

Notes

References

Aas J, Gessert CE, Bakken JS. Recurrent *Clostridium difficile* colitis: Case series involving 18 patients treated with donor stool administered via a nasogastric tube. Clin Infect Dis. 2003;36:580-585.

Aboudola S, Kotloff KL, Kyne L, et al. *Clostridium difficile* vaccine and serum immunoglobulin G antibody response to toxin A. Infect Immun. 2003;71:1608-1610.

Andrews PJ and Borody TJ. "Putting back the bugs": Bacterial treatment relieves chronic constipation and symptoms of irritable bowel syndrome. Med J Australia. 1993;159:633-634.

Arvola T, Laiho K, Toarkkeli S, et al. Prophylactic *Lactobacillus* GG reduces antibiotic-associated diarrhea in children with respiratory infections: A randomized study. Pediatrics. 1999;104:e64.

Bartlett J. Antibiotic-associated diarrhea. NEJM. 2002;346:334-339.

Bellomo G, Mangiagle A, Nicastro L, et al. A controlled double blind study of SF68 strain as a new biological preparation for the treatment of diarrhea in pediatrics. Curr Ther Res. 1980;28:927-936.

Biller JA, Katz AJ, Flores AF, et al. Treatment of recurrent *Clostridium difficile* colitis with *Lactobacillus* GG. J Pediatr Gastreoenterol Nutr. 1995; 21:224-226.

Black F, Andersen PL. Orskov J, et al. Prophylactic efficacy of lactobacilli on traveler's diarrhea. Travel Med. 1989;7:333-335.

Bleichner G, Benaut H, Mentec H, et al. *Saccharomyces boulardii* prevents diarrhea in critically ill tube-fed patients. A multicenter, randomized, double-blind placebo-controlled trial. Intens Care Med. 1997;23:517-523.

Borgia M, Sepe N, Brancato V, et al. A controlled clinical study on *Streptococcus faecium* preparation for the prevention of side reactions during long-term antibiotic treatments. Curr Ther Res. 1982;31:265-271.

Borody TJ. "Flora Power"-Fecal bacteria cure chronic *C. difficile* diarrhea. Am J Gastroenterol. 2000; 95:3028-3029.

Borody TJ. Infection with *Clostridim difficile*. Written for http://www.cdiffsupport.com 2002.

Bowden TA, Mansberger AR Jr., Lykins LE. Pseudomembranous enterocolitis: Mechanism of restoring floral homeostasis. Am Surg. 1981;47:178-183.

Buts JP, Corthier G, Delmee M. *Saccharomyces boulardii* for *Clostridium difficile* associated enteropathies in infants. J Pediatr Gastroenterol Nutr 1993; 16:419-425.

Buydens P, Debeuckelaere S. Efficacy of SF 68 in the treatment of acute diarrhea. A placebo-controlled trial. Scand J Gastroenterol. 1996;31:887-891.

Camarri E, Belvisi A, Guidoni G, et al. A double blind comparison of two different treatments for acute enteritis in adults. Chemotherapy. 1981;27:466-470.

Castagliuolo I, LaMont JT, Nikulasson, et al. *Saccharomyces boulardii* protease inhibits *Clostridium difficile* toxin A effects in the rat ileum. Infect Immun. 1996; 64:5225-32.

Clements ML, Levine MM, Ristaino PA, et al. Exogenous lactobacilli fed to man. Their fate and ability to prevent diarrheal disease. Prog Food Nutr Sci. 1983;7:29-37.

Colombel JF, Cortot A, Neut C, et al. Yoghurt with *Bifidobacterium longum* reduces erythromycin-induced gastrointestinal effects. Lancet. 1987;2:43.

Cunningham-Rundles S, Ahrne S, Bengmark S, et al. Probiotics and immune response. Am J Gastroenterol 2000;95:S22-5.

Eiseman B, Silen W, Bascom GS, et al. Fecal enema as an adjunct in the treatment of pseudomembranous enterocolitis. Surgery 1958;44:854-859.

Flotterod O, Hopen G. Refractory *Clostridium difficile* infection. Untraditional treatment of antibiotic-induced colitis. Tidsskr Nor Laegeforen. 1991;111:1364-1365.

Gorbach SL, Chang T-W, Goldin B. Successful treatment of relapsing *Clostridium difficile* colitis with *Lactobacillus* GG. Lancet.1987;2:1519.

Gotz V, Romankiewicz JA, Moss J, et al. Prophylaxis against ampicillin-associated diarrhea with a *Lactobacillus* preparation. Am J Hosp Pharm. 1979;36:754-757.

Guandalii S, Pensbene L, Zikri MA, et al. *Lactobacillus* GG administered in oral rehydration solution to children with acute diarrhea: A multicenter European trial. J Pediatric Gastroenterol Nutr. 2000;30:54-60.

Guarino A, Canani RB, Spagnuolo MI, et al. Oral bacterial therapy reduces the duration of symptoms and of viral excretion in children with mild diarrhea. J Pediatr Gastroenterol Nutr. 1997;25:516-519.

Gustafsson A, Lung-Tonnesen S, Berstad, et al. Faecal short-chain fatty acids in patients with antibiotic-associated diarrhoea, before and after faecal enema treatment. Scand J Gastroenterol. 1998;33:721-727.

Halpern GM, Prindiville T, Blackenburg M, et al. Treatment of irritable bowel syndrome with Lacterol fort: A randomized, double-blind, cross-over trial. Am J Gastroenterol. 1996;91:1579-1585.

Hilton E, Kolakowski P, Smith M, et al. Efficacy of *Lactobacillus* GG as a diarrheal preventative in travelers diarrhea. J Travel Med. 1996;4:41-43.

Hoyos AB. Reduced incidence of necrotizing enterocolitis associated with enteral administration of *Lactobacillus acidophilus* and *Bifidobacterium infantis* to neonates in an intensive care unit. Int J Infect Dis. 1999;3:197-202.

Isolauri E, Juntunen M, Rautanen T, et al. A human *Lactobacillus* strain (*Lactobacillus casei* sp strain GG) promotes recovery from acute diarrhea in children. Pediatrics. 1991; 88:90-97.

Isolauri E, Kaila M, Mykkanen H, et al. Oral bacteriotherapy for viral gastroenteritis. Dig Dis Sci. 1994;39:2595-2600.

Isolauri E, Kirjavainen PV, and Salminen S. Probiotics: A role in the treatment of intestinal infection and inflammation? Gut. 2002;50:iii54-iii59.

Kaila M, Isolauri E, Saxelin M, et al. Viable versus inactivated *Lactobacillus* strain GG in acute rotavirus diarrhoea. Arch Dis Child. 1995;72:51-53.

Kaila M, Isolauri E, Sopi E, et al. Enhancement of the circulating antibody secreting cell response in human diarrhea by a human *Lactobacillus* strain. Pediatric Res. 1992; 32:141-144.

Katelaris PH, Salam I, Farthing MJ. Lactobacilli to prevent travelers' diarrhea? N Engl J Med. 1995;333:1360-1361

Kimmey MB, Elmer GW, Surawicz CM, et al. Prevention of further recurrence of *Clostridium difficile* colitis with *Saccharomyces boulardii*. Dig Dig Sci. 1990;35:897-901.

Kollaritsch H, Holst H, Grobara P, et al. Prevention of traveler's diarrhea with *Saccharomyces boulardii*. Results of a placebo controlled double-blind study. Fortschr Med. 1993;111:52-156.

Kyne L, Warny, M. Qamar A, et al. Association between antibody response to toxin A and protection against recurrent *Clostridium difficile* diarrhoea. Lancet. 2001;357:189-193.

Leung DYM, Kelly CP, Boguniewicz, et al. Treatment with intravenously administered gamma globulin of chronic relapsing colitis induced by *Clostridium difficile* toxin. J. Pediatrics 1999; 118:633-637.

Levy J. Experience with live *Lactobacillus plantarum* 299v; A promising adjunct in the management of recurrent *Clostridium difficile* infection. Gasroenterology. 1997;112:A379.

Lodinova-Zadnikova R and Sonnenborn U. Effect of preventative administration of a nonpathogenic *Escherichia coli* strain on the colonization of the intestine with microbial patheogens in newborn infants. Biol Neonate. 1997;71:224-232.

Lund-Tonnesen S, Berstad A, Schreiner A, et al. *Clostridium difficile*-associated diarrhea treated with homologous feces. Tidsskr Nor Laegeforen. 1998;118:1027-1030.

Mahony DE, Lim-Morrison S, Faulkner G, et al. Antimicrobial activities of synthetic bismuth compounds against *Clostridium difficile*. Antimicrobial Agents Chemother 1999;43:582-588.

Majamaa H, Isolauri E, Saxeline M, et al. Lactic acid bacteria in the treatment of acute rotavirus gastroenteritis. J Pediatri Gastroenterol Nutr 1995;20:333-338.

Marteau P, Seksik P, and Jian R. Probiotics and intestinal health effects: A clinical perspective. Br J Nutr. 2002;88:S51-S57.

McFarland LV, Surawicz CM, Greenberg RN. A randomized placebo-controlled trial of *Saccharomyces boulardii* in combination with standard antibiotics for *Clostridium difficile* disease. JAMA. 1994; 271:1913-1918.

McFarland LV, Surawicz CM, Greenberg RN, et al. Prevention of beta-lactam-associated diarrhea by *Saccharomyces boulardii* compared to placebo. Am J Gastroenterol. 1995;90:439-448.

McFarland LV, Surawicz CM, Greenberg RN, et al. Recurrent *Clostridium difficile* disease: Epidemiology and clinical characteristics. Infect Control Hosp Epidemiol 1999;20:43-50.

Oberhleman RA, Gilman RH, Sheen P, et al. A placebo-controlled trial of *Lactobacillus* GG to prevent diarrhea in undernourished Peruvian children. J Pediatr. 1999;134:15-20.

Oksanen PJ, Salminen S, Saxelin M, et al. Prevention of traveler's diarrhea by *Lactobacillus* GG. Ann Med. 1990;22:53-56.

Pant AR, Graham SM, Allen SJ, et al. *Lactobacillus* GG and acute diarrhea in young children in the tropics. J Trop Pediatr. 1996; 42:162-165.

Paterson DL, Irdell J, Whitby M. Putting back the bugs: Bacterial treatment relieves chronic diarrhoea. Med J Aust. 1994;160:232-233.

Persky SE and Brandt J. Treatment of recurrent *Clostridium difficile*-associated diarrhea by administration of donated stool directly through a colonoscope. Amer J. Gastroenterol. 2000;95:3283-3285.

Pothoulakis C, Kelly CP, Joshi MA, et al. *Saccharomyces boulardii* inhibits *Clostridium difficile* toxin A binding and enterotoxicity in rat ileum. Gastroenterology. 1993;104:1108-1115.

Pozo-Olano JD, Warram JH, Gomez RG, et al. Effect of a lactobacilli preparation on traveler's diarrhea. A randomized, double blind clinical trial. Gastroenterol. 1978;74:829-830.

Qamar A, Aboudola S, Warny M, et al. *Saccharomyces boulardii* stimulates intestinal immunoglobulin A immune response to *Clostridium difficile* toxin A in mice. Infect Immun. 2001;69:2762-2765.

Rautanen T, Isolauri E, Salo E, et al. Management of acute diarrhoea with low osmolarity oral rehydration solutions and *Lactobacillus* strain GG. Arch Dis Child. 1998;79:157-160.

Raza S, Graham SM, Allen SJ. *Lactobacillus* GG promotes recovery from acute nonbloody diarrhea in Pakistan. Pediatr Infect Dis J. 1995;14:107-111.

Saavedra JM, Bauman NA, Oung I. Feeding of *Bifidobacterium bifidum* and *Streptococcus thermophilus* to infants in hospital for prevention of diarrhoea and shedding of rotavirus. Lancet. 1994;344:1046-1049,

Salminen E, Elomaa I, Minkkinen J, et al. Preservation of intestinal integrity during radiotherapy using live *Lactobacillus acidophilus* cultures. Clin Radiol. 1988;39:435-437.

Schwan A, Sjoin S, Trottestam U. Relapsing *Clostridium difficile* enterocolitis cured by rectal infusion of homologous faeces. Lancet. 1983;2:845.

Schwan A, Sjoin S, Trottestam U. Relapsing *Clostridium difficile* enterocolitis cured by rectal infusion of normal faeces. Scand J Infect Dis. 1984;16:211-215.

Seal D, Borriello SP, Barclay F. Treatment of relapsing *Clostridium difficile* diarrhoea by administration of a non-toxigenic strain. Eur J Clin Microbiol. 1987;6:51-53.

Seki H, Shiohara M, Matsumura T, et al. Prevention of antibiotic-associated diarrhea in children by *Clostridium butyricum* MIYAIRI. Pediatr Int. 2003;45:86-90.

Shornikova AV, Casa IA, Isolauri E, et al. *Lactobacillus reuteri* as a therapeutic agent in acute diarrhea in young children. J Pediatr Gastroenterol Nutr. 1997a;24:399-404.

Shornikova AV, Casa IA, Mykkanen H, et al. Bacteriotherapy with *Lactobacillus reuteri* in rotavirus gastroenteritis. Pediatr Infect Dis J. 1997b;16:1103-1107.

Shornikova AV, Isolauri E, Burkanova L, et al. A trial in the Karelian Republic of oral rehydration and *Lactobacillus* GG for treatment of acute diarrhoea. Acta Pediatr. 1997c;86:460-465.

Simakachorn N, Pichaipat V, Rithipornpaisarn P, et al. Clinical evaluation of the addition of lyophilized, heat-killed *Lactobacillus acidophilus* LB to oral rehydration therapy in the treatment of acute diarrhea in children. J Pediatr Gastroenterol Nutr. 2000;30::68-72.

Simenhoff ML, Dunn SR, Zollner GP. Biomodulation of the toxic and nutritional effects of small bowel bacterial overgrowth in end-stage kidney disease using freeze-dried *Lactobacillus acidophilus*. Miner Electrolyte Metab. 1996;22:92-96.

Siitonen S, Vapaatalo H, Salminen S, et al. Effect of *Lactobacillus* GG yoghurt in prevention of antibiotic-associated diarrhoea. Ann Med. 1990;22:57-59.

Surawicz CM, McFarland L, Elmer GW, et al. Treatment of recurrent *Clostridium difficile* colitis with vancomycin and *Saccharomyces boulardii*. Am J Gastrolenterol. 1989a;84:1285-1287.

Surawicz CM, McFarland LV, Greenburg RN, et al. The search for a better treatment for recurrent *Clostridium difficile* disease: Use of high-dose vancomycin combined with *Saccharomyces boulardii*. Clin Infect. Dis. 2000;31:1012-1017.

Surawicz CM, Elmer GW, Speelman P, et al. Prevention of antibiotic-associated diarrhea by *Saccharomyces boulardii*: A prospective study. Gastroenterology. 1989b;6:981-988.

Szajewska H, Kotowska M, Mrukowicz JZ. Efficacy of *Lactobacillus GG* in prevention of nosocomial diarrhea in infants. J Pediatr. 2001;138:361-365.

Tankanow RM, Ross MB, Ertel IJ, et al. A double-blind placebo-controlled study of the efficacy of Lactinex® in the prophylaxis of amoxicillin-induced diarrhea. DICP. 1990;24:382-384.

Thomas MR, Litin SC, Osmon DR, et al. Lack of effect of *Lactobacillus GG* on antibiotic-associated diarrhea: A randomized, placebo-controlled trial. May Clin Proc. 2001;76:883-889.

Tedesco FJ, Gordon D, Fortson WC. Approach to patients with multiple relapses of antibiotic-associated pseudomembranous colitis. Am J Gastroenterol. 1985;80:867-868.

Tvede M and Rask-Madsen J. Bacteriotherapy for chronic relapsing *Clostridium difficile* diarrhoea in six patients. Lancet. 1989;1:1156-1160.

Vanderhoof JA, Whitney DB, Antonson DL, et al. *Lactobacillus* GG in the prevention of antibiotic-associated diarrhea in children. J Pediatr 1999;135:564-568.

Vanderhoof JA, Young RJ, Murray N, et al. Treatment strategies for small bowel bacterial overgrowth in short bowel syndrome. J Pediatr Gastroenterol Nutr. 1998;27:155-160.

Van Niel CW, Feudtner C, Garrison MM. *Lactobacillus* therapy for acute infectious diarrhea in children: A meta-analysis. Pediatrics. 2002;109:678-684.

Witsell DL, Garrett CG, Yarbrough WG, et al. Effect of *Lactobacillus acidophilus* on antibiotic-associated gastrointestinal morbidity: A prospective randomized trial. J Otolarygol 1995;24:230-233.

Wunderlich PF, Braun L, Fumagalli I, et al. Double-blind report on the efficacy of lactic acid-producing *Enterococcus* SF68 in the prevention of antibiotic-associated diarrhoea and in the treatment of acute diarrhoea. J Int Med Res. 1989;17:333-338.

Chapter 6

Quenching the Fire
Probiotics and Inflammatory Bowel Disease

In the last chapter we saw how well probiotics work when treating diarrhea. Are probiotics equally effective in inflammatory bowel disease?

Collectively, the term inflammatory bowel disease (IBD) encompasses both ulcerative colitis and Crohn's disease. These diseases affect roughly 1.3 million individuals in North America alone (Loftus and Sandborn, 2002) and are characterized by chronically relapsing and remitting disease. Although the exact cause of inflammatory bowel disease is unknown, there are probably 3 essential factors: genetic susceptibility, gut bacteria, and immune responsiveness. Specifically, in susceptible individuals, inflammatory bowel disease occurs when there is a breakdown in the regulatory constraints of the immune system, allowing local gut bacteria to trigger an abnormal immune response (Shanahan, 2001).

Ulcerative colitis and Crohn's disease are similar in some respects. Both illnesses are extremely unpleasant and negatively impact the quality of one's life. Symptoms of both ulcerative colitis and Crohn's disease may include diarrhea, abdominal pain, rectal bleeding, fever, nausea, weight loss, fatigue, and loss of appetite. In extreme cases, malnutrition, dehydration, anemia, and even death may occur.

However, ulcerative colitis and Crohn's disease differ in several important ways. Ulcerative colitis is confined to the large intestine, while Crohn's disease may be found anywhere in the entire intestinal tract from mouth to rectum. Also, in ulcerative colitis, inflammation is restricted to the innermost (mucosal) layer of the intestine, while in Crohn's disease, inflammation can penetrate through the intestinal wall. Additionally, Crohn's disease is associated with high levels of pro-inflammatory type-1 helper (Th1) cytokines, like tumor necrosis factor-alpha (TNF-α), interferon-gamma (IFN-γ), and IL-12. Ulcerative colitis, on the other hand, is less related to specific cytokine-secretory patterns, although there may be a modified Th2 response, with deficient levels of IL-5 and IL-10 (See figure 6-1). Instead, ulcerative colitis, is triggered, in part, by environmental factors that break down normal regulatory constraints of the immune system. The low rates of ulcerative colitis in twins (6-14%) compared to Crohn's disease (44-50%) indicate that *environment*, more than genetics, favors development of ulcerative colitis (Farrell and Peppercorn, 2002).

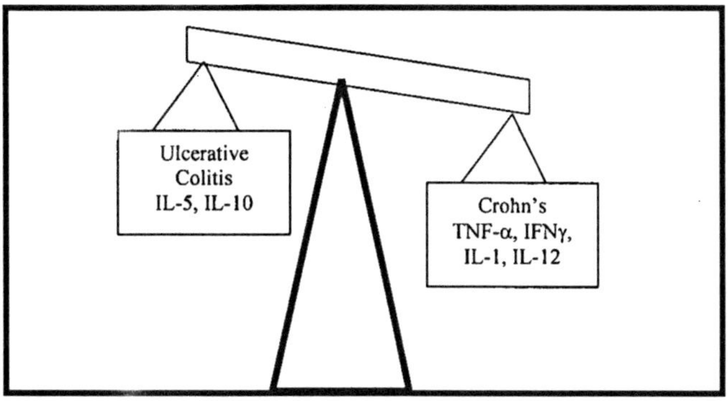

Figure 6-1. In Crohn's disease, inflammation may be caused, in part, by too much of the pro-inflammatory cytokines TNF-α, IFNγ, IL-1, and/or IL-12. Ulcerative colitis may be caused, in part, by too little of the non-inflammatory cytokines IL-5 and/or IL-10.

As we currently understand, inflammatory bowel disease involves a complex interaction between environment, genetic, immune, and microbial factors. For the purpose of this chapter, we will primarily be considering the role that gut bacteria (and probiotics) play in inflammatory bowel disease.

A great deal of evidence indicates gut bacteria either *initiate* or *perpetuate* inflammatory bowel disease. For example, inflammatory bowel disease usually flares up in areas of the bowel where the greatest number of bacteria is found (Farrell and LaMont, 2002). In fact, in both experimental animals and susceptible humans, inflammatory lesions only occur in the presence of gut bacteria (Farrell and LaMont, 2002; Harper et al., 1985; D'Haens et al., 1998). On the other hand, modification of gut bacteria, through use of antibiotics, or probiotics, or by diverting gut bacteria away from the bowel via **ileostomy**, improves symptoms and produces beneficial effects in both humans and experimental animals (Farrell and LaMont, 2003; Rutgeerts et al., 1991).

In inflammatory bowel disease, evidence of gut bacterial involvement goes even one step further. In both experimental animals and humans, evidence points heavily to a lack of oral tolerance to one's own normal gut flora. Essentially, the immune system mounts a faulty response, attacking normal flora that reside in the gut (Duchmann et al., 1995; Cong et al., 1998). Healthy people, on the other hand, are, of course, tolerant to their own gut bacteria.

As you will see, there are several different theories of what causes inflammatory bowel diseases. In fact, if you talked to 10 different gastroenterologists, you would probably get 10 different answers. Several years ago, inflammatory bowel disease was distinctly thought to be an autoimmune illness. Now, however, most leading theories involve gastrointestinal bacteria, in one way or another.

Regardless of the specific theory to which you subscribe, for the purpose of this chapter, it is important to understand that gut bacterial factors are intimately involved in all of the leading theories. According to two renowned gastroenterologists at Harvard Medical School, Richard Farrell and Thomas LaMont, there are currently four primary theories of inflammatory bowel disease:

(1) Inflammatory bowel disease is an appropriate reaction to a persistent bacterial infection in the gut
(2) Inflammatory bowel disease occurs when there are subtle alterations in bacterial composition within the gut
(3) Inflammatory bowel disease occurs as a natural response when the bowel mucosal lining is defective and continuously stimulated by gut bacteria
(4) Inflammatory bowel disease results from a loss of oral tolerance to normal gut bacteria (Farrell and LaMont, 2002).

In the next few pages, we will consider each of these theories in more detail.

Theories of Inflammatory Bowel Disease

Theory 1: Persistent bacterial infection in the gut

Throughout the years, many investigators have searched for a specific infectious agent in the feces of patients with inflammatory bowel disease. Depending upon whom you ask, you may be told that, so far, no specific pathogens have definitively been implicated in inflammatory bowel disease. Or, on the other hand, you may be informed that a specific microorganism has been identified as the underlying cause of Crohn's disease. In fact, there are numerous studies describing various disease-causing microorganisms found in fecal matter from patients with Crohn's disease, but these microbes are not found in feces from healthy folks or from individuals with ulcerative colitis.

With several hundred different species of bacteria living in our intestines, and as many as half of them not even identified, it is not out of the question that inflammatory bowel disease could result from gut colonization with an infectious agent. Indeed, new strains of disease-causing microorganisms are being identified all the time. So far, several microorganisms have surfaced as possible contributing factors to Crohn's disease, including strains of *Mycobacterium avium paratuberculosis, Listeria monocytogenes, Helicobacter hepaticus*, and even the virus that causes measles. Likewise, other microorganisms like *Clostridium difficile* and cytomegalovirus have sometimes been implicated in *relapses* of inflammatory bowel disease. (For a full list of suspected microorganisms, see Farrell and LaMont, 2002.) In fact, the presence of *C. difficile* may complicate treatment of inflammatory bowel disease. It has been reported to be almost impossible to eradicate *C. difficile* from patients with inflammatory bowel disease.

One individual who believes that Crohn's disease is caused by *Mycobacterium avium paratuberculosis* is an Australian gastroenterologist by the name of Thomas Borody. Dr. Borody heads up a digestive disease center and a probiotic research center in Sydney. According to Dr. Borody, if Crohn's disease patients are "given antimycobacterial drugs for 3 years, they are cured. No more symptoms, histology is negative." Dr. Borody makes the cure for Crohn's disease sound so matter-of-fact. He is certain that by the end of the decade, antimycobacterial antibiotics will be standard treatment for eradicating the disease. In fact, he likened current skepticism to that of the early 1990s when the medical community scoffed at researchers who announced that peptic ulcer disease is usually associated with the bacterium *Helicobacter pylori* — which is now accepted as fact.

In Borody's experience, sometimes patients with Crohn's disease benefit from human probiotic infusions (obtained from healthy fecal flora) if there is an indication that *Clostridium difficile* is present.

Additionally, human probiotic infusions are sometimes recommended after Dr. Borody's patients with Crohn's disease complete three years of antibiotic therapy. One obvious question that comes to mind is, why do antibiotics have to be given for so long? Three years is an awfully long time. The answer is: Antibiotics that we have to treat mycobacterial infections only kill microorganisms when they are actively dividing. Mycobacteria grow extremely slowly and only divide on the order of days, weeks, or even months. In order to eliminate all the bacteria, patients need to be treated for an extremely long period of time.

Theory 2: Subtle alterations in bacteria within the gut (dysbiosis)
Although there are many different animal models used to study inflammatory bowel disease, one constant factor that is absolutely required for full manifestations of the disease is the presence of gut flora. Inflammatory bowel disease can be created quite easily in experimental mice, rats, or guinea pigs. Some investigators cause intestinal inflammation in their experimental animals by giving specific antibiotic treatments that alter normal flora. Other scientists use experimental animals that have been genetically modified to have specific cytokine deficiencies. When these cytokine-deficient animals are kept in germ-free environments (thus, no bacteria in their guts) there is minimal gut inflammation. Inflammation develops when exposed to bacteria, but resolves when given antibiotics (that wipe out all normal gut flora). In these experimental animals, when gut bacteria are removed from the intestines, in some instances, inflammatory gut reactions are completely abolished (for details see Farrell and Lamont, 2002).

With more than 400 different bacterial strains living in our guts, the roles played by each and every species are largely unknown. However, as we've discussed in other segments of this book, the "forgotten organ" of gut flora is regulated by our diet, gut motility, our genetic characteristics, the acidic or alkaline properties of the intestine, and short-chain fatty acid fermentation products of resident bacterial species. Not surprisingly, subtle alterations in bacterial colonization and bacterial activities can have profound effects on the host's mucosa and immune response (Farrell and LaMont, 2002).

In support of this theory are two distinct observations. The first has to do with slight alterations in microbial gut colonization. In one study, a unique strain of *Escherichia coli* was found adhering to the intestinal mucosa of some patients with Crohn's disease and ulcerative colitis.

Other studies have implicated dysbiosis due to *increased* amounts of anaerobic gram negative bacteria like *Eubacterium* and *Peptostreptococcus* (Wensinck et al., 1991), increased amounts of *Escherichia coli* or *Bacteroides fragilis* (Keighley et al., 1978; Giaffer et al., 1991), or *decreased* numbers of lactobacilli and bifidobacteria (Giaffer et al., 1991; Favier et al., 1997) in inflammatory bowel disease. In theory, an imbalance of gut bacteria can be corrected with antibiotics which decrease the number of harmful bacteria, bowel rest, or fecal diversion. On the other hand, it is even more desirable to *increase* the number of protective "healthy" bacteria, by using probiotics (Kennedy et al., 2000).

The other observation has to do with inflammatory effects that occur due to toxins and harmful chemicals released by disease-causing bacteria. We already know from earlier chapters that many disease-causing strains of bacteria reek havoc in our intestines by secreting toxins that cause gut "leakiness" and disrupting our immune systems. As discussed in chapter 1, the short chain fatty acid butyric acid is a fermentation product produced by many gut bacteria. Butyric acid is the primary energy source used by epithelial cells lining our intestines and it also acts as an immune system modulator. At concentrations normally found in the body, butyric acid decreases pro-inflammatory activities of white blood cells (Chapman, 2001). As a result, bacteria that produce large quantities of butyric acid protect against bowel inflammation. On the other hand, bacteria that inhibit butyric acid production contribute to inflammatory bowel disease.

It turns out that some bacteria produce hydrogen sulfide, a chemical that blocks metabolism of butyric acid. Some have speculated that these bacteria which produce hydrogen sulfide, reduce levels of butyric acid, and therefore, increase intestinal permeability and impair healing. Some, but not all, researchers have found increased hydrogen sulfide-reducing bacterial species in feces from patients with ulcerative colitis (Pitcher et al., 2000).

In actuality, evidence for hydrogen sulfide as a toxin in inflammatory bowel disease is purely speculative (Pitcher et al., 2000). However, butyric acid supplements, have been used successfully in those with inflammatory bowel diseases. In experimental rat models of inflammatory bowel disease, butyric acid enemas prevent intestinal inflammation (Okamoto et al., 2000). Likewise, butyric acid enemas have also provided symptomatic relief in some individuals with ulcerative colitis (Steinhart et al., 1996).

> In 103 patients with ulcerative colitis who used short chain fatty acid enemas rectally for 6 weeks, there was a subset of individuals — particularly those with shorter episodes of intestinal inflammation — that experienced significant improvements in symptoms (Breuer et al., 1997).
>
> In fact, double blind, randomized, placebo-controlled clinical trials have now repeatedly demonstrated that: short chain fatty acid enemas (butyrate, propionate, acetate) improve ulcerative colitis (Vernia et al., 1995), butyric acid enemas are more effective than aminosalicylates alone for ulcerative colitis (Vernia et al., 2003), butyric acid enemas may improve ulcerative colitis in patients that have failed to respond to anything else (Steinhart et al., 1994), and butyric acid enemas are significantly more effective than placebo for radiation-induced intestinal inflammation (Vernia et al., 2000).

Butyric acid enemas have a foul odor. This makes it difficult for some folks to comply with therapy. As a result, some studies are examining the feasibility of delivering butyric acid to the intestine via capsules. The bacterium *Clostridium butyricum* strain M588 produces large amounts of butyric acid. In experimental rat models of ulcerative colitis, *Clostridium butyricum* did, in fact, produce large amounts of butyric acid which was recovered from the intestines, and this bacterium prevented intestinal inflammation and ulceration. This probiotic preparation, widely used in hospitalized patients in Japan as a preventative therapy to keep patients from acquiring *Clostridium difficile* during their hospital stay, may prove useful in humans to prevent progression of ulcerative colitis and maintain remission from active disease (Okamoto et al., 2000).

Many individuals with inflammatory bowel disease and even some patients with chronic, persistent *Clostridium difficile* colitis experience extra-intestinal symptoms — symptoms of disease outside their intestines. Other conditions frequently associated with chronic bowel inflammation include: bacterial abscesses in the liver, bacterial infections in the heart, arthritis, and inflammation of the uvea in the eye (potentially causing blindness if untreated). These extra-intestinal symptoms are caused by the uptake and distribution of bacterial components (cell wall proteins, toxins, etc.) throughout the body. Sometimes, these extra-intestinal symptoms improve when antibiotics are taken.

New therapies are being investigated to improve extra-intestinal symptoms associated with bowel inflammation. The enzyme mutanolysin, whose function is to degrade components of bacterial cell walls, has already been shown effective in preventing liver abscesses associated with inflammatory bowel disease. Mutanolysin does not have any antibiotic effects, but the enzyme does lower tumor necrosis factor-alpha (TNF-α) levels, a pro-inflammatory cytokine that is associated with inflammatory bowel disease. This data suggests that systemic exposure to components of gut bacteria contribute to extra-intestinal symptoms experienced by those with chronic inflammatory bowel diseases, again implicating gut bacteria as the underlying cause of Crohn's disease and ulcerative colitis (Lichtman et al., 1992; Farrell and LaMont, 2002).

Theory 3: Gut bacteria impair function of the intestinal mucosa, perpetuating inflammation

Many specific molecules on bacterial cell walls activate intestinal epithelial and immune cells to secrete inflammatory cytokines, damaging oxygen radicals, and other factors that cause localized inflammatory damage. Any time there is intestinal inflammation, increased intestinal permeability is also found. Interestingly, there is not only enhanced intestinal permeability in those with inflammatory bowel disease but also in *unaffected relatives* of patients with Crohn's disease (Hollander et al., 1986; May et al., 1993). This suggests that there is an intestinal defect of permeability *prior to* intestinal inflammation developing. In fact, it has been documented that intestinal leakiness precedes development of Crohn's disease (Irvine and Marshall, 2000). Additionally, increased intestinal leakiness also precedes reactivation of inactive Crohn's disease.

But what causes the leaky gut? Certainly infectious microorganisms themselves (*Escherichia coli, Vibrio cholerae*, or *Clostridium difficile*) can alter gut permeability. Likewise, the immune system's response to gut bacteria — through secretion of cytokines like IFN-γ or TNF-α — increases gut leakiness (Zolotarevsky et al., 2002). Some researchers have also suggested that individuals with Crohn's disease have "gastrointestinal leakiness" due to the presence of harmful bacteria secreting enzymes that degrade protective mucus layers in the gut (Quigley and Kelly, 1995).

While it is not entirely certain what the initial insult is that causes gut leakiness, it is clear that once the bowel becomes leaky, the presence of bacterial flora is the necessary component that perpetuates increased gut permeability (Farrell and LaMont, 2002). In Crohn's disease, intestinal inflammation may be stimulated by anaerobic microorganisms since we observe that antibiotics targeting these microorganisms alleviate the inflammation. On the other hand, symptoms of ulcerative colitis respond to antibiotics that treat both aerobic and anaerobic microorganisms, suggesting that several different species of gut bacteria play a role in this inflammatory bowel disease (Farrell and LaMont, 2002).

Importantly, not all gut bacteria induce or perpetuate gut inflammation. In fact, neither *Lactobacillus* nor *Bifidobacterium* evoke inflammatory effects. Numerous studies, in both animals and humans, indicate just the opposite — that these two strains can inhibit recurrent intestinal inflammation — thus, it is strains of these bacteria that have been widely used as probiotics for treating inflammatory bowel diseases.

Theory 4: Abnormal immune response to normal bacterial components (lack of oral tolerance)

One theory that attempts to explain the high incidence of inflammatory bowel disease in industrialized civilizations is based upon a *hygiene hypothesis*. Essentially, this theory suggests that when living in unsanitary conditions, our bodies respond by "turning on" specific genes that protect us from disease-causing bacterial invasion in the gut. This confers a "survival of the fittest" advantage in poorly sanitized living conditions because the immune system is on a heightened state of alert. However, in sanitary Western civilizations, these genes become a liability because they tend to respond against harmless normal gut flora (Farrell and LaMont, 2002). Essentially, lack of immune "education" causes an over-reaction, resulting in inflammatory damage and autoimmunity when our bodies react excessively against normal gut flora. Deliberately introducing bacteria, in the form of probiotics, may provide an immune "education" sufficient to challenge the immune system (Dunne et al., 1999) and prevent future over-activity.

The hygiene hypothesis has been supported in numerous studies. For example, many patients with Crohn's disease report having their own bedrooms as children. In contrast, healthy people who were surveyed were more likely to report sharing bedrooms or even beds with siblings while they were growing up. Additionally, individuals with Crohn's disease reported having hot water, indoor toilets, and central heating as children (Krishnan and Korzenik, 2002). These and other similar data suggest improved sanitation alters "immune education" by having decreased exposure to certain kinds of bacteria and parasites. One result of improved sanitation could be inflammatory bowel diseases, as overactive immune responses develop to normal gut bacteria.

Some of the genes important in this respect are genes that determine the balance between Th1-lymphocytes and Th-2 lymphocytes. You may recall that in allergic diseases there is a tendency toward Th-2 mediated cytokine responses, while in inflammatory disease of the bowel, there is a predominance of Th-1 mediated responses (See figure 6-2).

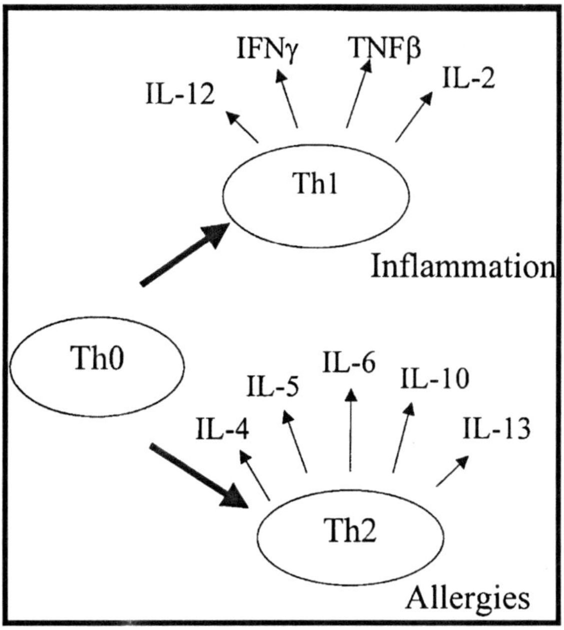

Figure 6-2. Type-0 helper lymphocytes differentiate either into Type-1 helper lymphocytes (Th1) or Type-2 helper lymphocytes (Th2). Early differentiation in infancy is largely controlled by specific types of bacteria present in the gastrointestinal tract as part of the normal flora. Th1 cells tend to secrete cytokines that are inflammatory in nature, while Th2 cells secrete cytokines that favor allergies.

IL-10 is a cytokine. It is not secreted by Th-1 pro-inflammatory cells, but instead is secreted by Th-2 cells that "balance out" or counteract inflammation. IL-10 suppresses inflammation by quelling excessive Th-1 responses. In the absence of IL-10, a harmless inflammatory response to gut normal flora becomes a harmful inflammatory state — suggesting inflammation is caused by an unbalanced cytokine milieu. When there is a lack of IL-10 (due to genetic deficiencies), intestinal inflammation rages out of control, presumably due to unopposed activation of Th-1 lymphocytes and scavenging macrophages (Farrell and LaMont, 2002).

Interestingly, intestinal worms that live inside human intestines under poor, unsanitary conditions, are a potent stimulus for secretion of Th-2 dominated anti-inflammatory responses (Farrell and LaMont, 2002) like IL-10. As a result, genetically modified intestinal worms could, in theory, be of potential benefit as a therapy for treating inflammatory bowel diseases. Early studies in humans have been encouraging (Farrell and LaMont, 2002), but becoming infected with worms in order to cure intestinal inflammation is not a very attractive proposal for most patients. But it does illustrate the point that I am trying to make, which is: exposure to intestinal "critters" alters the actions of our immune systems.

Like intestinal worms, certain strains of potentially harmful anaerobic gut bacteria also interact with our immune systems and trigger release of pro-inflammatory mediators like TGF-β1. If too much TGF-β1 is released in response to certain bacteria, it causes intestinal inflammation and fibrosis. In experimental mice, antibiotics — which kill bacteria — reduce levels of TGF-β1 (Mourelle et al., 1998). Thus, bacterial normal flora is a driving force behind the activities of our immune system. Simply by modifying normal gut flora, we can change cytokine activities within our immune systems.

Mice that lack T-cells (and therefore lack the ability to make pro-inflammatory cytokines) don't develop intestinal inflammation. On the other hand, when T-cells from mice with inflammatory bowel disease are transferred to healthy mice, inflammatory bowel disease is also transferred to the previously undiseased mice (Cong et al., 1998). Thus, it is logical to speculate that the main abnormality driving intestinal inflammation is an exaggerated response to normal gut bacteria. In other words, inflammatory bowel disease may be due to a lack of oral tolerance to one's own gut flora.

As we learned in chapter 3, in the normal gastrointestinal tract, a specific subset of T cells, termed CD4+ cells, are always stimulated —

always on a heightened state of alert to attack foreign invading microorganisms. So why doesn't everyone suffer from excessive gut inflammation and injury? The answer is, in part, first due to local production of suppressive cytokines released by the intestinal cells. Specifically, *regulatory* cytokines like IL-10 are present to *modify* the activities of the immune system — essentially, IL-10 "turns off" inflammation (by suppressing activities of pro-inflammatory cytokines) before inflammation gets out of control. Secondly, in normal individuals, after activation by bacteria and other invaders, CD4+ T cells undergo a programmed cell death (called apoptosis) and die before they can cause significant damage (Monteleone et al., 2002). In Crohn's disease, CD4+ cells "forget" to undergo apoptosis — essentially, they don't die when they're supposed to, so inflammation gets continually perpetuated. In inflammatory bowel disease, not only are individuals hyperreactive to their own normal intestinal bacteria, but the cells that drive this inappropriate hyperactivity refuse to die!

As a result of persistent CD4+ activation in Crohn's disease, these cells produce large amounts of pro-inflammatory cytokines, specifically IFN-γ. IFN-γ is a major cause of intestinal tissue damage and inflammation (Monteleone et al., 2002). IFN-γ facilitates release of other pro-inflammatory cytokines like IL-1, IL-6, and TNF-α, all of which perpetuate inflammation. In tissues taken from patients with Crohn's disease, TNF-α is released in significant quantities from diseased portions of the intestines (Borruel et al., 2002). Recently, through a breakthrough in inflammatory bowel disease genetics, a specific gene, called NOD2, was identified. This gene plays a role in detection and recognition of bacteria and has a part in inflammatory responses (Hart et al., 2003). Abnormalities within this gene may play a part in abnormal immune responsiveness to gut flora in Crohn's disease (Watts and Satsangi, 2002).

Many studies support the idea that persistent inflammation in the intestines is due to inappropriate activity of immune cells, rather than being a property that is inherent to the gut itself. In a mouse strain that spontaneously develops intestinal inflammation, T cells are overly reactive to gut bacterial flora, secreting pro-inflammatory cytokines like IL-2 and IFN-γ. As mentioned previously, if these supersensitive T cells are transferred into a strain of healthy mice, the healthy mice then also develop intestinal inflammation (Cong et al., 1998). Similar examples in humans also illustrate that the underlying problem in inflammatory bowel disease stems from overactive immune cells. One woman with Crohn's disease had a transplantation of her entire small intestines, hoping that the transplant would cure her Crohn's disease. However, despite massive immunosuppressive medications, within 6 months of surgery, Crohn's disease returned (Sustento-Reodica et al., 1997). This indicates that Crohn's disease isn't a disease of the intestine *per se*, but is, instead, a disease of the immune system reacting against the intestine or the components (normal flora) of the intestine. On the other hand, bone marrow transplantation — essentially transplanting immune cells from healthy people into those with Crohn's disease — has cured 4 out of 5 (80%) former Crohn's disease patients. Following bone marrow transplantation, these individuals have remained in long-term remission from inflammatory bowel disease (Lopez-Cubero, 1998). These studies probably provide some of the strongest evidence to date for inflammatory bowel disease being a disease of abnormal immune responses rather than a disease of the gut *per se*.

Common Therapies for Inflammatory Bowel Disease

Many different prescription products have been used with varying degrees of success over the years to either treat flare-ups or to try to maintain remission. At the present time, anti-inflammatory agents like 5-aminosalicylates, azathioprine, 6-mercaptopurine, cyclosporine, and prednisone or antibiotics like metronidazole or vancomycin are the main prescription products used to treat inflammatory bowel disease. Interestingly, each of the above mentioned drugs (except for prednisone) has some anti-microbial actions, pointing to the idea that intestinal inflammation is almost certainly related directly or indirectly to a problem with gut bacteria. However, each of these therapies is associated with potential for severe, even life-threatening adverse effects.

Antibiotics offer some benefits in inflammatory bowel disease by (a) reducing the overall numbers of bacteria in the intestine, (b) entirely eliminating specific infectious bacterial populations, (c) diminishing tissue invasion and abscess formation, and (d) preventing bacterial translocation out of the intestines to other parts of the body (Farrell and LaMont, 2002). However, continuous antibiotic therapy also comes with the risk of harmful side effects, antibiotic-resistant microorganisms emerging, and the potential overgrowth of disease-causing strains like *Clostridium difficile* (Farrell and LaMont, 2002). Additionally, many folks cannot tolerate antibiotics due to allergic reactions.

Immunosuppressants

The use of 5-aminosalicylates, namely sulfasalazine and its chemical derivatives (balsalazide and olsalazine) are the main treatments for (a) inducing remission in mild-to-moderate ulcerative colitis and (b) keeping patients in remission. These are first line prescription drugs, usually used for at least 4-6 weeks to determine their efficacy. However, approximately 30% of individuals cannot tolerate these drugs because of side effects: nausea, vomiting, anorexia, allergies, headaches, rashes, fever, pancreatitis, kidney disease, liver disease, male infertility, and blood diseases. These drugs primarily have anti-inflammatory actions, probably, in part, due to inhibiting the activities of some pro-inflammatory cytokines (Jani and Regueiro, 2002).

Steroids, with potent anti-inflammatory and immunosuppressive activities, are widely used to treat active Crohn's diseases and ulcerative colitis. Steroids can induce remission in patients with moderate-to-severe inflammatory bowel disease, but steroids are not effective for maintaining remission. Steroids decrease levels of many pro-inflammatory cytokines (IL-1, IL-2, IL-4, IL-5, IL-6, IL-8, and IFN-γ) (Jani and Regueiro, 2002). Interestingly, various strains of probiotic bacteria also suppress lymphocyte and cytokine production in T cells and are as effective as the steroid dexamethasone (used at a concentration of 10 umol/L) in inflammatory bowel disease (Isolauri et al., 2001). Numerous adverse effects associated with steroids prevent folks from relying excessively upon these drugs. Common short term side effects include: fluid retention, weight gain, and blurred vision, but serious, long-term side effects include osteoporosis, cataracts, and loss of muscle mass. Recently, a new steroid called budesonide (Entocort EC®) was approved for use in those with inflammatory bowel disease in the United States. In theory, budesonide's actions are confined only to the intestines due to rapid, localized metabolism in the gut. As such, with budesonide, there may be fewer adverse effects in individuals who require steroids to keep symptoms of inflammatory bowel disease under control.

Roughly 16% of affected individuals cannot tolerate either aminosalicylates or steroids, so in these individuals the drug azathioprine is sometimes useful to prevent acute flare-ups of Crohn's disease or ulcerative colitis. Additionally, azathioprine has the advantage of being able to help individuals remain in remission. Azathioprine (a) modulates the immune system and directly reduces inflammation and (b) suppresses the actions of T cells and natural killer cells. Sometimes adding azathioprine to steroids, allows steroid dosages to be reduced. This may help to prevent some steroid-associated adverse effects. Side effects of azathioprine include allergic reactions (15%), bone marrow suppression, infection, and hepatitis.

Very recently, drugs that block the actions of specific inflammatory cytokines have been introduced for treating inflammatory bowel disease. One such therapy approved for use in the United States is a drug that is actually an antibody that targets TNF-α. By neutralizing the pro-inflammatory actions of TNF-α, two-thirds of inflammatory bowel disease patients who don't respond to anything else, experience healing of their intestinal mucosa and reduced intestinal inflammation (Kamm, 2001). However, this drug called infliximab (Remicade®) can also be quite toxic for some folks, making them more susceptible to severe infections like tuberculosis or even contributing to the development of cancers.

Probiotics in Inflammatory Bowel Disease

How probiotics work

From the previous section, we learned that drugs used for treating inflammatory bowel disease do so by either acting as antimicrobials or by altering activities of the immune system. However, these prescription drugs come with a host of nasty side effects. Wouldn't it be great if we had a therapy that worked as both an antimicrobial and an immune-regulator without all the side effects? Well, thanks to probiotics, we do! Of all emerging treatments for inflammatory bowel disease, probiotics are the most promising.

Probiotics restore homeostasis in the gut in many ways. Many probiotics increase gut acidity by producing short chain fatty acids — an effect that directly inhibits the growth of disease-causing bacteria. *Lactobacillus salivarius* and other probiotics secrete antimicrobial substances (called bacteriocins) that inhibit growth of disease-causing bacteria like *Listeria* and *Salmonella* (Hart et al., 2003). Some lactobacilli also stimulate gastrointestinal mucus production, which makes it difficult for disease-causing bacteria to attach to the intestinal wall (Hart et al., 2003). Probiotics alleviate inflammation in the gut by competing with disease-causing bacteria for binding sites and essential nutrients. Probiotic bacteria also *stimulate* production of anti-inflammatory cytokines in the gut epithelium (Hart et al., 2003), and probiotics *decrease* secretion of pro-inflammatory cytokines (Borrel et al, 2002).

> Gram-positive probiotic bacteria do not stimulate the pro-inflammatory cytokine IL-8, like other bacteria do (Lammers et al., 2002). Furthermore, two strains of probiotics, *Lactobacillus casei* and *Lactobacillus bulgaricus*, *decrease* the release of pro-inflammatory cytokines like TNF-α from intestinal tissue taken from patients with Crohn's disease (Borruel et al., 2002). On the other hand, when the same tissues were exposed to certain strains of *Escherichia coli* more TNF-α was released — consistent with the theory that there is a lack of tolerance to common normal flora in some patients with inflammatory bowel disease (Borruel et al., 2002).

Additionally, probiotics enhance the immune system by activating macrophages and natural killer cells to increase phagocytic and lymphocytic activities (Hart et al., 2003; Farrell and LaMont, 2000). Probiotic bacteria also increase IgA antibody levels (Malin et al., 1996), enhancing mucosal resistance to disease-causing invaders.

> In fact, in 14 children with Crohn's disease, *Lactobacillus* GG significantly increased the number of IgA antibody secreting cells, indicating that this probiotic could be a useful therapy in Crohn's disease (Malin et al., 1996).

Animal data

Before we discuss human clinical trials, let's consider the effects of probiotics in experimental animal models of intestinal inflammation. Acetic acid is one of many chemicals that is sometimes used to cause intestinal inflammation in mice.

> When *Lactobacillus reuteri* is given immediately after acetic acid, the probiotic prevents intestinal inflammation and causes minimal changes in intestinal leakiness (Fabia et al., 1993).

> In another mouse model of intestinal inflammation, milk containing 3 different probiotic strains *Lactobacillus acidophilus, Bifidobacterium breve*, and *Bifidobacterium bifidum* also reduced intestinal inflammation (Matsumoto et al., 2001).

In fact, numerous other strains of lactobacilli (like *Lactobacillus plantarum*) and combination "cocktails" of many different probiotic strains (such as VSL#3®, discussed in detail later) have reduced the severity of intestinal inflammation in experimental animal models. In addition to acetic acid, another commonly used animal model of inflammatory bowel disease is IL-10-deficient mice.

You may recall, IL-10 is a cytokine that "turns off" inflammation, so in animals that lack IL-10 intestinal inflammation is quite severe. Probably the most interesting finding in these mice is that they develop chronic inflammation of the entire intestinal tract, *unless* they are kept under strict germ-free conditions. Intestinal inflammation develops *only* when there are bacteria in their guts. Furthermore, the specific species of bacteria that comprise the mouse's normal flora determines the extent and severity of symptoms (Kuhn et al., 1993). As a result, IL-10-deficient mouse strains have become a key model for studying human diseases like ulcerative colitis and Crohn's disease.

In experiments using IL-10-deficient mice to study intestinal inflammation, numerous probiotics have demonstrated potent ability to decrease gut inflammation and injury.

> A probiotic product known as VSL#3® not only reduced intestinal inflammation in these mice, but the probiotic also reduced intestinal leakiness by inhibiting secretion of pro-inflammatory cytokines like TNF-α and IFN-γ (Madsen et al., 2001).
>
> Likewise, in the same IL-10-deficient mouse model, *Lactobacillus plantarum* 299v significantly reduced intestinal inflammation (Schultz et al., 2002) as did *Lactobacillus reuteri* (Madsen et al., 1999).
>
> In this mouse model, *Lactobacillus reuteri* prevented other gut bacteria from attaching to the intestines, restored the total number of *Lactobacillus* microorganisms to normal levels, and minimized gut injury (Madsen et al., 1999).
>
> Additionally, in the same IL-10-deficient mouse model, administration of lactulose, a prebiotic (covered in chapter 10) increased the total number of lactobacilli, decreased the number of bacteria adhering to the intestines, and significantly diminished intestinal injury (Madsen et al., 1999).

It is important to remember that in animal models of intestinal inflammation, just like in human inflammatory bowel conditions, all probiotic strains are *not* created equally. It is not only the *dose* of probiotic, but also the *strain* of probiotic that determines efficacy. In this regard, *Lactobacillus reuteri* R2LC is much more effective at reducing intestinal inflammation in rats than *Lactobacillus rhamnosus* GG (Holma et al., 2001). However, in further studies, *Lactobacillus plantarum* was even more effective at reducing inflammation and restoring normal intestinal function than *Lactobacillus reuteri* (Mao et al., 1996).

Results from this next study illustrate specific reasons why all probiotic strains are not created equal. Recently, in a mouse experimental model of inflammatory bowel disease, the probiotic strains *Lactobacillus salivarius* and *Bifidobacterium longum infantis* were found to suppress intestinal inflammation (Dunne et al., 1999). Additionally, this combination of probiotics improved the appearance of mice during the six week study period and reduced their weight loss. Okay, so far those findings are not particularly unexpected, given what we already know about probiotics. However, here's the key: During the course of the study, a heat-stable, acid resistant, antimicrobial compound was isolated as a by-product of *Lactobacillus salivarius*. This antimicrobial component is unlike any other antimicrobial factor previously identified. It inhibits growth of a wide variety of gram-positive and gram-negative bacteria, with the exception of closely related lactic acid bacteria like *Lactobacillus acidophilus* or *Lactobacillus reuteri* (Dunne et al., 1999).

This new information is critical for several reasons. Firstly, it tells us that *Lactobacillus salivarius* produces a toxin that kills other bacterial species. We can infer from the data that the toxin is killing whatever species of bacteria is responsible for the development of inflammatory disease. Secondly, this new compound can help scientists design a new class of antibiotic compounds for use in intestinal disorders. Thirdly, this toxin selectively spares closely-related "healthy" bacteria.

Certainly prolonged illnesses with inflammatory bowel disease increases the likelihood of colorectal cancer later in life, so it is interesting that in several mouse models of inflammatory bowel disease, supplementation of *Lactobacillus salivarius* not only reduced intestinal inflammation, but also reduced the incidence of colon cancer in these animals, too (O'Mahony et al., 2001; Kamm, 2001). Additionally, in mice that received this probiotic, the numbers of clostridia and enterococci were substantially reduced, indicating a new balance of intestinal bacteria (Kamm, 2001).

Human data

Quite possibly the earliest studies in humans that definitively noted a relationship between gut flora and improvements in inflammatory bowel disease were published in 1989 when two different groups of investigators — one in Kansas City, Kansas, and the other in Australia — published reports that they had used human feces to "cure" inflammatory bowel disease. The first report was from a physician, who himself, had continuously active ulcerative colitis. He decided to replace his "diseased" gut flora with flora from a healthy donor. The report was published 6 months after the procedure and he was still symptom-free (Bennet and Brinkman, 1989).

A subsequent report came out only a few months later from Dr. Borody and colleagues, at the Centre for Digestive Disease in Australia. They replaced bowel flora in 55 "sick" individuals with fecal flora from healthy persons. After receiving the human probiotic infusions, 20 patients were deemed to be "cured" and 9 patients experienced fewer symptoms (Borody et al., 1989). (It should be noted that not all 55 patients in this study had been diagnosed with inflammatory bowel disease. Some patients did have confirmed ulcerative colitis or Crohn's disease, but others had symptoms of irritable bowel syndrome or evidence of *C. difficile*.)

Certainly not all patients will agree to undergo human fecal infusions to replace their entire flora, so individual species of bacteria have been used as probiotics, often with great benefit, for those with inflammatory bowel disease. One such strain actually surprises many people — it is a nondisease-causing *Escherichia coli* strain Nissle 1917 (Mutaflor®) and has been used as a probiotic in both ulcerative colitis and Crohn's disease (Malchow, 1997; Rembacken et al., 1999).

> In a double-blind randomized placebo controlled clinical trial, *Escherichia coli* Nissle strain 1917 was useful for maintaining remission in individuals with Crohn's disease. The relapse rate was considerably lower (33% versus 66%) in the probiotic group. Importantly, this probiotic minimized the need for glucocorticoids (Malchow, 1997). This last point translates into fewer side effects for patients.

> In another study of 116 patients with ulcerative colitis, *Escherichia coli* Nissle 1917 was compared to mesalamine, a commonly used prescription drug. In this study, 73% of patients on mesalamine relapsed during the 12 month study period versus 66% of those receiving the probiotic. When we consider that about 70% of patients with ulcerative colitis will relapse during a 12-month period when given no treatment at all, in this study the probiotic doesn't appear particularly effective in preventing relapses (Rembacken et al., 1999).

Keep in mind that this study used patients with ulcerative colitis, whereas the previous study was conducted using folks with Crohn's disease. On the basis of these two studies alone, one might conclude that the efficacy of *Escherichia coli* could reflect different underlying causes for the two disease processes. However, in several other studies this strain of *E. coli* was found to be just as effective at maintaining remission in ulcerative colitis as the prescription drug mesalamine, which is the "gold standard" to which new drugs are often compared (Rembacken et al., 1999; Kruis et al., 1997). Some have been critical of these studies for various reasons, including the small size of the trials. However, at the very least, these studies are provocative enough to warrant further investigations (Marteau et al., 2002). In fact, the latest clinical trial was the most conclusive (Marteau et al., 2002)

> Two hundred twenty-two patients with ulcerative colitis were treated for one year with either the *Escherichia coli* probiotic or mesalamine. At the end of the year, 36% of patients in the probiotic group and 33% of patients in the mesalamine group had relapsed. From a statistical perspective, the results of this trial illustrate that treatment effects with either *Escherichia coli* Nissle 1917 or mesalamine are equivalent. For individuals who are allergic to mesalamine or who cannot tolerate its side effects, this probiotic may be a safe and effective alternative (Kruis et al., 2001).

As I was writing this chapter, a press release was issued that described data presented by Israeli physicians at a Digestive Disease Week conference in Orlando, FL, using another strain of *Escherichia coli,* strain ATCC20226 (trade name Probactrix®), in patients with inflammatory bowel disease. This strain of *Escherichia coli* is not yet marketed in the United States, however it is available in Russia and Israel.

> Out of 6 patients with inflammatory bowel disease who took 20-40 milliliters of the probiotic (containing 100 million organisms per milliliter) for four to six weeks, 3 patients experienced not only a significant reduction in abdominal symptoms, but also had significant decreases in intestinal inflammation after treatment (The BioBalance Corporation©).

Other probiotics have also been useful in treating ulcerative colitis. Take a look at the following former ulcerative colitis patient's story.

> In 1992, RG was a 10 year old girl with severe ulcerative colitis. She was anemic from blood loss, was losing weight (weighed only 69 pounds), had stopped growing, was pale and frail, and was passing 10 bloody stools every day. Numerous pharmacotherapies had been tried, and though her disease waxed and waned, symptoms always recurred.
>
> After "cleansing her bowel" with antibiotics and 2 antifungals every 4 hours for two days, she was started on several different probiotic strains including two non-disease-causing strains of *Escherichia coli, Lactobacillus acidophilus strain DDS-1, Lactobacillus bulgaricus strain LB-51, and Bifidobacteria bifidum Malyoth strain* (McCann et al., 1997).
>
> After 6 weeks of probiotic therapy, no more blood was detected in her stools. A year after initiating probiotics, an endoscopy and biopsy were completely normal, she had gained 20 pounds, grew 4 inches, and all laboratory tests were completely normal. Most exciting of all, this child has continued on the same probiotic therapy and has had no relapses in more than 10 years!

Another probiotic to which I've referred to earlier in the chapter, VSL#3®, is a preparation of 450 billion live microorganisms in each 6-gram dose. This probiotic is often effective in maintaining remission in ulcerative colitis and Crohn's disease. This product is comprised of 4 different strains of *Lactobacillus* (*L. casei, L. plantarum, L acidophilus, L. bulgaricus*), 3 strains of *Bifidobacterium* (*B. longum, B. breve, B. infantis*), and 1 strain of *Streptococci* (*S. thermophilus*). VSL#3® has three key characteristics that set it apart from most other products on the market: a high bacterial concentration in each dose (450 billion), multiple (8) species of bacteria whose actions complement each other and act synergistically, and the product is manufactured by a reputable pharmaceutical company.

> Fifteen of twenty patients (75%) with ulcerative colitis remained in remission for 12 months when 3 grams of VSL#3® was administered twice daily. During the year of treatment feces became more acidic which suppresses growth of harmful bacteria, and no significant adverse effects were reported (Venturi et al., 1999). This probiotic may be an essential therapy in individuals who are allergic or unable to tolerate side effects of prescription drugs like 5-aminosalicylic acid.

Here is one ulcerative colitis patient's success story with VSL#3®.

> A five year old boy, J.A., had anemia, a low grade fever, and cramping. He passed as many as 10 bloody, loose bowel movements every day. Prescription drugs for inflammatory bowel disease had failed and were not effective.
>
> At 10 years of age, an experimental rectal enema of donor feces was given to the child, and the child had normal stools for approximately 10 days! Encouraged by those results, antibiotics were given to try to eliminate his intestinal flora, followed by both oral and rectal administration of 12 different strains of bacteria normally found in the large intestines. After the third attempt to re-colonize the intestines with healthy flora, the child experienced a full remission for 3 years!
>
> However, the patient again relapsed and spent several more years with minimal weight gain, frequent mucous-filled and bloody stools, lack of energy, and poor appetite. By this point, ulcerative colitis had been confirmed.
>
> At 18 years of age, multiple antibiotics were again given to eliminate his unhealthy gut flora, followed by large doses of VSL#3® to re-colonize his intestines with healthy bacteria. After initiating therapy with VSL#3®, all symptoms of ulcerative colitis gradually disappeared over a four month period of time. Additionally, this young man began passing solid stools only once each day. Still taking VSL#3®, his stools are no longer bloody or mucous-filled, his appetite is normal for a male teenager, and an endoscopy of his intestines is completely normal.

VSL#3® isn't just successful in treating ulcerative colitis. It has been used with great success for other types of inflammatory bowel disease, too.

> In 40 patients with Crohn's disease, patients received either mesalamine or VSL#3® for one year. After 12 months, the risk of severe relapse was 20% in the probiotic group compared to 30% in the group receiving mesalamine (Campieri et al., 2000).

VSL#3® is also effective for maintaining remission in pouchitis (Gionchetti et al., 2000a). Pouchitis is inflammation of the surgical "pouch" (the pouch is created to hold stools) after ileal pouch-anal anastomosis (an artificial connection between the ileum and the anus, created when the large intestines are surgically removed because of disease). This inflammation is acquired as a post-surgical complication. The intention of the surgery is to remove diseased portions of the bowel in those with severe ulcerative colitis. Unfortunately, pouchitis is a major long-term complication associated with this surgical procedure. About half of all patients with a pouch end up with inflammation at some point. Most folks respond to antibiotics, but 10-15% are forced to deal with recurrent or chronic symptoms. Some studies suggest that these individuals have less-than-optimal numbers of lactobacilli and bifidobacteria in their guts (Hart et al., 2003).

VSL#3® is not only effective for maintaining remission of pouchitis, but also for *preventing* pouchitis from developing in the first place.

> The risk of developing pouchitis within the first year after surgery is significantly less (10% versus 40%) in those individuals using VSL#3® (Gionchetti et al., 2000b).

There are two remarkable things about the studies that used VSL#3®. First, the probiotic is very clearly efficacious in suppressing intestinal inflammation. There is no doubt about the clarity of that data. Secondly, these studies were the first clinical trials to use a preparation that contained so many different probiotic strains (Schultz and Sartor, 2000).

> Another small study in only 10 patients indicated that a combination of *Lactobacillus* GG with a prebiotic (in this case fructooligosaccharide) may be effective in folks with chronic pouchitis. In this study, symptoms of pouchitis completely disappeared in all 10 patients within one month of treatment (Hart et al., 2003; Friedman and George, 2000).

Probiotics are safe for children and certainly a better alternative than steroids, especially in youngsters:

> *Lactobacillus* GG was also used in a study of 4 children with Crohn's disease. In this small, preliminary, **open-label** study, *Lactobacillus* GG improved symptoms throughout the 24 weeks of therapy, 3 patients were able to reduce their steroid doses by 50%, and intestinal permeability improved significantly (Gupta et al., 2000).

The probiotic yeast, *Saccharomyces boulardii* has also been used as a therapy to treat Crohn's disease.

> As early as 1993, 20 individuals with moderately active inflammation were randomly assigned to receive either *Saccharomyces boulardii* (750 mg) or placebo for 7 weeks. Only those in the probiotic group had a significant reduction in disease severity (Plein and Hotz , 1993).
>
> In a year long, double-blind, randomized, controlled trial of 32 patients with Crohn's disease patients receiving one gram of *Saccharomyces boulardii* plus mesalamine rarely relapsed (1 in 16 or 6.25%) compared to those receiving mesalamine alone (6 in 16 or 37.5%) (Guslandi et al., 2000). The benefits of the probiotic were shown not only in a reduction of diarrheal episodes, but also in a reduction of abdominal pain, improved hematocrit levels, and general improvement in well-being.

These promising trials clearly need to be confirmed with more patients. A very recent publication also illustrated the effectiveness of a bifidobacteria-fermented milk supplement as a dietary aid for treating ulcerative colitis.

> During a year long study, only 3 of 11 ulcerative colitis patients using a probiotic-fermented milk product suffered a flare-up of symptoms, while 9 of 10 patients who drank the placebo product developed symptomatic disease (Ishikawa et al., 2003).

I would be remiss if I didn't let you know that not every clinical trial using probiotics to treat inflammatory bowel disease has had such positive outcomes. In a randomized, double-blind, placebo-controlled trial *Lactobacillus* GG was given following surgical removal of the diseased portion of the gut. It was thought that the probiotic would prevent new lesions from appearing or would reduce their severity. However, that theory did not hold true (Prantera et al., 2002). There are several potential reasons for the lack of beneficial effects in this study: one bacterial strain alone may not exert a competitive beneficial action in the human intestine (contrast with the many strains in VSL#3®), the bacterial concentration may have been too low in this study, and, as we know, one probiotic may not be effective in all patients or even in the same patient during all stages of disease (Prantera et al., 2002).

Genetically-engineered Probiotics?

A unique role for probiotics could result if probiotic bacteria are genetically engineered to deliver anti-inflammatory or immunomodulatory cytokines *directly* to intestinal cells. For example, one group of researchers genetically designed a probiotic strain of *Lactococcus lactis* to secrete the cytokine, IL-10 (Steidler, 2000). IL-10 is normally produced by T cells, B cells, macrophages, and monocytes. As mentioned earlier, IL-10 plays an essential role in controlling intestinal inflammation. IL-10 suppresses secretion of numerous pro-inflammatory cytokines like IL-2, IFN-γ, IL-1, IL-6, IL-8, and TNF-α (van Deventer et al., 1997).

In experimental mice with intestinal inflammation, administration of IL-10-secreting-*Lactococcus* reduced inflammation by 50%. Additionally, this specially engineered probiotic *prevented* the development of intestinal inflammation in mice that were genetically deficient in secreting their own IL-10 (van Deventer et al., 1997).

In theory, this approach could be used to deliver any one of several different therapeutic molecules. With its central role in regulating gut inflammation, IL-10 is a good choice for initial studies. Certainly there are safety concerns that need to be addressed before this type of therapy could be used in humans. However, potential advantages of this strategy to treat inflammatory bowel diseases include avoidance of side effects and avoidance of the high cost that would be associated with administering IL-10 intravenously. Additionally, considerably lower dosages could be used if IL-10 is administered locally to the inflamed areas of the gut, rather than delivered in an injectable form. Although still years from being commercially available, the idea of genetically modifying probiotics to secrete anti-inflammatory chemical mediators is a novel one and should be explored further by the scientific and medical communities.

*Pre*biotics in Inflammatory Bowel Disease

Prebiotics are food ingredients that are not broken down by the human body. They are, instead, food for bacteria — an energy source for the many bacteria living in the large intestines. Fructooligosaccharides (FOS) are found in garlic, onion, artichoke, asparagus, bananas, and tomatoes, and are among the most widely studied prebiotics. FOS are selectively fermented and utilized by bifidobacteria and perhaps some lactobacilli. In healthy volunteers, dietary supplementation with prebiotics increases the numbers of bifidobacteria in feces and inhibits the growth of other bacterial species (Kennedy et al., 2000). FOS and other undigestible sugars like lactosucrose and lactulose, not only promote growth of bifidobacteria and lactobacilli by serving as food substrates but are also metabolized into short chain fatty acids. As you recall, short chain fatty acids are an important energy source for intestinal cells, creating an acidic environment that suppresses the growth of anaerobic bacteria like *Bacteroides* (Kennedy et al., 2000).

In both experimental animal models of intestinal inflammation and in a preliminary experiment in humans with inflammatory bowel disease, prebiotics had protective and therapeutic effects (Kennedy et al., 2000). However, at the present time, there are no properly controlled clinical trials to fully evaluate the utility of prebiotics in treating inflammatory bowel disease.

Conclusion

At the present time, all four major theories of inflammatory bowel disease focus on a disrupted normal flora as a major contributing cause. Whether inflammatory bowel disease is caused by (a) an appropriate reaction to a persistent bacterial infection in the gut, (b) a subtle alteration in bacterial flora within the gut (c) a natural response to continuous stimulation by gut bacteria, occurring to a severe extent only when the bowel mucosal lining is defective, (d) a lack of oral tolerance to normal gut bacteria, or (e) a combination of these factors, what is clear is that gut flora does play a role. As a result, changes in gut flora from using probiotics may create a more favorable environment and may alleviate symptoms of inflammatory bowel disease for many individuals. However, keep in mind, since we as individuals are not created equally — each one of us having our own unique flora — the probiotic approach that works for one person may not work for another. A different probiotic product, a greater number of bacteria, or a combination of various probiotics may be the key.

Notes

Notes

References

Bennet JD and Brinkman M. Treatment of ulcerative colitis by implantation of normal colonic flora. Lancet. 1989;1:164.

Borody TJ, George L, Andrews P, et al. Bowel-flora alteration: A potential cure for inflammatory bowel disease and irritable bowel syndrome? Med J Austral. 1989;150:604.

Borruel N, Carol M, Casellas F, et al. Increased mucosal tumor necrosis factor α production in Crohn's disease can be downregulated *ex vivo* by probiotic bacteria. Gut. 2002;51:659-664.

Breuer RJ, Soergel KH, Lashner BA, et al. Short chain fatty acid rectal irrigation for left-sided ulcerative colitis: A randomised, placebo controlled trial. Gut. 1997;40:485-491.

Campieri M, Rizzello F, Venturi A, et al. Combination of antibiotic and probiotic treatment is efficacious in prophylaxis of post-operative recurrence of Crohn's disease: A randomized controlled study versus mesalamine. Gastroenterol. 2000;118:G4179.

Chapman MAS. The role of the colonic flora in maintaining a healthy large bowel mucosa. Am R Coll Surg Engl. 2001;83:75-80.

Cong Y, Brandwein SL, McCabe RP. CD4+ cells reactive to enteric bacterial antigens in spontaneously colitic C3H/HeJbir mice: Increased T helper cell type I response and ability to transfer disease. J Exp Med. 1998;187:855-864.

D'Haens GR, Goboes K, Peeters M, et al. Early lesions of recurrent Crohn's disease caused by infusion of intestinal contents in excluded ileum. Gastroenterol. 1998;114:262-267.

Duchmann R, Kaiser I, Hermann E, et al. Tolerance exists towards resident intestinal flora but is broken in active inflammatory bowel disease (IBD). Clin Exp Immunol. 1995;102:448-455.

Dunne C, Murphy L, Flynn L, et al. Probiotics: From myth to reality. Demonstration of functionality in animal models of disease and in human clinical trials. Antonie Leeuwenhoek. 1999;76:279-292.

Fabia R, Ar-Rajab A, Johansson MI, et al. The effect of exogenous administration of *Lactobacillus reuteri* R2LC and oat fiber on acetic acid-induced colitis in the rat. Scand J Gastroenterol. 1993;28:15-162.

Farrell RJ and LaMont JT. Microbial factors in inflammatory bowel disease. Gastroenterol Clinics North Am. 2002;31:41-62.

Farrell RJ and Peppercorn MA. Ulcerative colitis. Lancet. 2002;359:331-340.

Favier C, Neut C, Mizon C, et al. Fecal beta-D-galactosidase production and Bifidobacteria are decreased in Crohn's disease. Dig Dis Sci. 1997;42:817-822.

Friedman G and George J. Treatment of refractory "pouchitis" wth prebioic and probiotic therapy [abstract]. Gastroenterol. 2000;118:4167.

Giaffer MH, Holdsworth CD, Duerden BI. The assessment of faecal flora in patients with inflammatory bowel disease by a simplified bacteriological technique. J Med Microbiol. 1991;35:238-243.

Gionchetti P, Rizzello F, Venturi A, et al. Oral bacteriotherapy as maintenance treatment in patients with chronic pouchitis: A double-blind, placebo-controlled trial. Gastroenterol. 2000a;119:305-309.

Gionchetti P, Rizzello F, Venturi A, et al. Prophylaxis of pouchitis onset with probiotic therapy: A double-blind, placebo controlled trial. Gastroenterol. 2000b;118:G1214.

Gupta P, Andrew H, Kirschnet B, et al. Is *Lactobacillus* GG helpful in children with Crohns disease? Results of a preliminary, open-label study. J Ped Gastrenterol Nutr. 2000;31:453-457.

Guslandi M, Mezzi G, Sorghi M, et al. *Saccharomyces boulardii* in maintenance treatment of Crohn's disease. Dig Dis Sci. 2000;45:1462-1464.

Harper PH, Lee EC, Kettlewell MG, et al. Role of the faecal stream in the maintenance of Crohns colitis. Gut. 1985;26:279-284.

Hart AL, Stagg AJ, Kamm MA. Use of probiotics in the treatment of inflammatory bowel disease. J Clin Gastroenterol. 2003:36:111-119.

Hollander D, Vadheim CM, Brettholz E, et al. Increased intestinal permeability in patients with Crohn's disease and their relatives: A possible etiologic factor. Ann Intern Med. 1986;105:883-885.

Holma R, Salmenpera P, Lohi J, et al. Effects of *Lactobacillus rhamnosus* GG and *Lactobacillus reuteri* R2LC and oat fiber on acetic acid-induced colitis in rats. Scand J Gastroenterol. 2001;36:630-635.

Irvine EJ and Marshall JK. Increased intestinal permeability precedes onset of Crohn's disease in a subject with familial risk. Gastroenterol. 2000;119:1740-1744.

Ishkawa H, Akedo I, Umesaki Y, et al. Randomized controlled trial of the effect of bifidobacteria-fermented milk on ulcerative colitis. J Am Coll Nutr. 2003;22:56-63.

Isolauri E, Sutas Y, Kankaanpaa P, et al. Probiotics: Effects on Immunity. Am J Clin Nutr. 2001;73:444S-450S.

Jani N and Regueiro MD. Medical therapy for ulcerative colitis. Gastroenterol Clin N Am. 2002;31:147-166.

Kamm MA. New therapeutic possibilities in inflammatory bowel disease. Eur J Surg. 2001;Suppl 586:30-33.

Keighley MR, Arabi Y, Dimock F, et al. Influence of inflammatory bowel disease on intestinal flora. Gut. 1978;19:1099-1104.

Kennedy RJ, Kirk SJ, Gardiner KR. Promotion of a favorable gut flora in inflammatory bowel disease. J Parenteral Enteral Nutr. 2000;24:189-195.

Krishnan A and Korzenik JR. Inflammatory bowel disease and environmental influences. Gastroenterol Clin N Am. 2002;31:21-39.

Kruis W, Fric P, Stolte M, and the Mutaflor® study group. Maintenance of remission in ulcerative colitis is equally effective with *Escherichia coli* Nissle 1917 and with standard mesalamine. Gastroenterol. 2001;120:A139.

Kruis W, Schutz E, Fric P, et al. Double-blind comparison of an oral *Escherichia coli* preparation and mesalamine in maintaining remission of ulcerative colitis. Aliment Pharmacol Ther. 1997;11:853-858.

Kuhn R, Lohler J, Rennick D, et al. Interleukin-10-deficient mice develop chronic enterocolitis. Cell. 1993;75:263-274.

Lammers KM, Helwig U, Swennen E, et al. Effect of probiotic strains on interleukin 8 production by HT29/19A cells. Am J Gastroenterol. 2002;97:1182-1186.

Lichtman SN, Okoruwa EE, Keku J, et al. Degradation of endogenous bacterial cell wall polymers by the muralytic enzyme mutanolysin prevents hepatobiliary injury in genetically susceptible rats with experimental intestinal bacterial overgrowth. J Clin Invest. 1992;90:1313-1322.

Loftus EV and Sandborn WJ. Epidemiology of inflammatory bowel disease. Gastroenterol Clin N Am. 2002;31:1-20.

Lopez-Cubero SO, Sullivan KM, McDonald GB. Course of Crohn's disease after allogeneic marrow transplantation. Gastroenterol. 1998;114:433-440.

Madsen K, Cornish A, Soper P, et al. Probiotic bacteria enhance murine and human intestinal epithelial barrier function. Gastroenterol. 2001;121:580-591.

Madsen KL, Doyle JS, Jewell LD, et al. Lactobacillus species prevents colitis in interleukin 10 gene deficient mice. Gastroenterol. 1999;116:1107-1114.

Malchow HA. Crohn's disease and *Escherichia coli*. A new approach in therapy to maintain remission of colonic Crohns' disease? J Clin Gastroenterol. 1997;25:653-658.

Malin M, Suomalainen H, Saxelin M, et al. Promotion of IgA immune response in patients with Crohn's disease by oral bacteriotherapy with *Lactobacillus* GG. Ann Nutr Metab. 1996;40:137-145.

Mao Y, Nobaek S, Kasravi B, et al. The effects of Lactobacillus strains and oat fiber on methotrexate-induced enterocolitis in rats. Gastroenterol. 1996;111:334-344.

Marteau P, Seksik P, Jian R. Probiotics and intestinal health effects: A clinical perspective. Br. J Nutr. 2002;88:S51-S57.

May GR, Sutherland LR, Meddings JB. Is small intestinal permeability really increased in relatives of patients with Crohn's disease? Gastroenterol. 1993;104:1627-1632.

McCann ML, Buck RA, Trenev N. Probiotics to treat and prevent relapses in inflammatory bowel disease (IBD) [abstract]. JACI. 1997:991 #358.

MimuraT, Rizzello F, Schreiber S, et al. Once daily high dose probiotic therapy maintains remission and improves quality of life in patients with recurrent or refractory pouchitis: A randomised, placebo-conrolled, double-blind trial [abstract]. Gastroenterol. 2002;122:667.

Monteleone I, Vavassori P, Biancone L, et al. Immunoregulation in the gut: Success and failures in human disease. Gut. 2002;50:iii60-iii64.

Mourelle M, Salas A, Guarner F, et al. Stimulation of transforming growth factor geta1 by enteric bacteria in the pathogenesis of rat intestinal fibrosis. Gastroenterol. 1998;114:519-526.

Okamoto T, Sasaki M, Tsujikawa T, et al. Preventative efficacy of butyrate enemas and oral administration of *Clostridium butyricum* M588 in dextran sodium sulfate-induced colitis in rats. Gastrenterol. 2000;35:341-346.

O'Mahony L, Feeney M, O'Halloran S, et al. Probiotic impact on microbial flora, inflammation and tumor development in IL-10 knockout mice. Aliment Pharmacol Ther. 2001;15:1219-1225.

Pitcher MC, Beatty ER, Cummings JH. The contribution of sulphate reducing bacteria and 5-aminosalicylic acid to faecal sulphide in patients with ulcerative colitis. Gut. 2000;46:64-72.

Plein K and Hotz J. Therapeutic effects of *Saccharomyces boulardii* on mild residual symptoms in a stable phase of Crohn's disease with special respect to chronic diarrhea - a pilot study. Z Gastroenterol. 1993:31:129-134.

Prantera C, Scribano ML, Falasco G, et al. Ineffectiveness of probiotics in preventing recurrence after curative resection for Crohn's disease: A randomised controlled trial with *Lactobacillus* GG. Gut. 2002;51:405-409.

Quigley ME and Kelly SM. Structure, Function, and Metabolism of Host Mucus Glycoproteins. In Gibson CR and MacFarlance GT, eds. Human Colonic Bacteria: Role in Nutrition, Physiology, and Pathology. CRC Press, Boca Raton, FL, 1995.

Rembacken BJ, Snelling AM, Hawkey PM, et al. Non-pathogenic *Escherichia coli* versus mesalamine for the treatment of ulcerative colitis: A randomised trial. Lancet. 1999;354:635-639.

Rutgeerts P, Goboes K, Peeters M, et al. Effect of faecal stream diversion on recurrence of Crohn's disease in the neoterminal ileum. Lancet. 1991;338:771-774.

Schultz M and Sartor RB. Probiotics and inflammatory bowel disease. Am J Gastroenterol. 2000;95:S19-S21.

Schultz M, Veltkamp C, Dieleman LA, et al. *Lactobacillus plantarum* 299V in the treatment and prevention of spontaneous colitis in interleukin-10-deficient mice. Inflamm Bowel Dis. 2002;8:71-80.

Shanahan F. Inflammatory bowel disease: Immunodiagnostics, immunotherapeutics, and ecotherapeutics. Gastroenterol. 2001;120:622-635.

Steidler L, Hans W, Schotte L, et al. Treatment of murine colitis by *Lactococcus lactis* secreting interleukin-10. Science. 2000;289:1352-1355.

Steinhart AH, Brzezinski A, Baker JP. Treatment of refractory ulcerative proctosigmoiditis with butyrate enemas. Am J Gastroenterol. 1994;89:179-183.

Steinhart AH, Hiruki T, Brzezinski A, et al. Treatment of left-sided ulcerative colitis with butyrate enemas: A controlled trial. Aliment Pharmacol Ther. 1996;10:729-736.

Susteno-Reodica N, Ruiz P, Rogers, A, et al. Recurrent Crohn's disease in transplanted bowel. Lancet. 1997;349:688-691.

Van Deventer SJH, Elson CO, Fedorak RN. Multiple doses of intravenous interleukin 10 in steroid-refractory Crohn's disease. Gastroenterol. 1997;113:383-389.

Venturi A, Gionchetti P, Rizzello F, et al. Impact on the composition of the faecal flora by a new probiotic preparation: Preliminary data on maintenance treatment of patients with ulcerative colitis. Aliment Pharmacol Ther. 1999;13:1103-108.

Vernia P, Annese V, Bresci G, et al. Topical butyrate improves efficacy of 5-ASA in refractory distal ulcerative colitis: Results of a multicentre trial. Eur J Clin Invest. 2003;33:244-248.

Vernia P, Fracasso PL, Casale V, et al. Topical butyrate for acute radiation proctitis: Randomized crossover trial. Lancet. 2000;356:1232-1235.

Vernia P, Marcheggiano A, Caprilli R, et al. Short-chain fatty acid topical treatment in distal ulcerative colitis. Aliment Pharmacol Ther. 1995;9:309-313.

Watts DA and Satsangi J. The genetic jigsaw of inflammatory bowel disease. Gut. 2002;50:iii31-iii36.

Wensinck F, Custers-van Lieshout LMC, Poppelaars-Kustermans PA, et al. The faecal flora of patients with Crohn's disease. J Hyg. 1981;87:1-12.

Zolotarevsky Y, Hecht G, Koutsouris A, et al. A membrane-permeant peptide that inhibits MLC kinase restores barrier function in *in vitro* models of intestinal disease. Gastroenterol. 2002;23:163-172.

Chapter 7

Why Does My Food Make Me Sick? Probiotics and Allergic Diseases

While it may seem like a rather new idea to us that the bacteria in our guts could possibly play a role in allergies, as early as 1924 a correlation was noted between disrupted normal flora and chronic allergic diseases. Specifically, an overabundance of anaerobic clostridial species, which normally make up a rather small portion of the total gut flora, was associated with chronic eczema and asthma (Olhagen and Mansson et al., 1968). For those who suffer from hives and rashes when they eat certain foods and the 5 million children in the United States with asthma, is it possible that probiotics hold the answer to relieving their discomfort? This is what we are going to find out in the current chapter.

It has been estimated that 1 in 3 children in the Western world have an allergic condition (Alm et al., 1999). That means 33% of children develop at least one of the following: eczema (skin rash), food allergies, hay fever, or asthma.

What are allergies? Allergies are really inappropriate immune responses to environmental or food allergens. Allergic conditions involve activation of Th2-type T cells which release IL-4, IL-5, and IL-6. These cytokines work together to produce IgE allergic antibodies and recruit white blood cells (called eosinophils) that ingest foreign particles and play a role in allergic reactions.

On the other hand, the cytokine IFN-γ, produced by Th1-type T cells, suppresses allergic responses by inhibiting Th2 cells and interfering with IgE production (See figure 7-1). So, we find, yet again, that within the immune system, there are two competing forces — in other words — a system of checks and balances that can modulate immune responses. In this chapter we are going to explore *why* there has been a dramatic increase in allergies during the past two generations and, most importantly, what can we do about it?

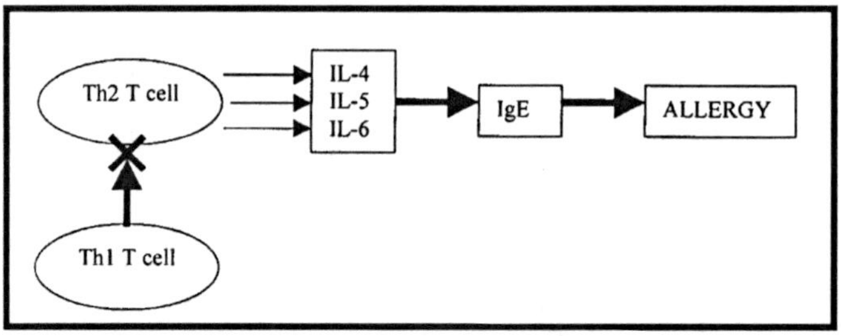

Figure 7-1. Th2 T cells secrete cytokines that stimulate allergic responses. On the other hand, Th1 T cells secrete cytokines that inhibit "allergic" activities of Th2 T cells.

Hygiene Hypothesis

Certainly, hereditary factors play a role in developing allergies, but the dramatic increase in prevalence during the past 50 years suggests that non-hereditary factors must also play a role. The incidence of allergy is much higher in Western civilizations than in Eastern Europe (Wold et al., 1998), and the increasing incidence seems to have started with people born in the 1960s. One leading theory is the "hygiene hypothesis".

The hygiene hypothesis suggests that if infants are *not* exposed to microbes early in life, they have an increased tendency to develop allergies. In other words, immature immune systems will develop Th2-dominated allergic tendencies if there is insufficient stimulation of the immune system. How does an infant's immune system get "stimulated" without causing harm to the newborn? An infant's immune system is stimulated through acquisition of gut bacteria, of course. Specifically, normal gut flora stimulates the release of Th1 cytokines.

When an infant acquires gut flora, the immune system gets "educated". "Healthy" flora is associated with a "good education". On the other hand, when there are excessively sterile conditions or heavy antibiotic use, the immune system fails to get a good "education" and over-reacts, causing allergies. Of course we all want our children to be "well-educated". If we feed healthy bacteria to our infants, in the form of probiotics, we can provide them with a "good education" and prevent allergies from developing (Dunne et al., 1999). Certainly, the bacteria living in our digestive tracts are far from inert parasites. Rather, the bacteria living within us are more like a "forgotten organ" that actively communicates with our immune system.

During the spring of 2003, I was given a clipping from a Florida newspaper — source uncertain — describing the hygiene hypothesis in our everyday lives. The article cited a study sponsored by the National Institute of Allergy and Infectious Disease which illustrates that growing up sheltered from "germs" in excessively clean homes makes us more susceptible to allergies. A total of 450 children, having had two or more cats and/or dogs during their first year of life, were half as likely to have allergies at 6 and 7 years of age, compared to children that had no pets. When the children with pets were exposed at young ages to "germs" in their pet's saliva or stools, their immune systems were triggered in such a way that a host of common allergens (dust mites, ragweed, grass) were not perceived as "allergic".

Why does the immune system favor Th-2 allergic responses in infancy? During pregnancy, the immune system develops a tendency away from Th1 inflammatory responses and, instead, leans towards Th2 responses. This is to protect the developing fetus. In newborns, Th2 allergic responses are universal. The hygiene hypothesis of allergic diseases relies on the assumption that exposure to specific bacterial strains is the key modulator of the immune system. With exposure to bacteria, especially gut flora, the immune system is stimulated in such a way that immune responsiveness is directed away from Th2 allergic responses. This is because bacterial exposure causes the following immune activities: (1) IgE allergic antibody production halts and (2) secretion of IgA antibodies (the type of antibodies that lines the inside of the intestines) increases. These factors together reduce allergic responsiveness. In other words, exposure to bacteria — whether by external infections or via gut normal flora — provide stimuli to protect against allergic diseases. Clearly, with vaccinations, antibiotics, and reduced family sizes, today's infants simply aren't exposed to the same "germs" that they were two generations ago. As a result of improved hygiene, the "relative lack" of bacterial exposure fails to shift the immune system away from Th2-allergic responses that dominate at birth.

One way investigators study the hygiene hypothesis is by comparing incidence of allergies in folks that live in industrialized societies to folks living a more "anthroposophic" way of life. The term anthroposophic is a fancy word that refers to a type of holistic approach in which entire societies use organic farming and restrict the use of antibiotics, fever-suppressing medications, and vaccinations. The prevalence of allergies is substantially lower in children reared under anthroposophic ways of life than in children from other Western families, suggesting that lifestyle factors — specifically, exposure to more bacteria — lessens the risk of contracting allergic diseases in childhood (Alm et al., 1999). In these anthroposophic societies, 13% of children have a history of allergies versus 25% of other Western children. Only half of the children raised in anthroposophic conditions have ever received antibiotics or fever-suppressing drugs compared to 90% of other children. These children have vastly different diets compared to most of us. Fermented vegetables and organic foods are consumed by 63% of anthroposophic children, compared to 4.5% of other children and breast feeding is of longer duration for anthroposophic children versus other children (5.7 months versus 4.3 months) (Alm et al., 1999).

Data from immune studies have shown that different infections can either promote allergies (respiratory syncytial virus) or prevent allergies (measles, hepatitis A, tuberculosis) (Alm et al., 1999). Yet, it seems unlikely that a stimulus that is potentially harmful is necessary for the immune system to mature properly. Therefore, it is probably the normal flora of the gastrointestinal tract that serves as the primary signal for immune maturation, not disease-causing invaders (Bjorksten et al., 2001). If microbial stimulation is, indeed, the driving force behind immune system maturity, altered lifestyles and dietary changes during the past 50 years in Western civilization are quite likely the driving force behind the high prevalence of allergies that we see today. In practical terms, this means that fewer childhood infections — due to use of vaccinations and antibiotics — are responsible for the recent increase in allergic diseases.

The immunological role of intestinal gut bacteria has also been explored in other societies. In certain parts of Europe, lifestyles today still resemble those of Western Europe in the 1960s. Regions of Estonia, the former German Democratic Republic, and Poland are ideal for these types of studies, especially since there is still a lower incidence of allergies in these areas compared to the rest of the Western world. For example, children in Estonia have lower rates of allergies than children from Sweden (Sepp et al., 1997). Interestingly, comparisons between children's gut flora identified significant differences in these two populations. Substantially more lactobacilli ("healthy bacteria") and *Eubacterium* are present in Estonian children (with low incidence of allergies) compared to their Swedish counterparts. In contrast, clostridia, especially *Clostridium difficile* ("disease-causing bacteria") were much more common in Swedish children (with high incidence of allergies) than Estonian infants. These differences may stem from different dietary preferences or from differing sanitation conditions between the countries.

One possible suggestion is that *Lactobacillus plantarum* may play a role in the low incidence of allergies in Estonian children. This bacterium is commonly found in fermented vegetables. The Estonian diet is still largely based on locally produced foods and varying lactic acid fermented products are common dietary staples, even among small children. Thus, diets rich in fermented vegetables may affect intestinal flora and play a substantial role in preventing allergic diseases. It may be that *Lactobacillus plantarum* colonizes inside the human intestines and alters the growth of other bacterial strains. On the other hand, *Clostridium difficile*, which is more frequent in those living a "sterilized" lifestyle, can invade intestinal mucosa and cause inflammation. Gut inflammation and associated "leakiness" and "intestinal permeability" facilitate penetration of innocuous antigens from the gut into the blood stream — triggering allergic responses. Thus, it is tempting to speculate that a correlation exists between intestinal colonization with lactobacilli/eubacteria in "old world" diets and low allergy rates *versus* intestinal colonization with clostridial flora in those eating "conventional" diets and high rates of allergic diseases.

Many other groups of investigators have explored correlations between gut bacteria (species and number) in allergic versus non-allergic children.

> Researchers compared two year old children in Sweden and Estonia and found that allergic children — in both Sweden and Estonia — possessed fewer lactobacilli and bifidobacteria compared to non-allergic children, but were more likely to be colonized by coliforms and *Staphylococcus aureus*. The flora in the allergic children was similar to what might be expected after a course of antibiotics (Bjorksten et al., 1999).

> In a different study, newborn infants in both Estonia and Sweden were followed for the first two years of their lives. Compared to healthy infants, children who developed allergies were less likely to have been colonized with enterococci during their first month of life and less likely to have been colonized by bifidobacteria during their first year of life. Additionally, allergic infants had higher levels of clostridia at 3 months of age, a higher incidence of *Staphylococcus aureus* at 6 months of age, and a lower colonization with *Bacteroides* at 1 year of age (Sepp et al., 1997).

> Still another group of researchers studied fecal bacteria from 27 infants with allergies and 10 healthy infants. Again, there was a tendency for allergic infants to have lower bifidobacteria concentrations compared to healthy babies (Kirjavainen et al., 2001).

> In another study conducted in Denmark, investigators found that even among adults, exposure to certain types of infections (hepatitis A virus, *Helicobacter pylori*, and *Toxoplasma gondii*), which are considered indicators of poor hygiene, correlates with a lower incidence of allergies. While, on the other hand, exposure to intestinal bacteria like *Clostridium difficile*, *Campylobacter jejuni*, and *Yersinia enterocolitica* is associated with a higher likelihood of allergies (Linneberg et al., 2003).

When all this data is compiled, we see that there is a clear correlation between allergies and the gut floral composition in infants. Even more importantly is the fact that discrepancies in microbial composition (in allergic versus non-allergic infants) were apparent *before* allergy symptoms appeared (Bjorksten et al., 2001). The underlying thread tying these studies together is that allergic children tend to have fewer "healthy" bacteria in their guts than non-allergic children — even from infancy *before* allergies are apparent.

The obvious question is *how* do allergic children acquire a relative lack of bifidobacteria and lactobacilli in their guts in the first place? While this is not entirely clear, certainly consumption of processed, sterilized foods in Western societies has an impact, as does altered maternal vaginal flora, and strict hygiene during birthing (Bjorksten et al., 1999). Additionally, antibiotics, often given early in infancy, suppress growth of anaerobic species of bacteria, allowing disease-causing bacteria to overgrow. Unfortunately for those infants who acquire less-than-optimal gut flora, the flora that is acquired early in life is relatively stable — it takes up permanent residence in the intestines. Once the flora is established in infancy, it is difficult to alter on a permanent basis, unless *major* dietary changes are made (Bjorksten et al., 1999).

Why "Healthy" Bacteria Are So Important

Role for bifidobacteria

One significant feature about bifidobacteria is that these bacteria are gram-positive microorganisms. Gram-positive bacteria are potent inducers of Th1 cytokines like IL-12 and IFN-γ. These cytokines "shift" the immune system away from Th-2 allergic activities. On the other hand, gram-negative bacteria are potent stimulators of Th2 cytokines. Therefore, it could be suggested that an insufficient amount of gram-positive-bacterial-mediated stimulation (lack of Th1 activity) allows a newborn's immune system to continue favoring Th2 allergic responses (See figure 7-1). Part of this shift in immune activities involves the acquisition of 'oral tolerance' or the ability to tolerate and NOT react or be allergic to normal antigens.

Role for Escherichia coli

Interestingly, gram-negative bacteria like *Escherichia coli* and other related species (known as enterobacteria) possess lipopolysaccharides as components of their cell membranes. Lipopolysaccharides are known to increase the capacity of oral tolerance. In modernized countries, gastrointestinal colonization with enterobacteria occurs later than in infants born in developing countries (Wold et al., 1998).

> For example, 25% of Swedish infants don't acquire any enterobacteria during the first week of life, compared to developing countries where enterobacteria are established in infant's intestines by the third day of life. Additionally, only one strain of *Escherichia coli* is found as part of gut flora in children living in Western cultures, while in developing countries, by six months of age, infants are colonized by several different *Escherichia coli* strains (Wold et al., 1998).

By the time Western infants are finally colonized by *Escherichia coli* and other enterobacteria, the gut flora has already become established with other bacterial species. As a result, enterobacteria are unable to reach the high numbers that they would have achieved in the absence of competition. Lower than optimal enterobacteria numbers in the gastrointestinal tract hamper the influence of these bacteria over the developing immune system and impair acquisition of oral tolerance (Wold et al., 1998).

Role for lactobacilli

Using experimental animals, it has been found that lactobacilli can change the patterns of cytokine secretion and inhibit IgE allergic responses also.

> For example, *Lactobacillus casei*, has long been known to enhance production of IFN-γ. A recent study demonstrated that even heat-killed *Lactobacillus casei* increases IFN-γ and IL-12 production in experimental mice, while simultaneously inhibiting secretion of the pro-allergic IL-4 and IL-5 cytokines. IL-12 is well known to enhance the immune system, prevent allergic diseases, facilitate anti-tumor actions, and potentiate host resistance to infections (Shida et al., 1998). IL-12 causes Th1 cells to produce IFN-γ. IFN-γ inhibits Th2 allergic responses. Additionally, IL-12 suppresses production of allergic IgE antibodies. All together, *Lactobacillus casei* acts in several different ways to prevent allergic responses.
>
> Another experimental study investigated the immune-modulating activity of *Lactobacillus plantarum* L-137 in a mouse model of food allergy. In these studies, heat-killed *Lactobacillus plantarum* stimulated IL-12 and suppressed allergic IgE antibodies (Murosaki et al., 1998). Again, this study illustrates the value of using probiotics as therapeutic tools for controlling allergic diseases.
>
> *Lactobacillus plantarum* may be particularly beneficial for treating allergic disorders because this *Lactobacillus* suppresses IL-5, a pro-allergic cytokine, in mice genetically engineered to be allergic to dust mites (Kruisselbrink et al., 2001).
>
> Perhaps the most interesting finding of recent studies is that a closely related lactobacilli strain, *Lactobacillus johnsonii*, does not have the same immune modulating effects as *Lactobacillus casei* (Shida et al., 1998) or *Lactobacillus plantarum*.

Results from this last study make it clear that probiotics are not all created equally. While some lactic acid bacteria curb hypersensitive allergic reactions, other probiotic strains do not have the same effects. However, at least some strains of lactobacilli stimulate secretion of cytokines that down regulate activities of Th-2 allergic cytokines. Thus, gut flora probably plays a big part in determining allergic responsiveness.

As we've already discussed, the hygiene hypothesis of allergies says that reduced microbial stimulation of the gut during infancy and early childhood slows immune system maturation and delays the necessary balance between Th1- and Th2- immunity — shifting it in favor of allergic responses. While we call it a "hypothesis" or "educated guess" the truth is, we clearly observe this phenomenon occurring in germ-free newborn rodents. In germ-free animals, there is, by definition, no bacteria in their guts. These animals tend to be hyper-allergic and in these animals, there is no shift away from Th-2 allergic responses. As a result, oral tolerance to normal antigens is delayed. However, oral tolerance, *can be restored* in these animals *by introducing normal gut flora at the neonatal stage of life* (Sudo et al., 1997), but not at any later developmental stage. If normal gut flora is introduced to these animals later in life, the necessary Th2-to-Th1 immune shift does not occur and oral tolerance to normal antigens can not be restored. Thus, gut bacterial flora is absolutely necessary for oral tolerance in experimental animal models. So far, it looks like intestinal normal flora can also affect development and priming of the human immune system early in childhood, similar to what is seen in rodents.

Of course, we don't rear our children under germ-free conditions, so we can't exactly extrapolate the rodent data to human data. Instead, investigators studied newborns that were prone to developing allergies — by virtue of the fact that their parents or siblings had a history of allergic diseases. Once a suitable group of pregnant women was identified, normal gut flora was supplemented with *Lactobacillus rhamnosus* strain GG for four weeks prior to birth and continued post-natally in the mother or infant for 6 months. You know what? Just like in the rodent study described above, this study also found that by introducing healthy gut flora in human newborns, oral tolerance was restored and children had fewer allergies. Participants in this study have now been followed for four years. Results indicate that 14 of 53 children that received the probiotic have developed eczema compared with 25 of 54 children who received placebo. There is nearly a 50% reduction in the incidence of eczema in children who were given probiotics for the first six months of life. These results indicate that this strain of lactobacillus prevents eczema beyond infancy and into early childhood (Kalliomaki et al., 2001; Kalliomaki et al., 2003).

The Role of "Leaky Guts" in Allergies

Lots of things can make the gut "leaky" including bacteria, foods, and cytokines. When infants acquire unhealthy gut bacteria flora, not only are they at risk of developing allergies due to deprivation of Th-1-mediated-counterregulatory signals against Th2-mediated allergic responses, but they are also at risk for allergies due to increased gut "leakiness".

Under normal conditions, most bacteria living in the gastrointestinal tract don't ever come into direct contact with intestinal epithelial cells. Mucus, peristalsis, IgA antibodies — all of these mechanisms — prevent bacteria from binding to epithelial cells and protect from disease-causing bacterial invasion. However, some drugs that suppress the immune system, like steroids, can significantly disrupt these protective mechanisms. Dexamethasone, a commonly prescribed steroid, reduces IgA secretions and increases gastrointestinal permeability. Both of these actions result in increased bacterial adherence to the intestine and allow migration of gut bacteria out of the intestine into other body tissues (Spitz et al., 1994).

When bacteria bind to the intestinal wall, gut permeability increases since inflammatory cytokines are released. The inflammatory cytokine IFN-γ is also known to disrupt the normally "tight" junctions between epithelial cells — thus increasing gut permeability and making it extra "leaky". Gut permeability can also be increased by bacteria that release their own inflammatory toxins. Inflammatory cytokines or inflammatory toxins increase intestinal permeability by disrupting the normally tight junctions between intestinal epithelial cells. In infancy, *Escherichia coli*, *Vibrio cholerae*, *Bacteroides*, and *Clostridium* can all cause gut leakiness (Kirjavainen et al., 2002; Boedeker, 1994), and these bacteria may increase the likelihood of allergies. In fact, as discussed above, numerous studies in children have found an association between gut clostridia and allergies.

Food allergens such as proteins in cow's milk or egg whites, also cause gut inflammation in sensitive individuals. Once sensitized to the allergen, the intestines respond by releasing more inflammatory mediators, causing even more intestinal "leakiness" (Pelto et al., 1998), thereby perpetuating the allergic response.

Regardless of the initial cause of gut leakiness, increased permeability in the gut causes two main problems. First, when the gut is leaky, large, potentially allergic food antigens can be absorbed, which means antigens leave the gut and enter the blood stream. When large food proteins are encountered in the blood stream, the immune system mounts a vigorous defense against what it perceives to be a "foreign invader" and the result is severe, even life-threatening food allergies (See figure 7-2). Second, diarrhea can be an obvious manifestation of allergic responses in the gut (Heyman and Desjeux, 2000).

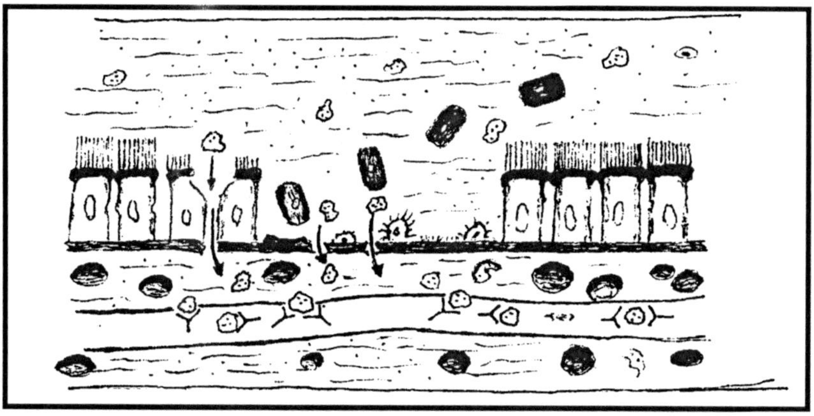

Figure 7-2. When the gut is "leaky", large proteins penetrate easily through epithelial cells and enter the blood stream. Once large proteins are in blood vessels, the immune system reacts vigorously by attacking with IgE antibodies (depicted by "Y"). This is what causes food allergies to occur.

While on the subject of "leaky" guts, it is necessary to mention that the mucosal barrier is never an absolute barrier. Selective uptake of nutrients and ions is always permitted, but substances larger than a few microns in size should be excluded from being absorbed — that is to say, under normal conditions, only very small particles should leave the gastrointestinal tract and enter the blood stream. Also, it is important to point out that while we've only considered a handful of things that influence mucosal structure and function, there are many factors that influence gut leakiness including: malnutrition, rotaviral infections, bacterial toxins, immunosuppressive drugs, and chronic exposure to dietary antigens early in life. Any one of these things can increase the gut's permeability, cause harmful antigens to be absorbed, impair immune responses, and lead toward a tendency to develop allergic diseases. Fortunately, as we will see, probiotics are remarkably able to regulate a dysregulated system.

> In experimental rats infected with rotavirus, there is dysfunction of the small intestine's epithelial barrier. This leads to increased permeability and increased absorption of antigens. However, when *Lactobacillus* GG is given to such rats, the probiotic counteracts dysfunction, decreases intestinal permeability, and stabilizes the gastrointestinal tract. This type of stabilizing effect demonstrates the important role played by intestinal bacteria in maintaining homeostasis (Isolauri et al., 1993).

Interestingly, it is *normal* for infants to have high gut permeability, immediately after birth. In experimental mice, *gut closure*, in which intestinal permeability decreases to the adult level, occurs at 21 days of age. The precise timing of gut maturation has not been determined in humans. However, it is clear that there is a period of intestinal permeability in infancy, during which time, immune defenses are still too immature to handle "adult foods." Exposing infants to dietary antigens too early in life often ends in severe food allergies.

It is also apparent that chronic exposure to dietary antigens early in life (for example, cow's milk or eggs) can delay gut closure, increasing the likelihood of food allergies (Arvola et al., 1992; 1993). For this reason, it is often recommended to delay using cow's milk or cow's milk-derived formulas in infants at high risk for developing allergies. Yet, even when gastrointestinal permeability is increased by food antigens, probiotics like *Lactobacillus* GG can counteract these permeability disorders (Isolauri et al., 1993).

Remarkably, leaky gut situations can be successfully managed by using probiotic bacteria. Probiotics *improve digestion* of dietary antigens in the intestines to down-regulate the allergic response. Probiotics *alter secretion of cytokines* and other inflammatory mediators. Probiotics produce short chain fatty acids which *improve the function of the intestinal epithelium.* Additionally, some probiotic lactobacilli and bifidobacteria *enhance IgA antibody secretion* which strengthens the gut mucosal barrier. (Laiho et al., 2000).

Relationship Between Gut Bacteria and Allergies

Investigators have attempted to characterize the relationship between gut bacteria and allergies. One group of researchers found that infants with eczema were more likely to be colonized with *Escherichia coli* and *Bacteroides* species than infants without a history of allergies (Kirjavainen et al., 2002). Additionally, in this study, the amount of allergic IgE antibodies in the blood directly correlated with the numbers of *Escherichia coli*, making it tempting to speculate that *Escherichia coli* may evoke an inflammatory response in the gut, leading to increased gut permeability, and a greater likelihood of allergies. If so, it is interesting to note that, in a recent study, *Bifidobacterium lactis* — a probiotic — prohibited growth of *Bacteroides* and *Escherichia coli* during weaning (Kirjavainen et al., 2002) and may have favorable effects in infants prone to allergies.

Another group of investigators also attempted to determine if there was an association between bacterial species present in the gut and development of allergies later in life. To ascertain this, the major gut bacterial species present in 76 infants was determined periodically during the first year of life, while also following the development of allergies in these children. The most significant finding of these researchers was that at 3 weeks of age, infants who developed allergies had lower numbers of bifidobacteria and higher counts of clostridial species in their guts (Kalliomaki et al., 2001a). Distinct differences in gut bacteria preceded development of allergies, indicating a crucial role for gut flora in helping the immune system to mature into a non-allergic mode. Recent studies clearly indicate that when gut bacteria are disrupted, *allergies can only be prevented when the normal bacterial flora is replaced early in the neonatal period* (Sudo et al., 1997).

Role of Probiotics in Allergies

Lactobacilli

If, in fact, a disturbance in intestinal bacteria plays a role in allergies, it is important to understand which bacteria are the necessary "good guys". To date, the benefits of lactic-acid secreting bacteria have been the most widely studied. *Lactobacillus* GG has been shown to modify the immune system. This bacteria does so by (1) altering cytokine production, (2) stimulating phagocytosis, and (3) increasing activity of IgA antibody secretion (Pelto et al., 1998). Indeed, probiotics must stimulate the immune system nonspecifically to down-regulate allergic reactions.

Lactobacilli supplementation has received a great deal of attention in the management of allergic diseases. In a 1997 double-blind, placebo controlled study, *Lactobacillus* GG was given to 10 breast fed infants who had both eczema and milk allergies. During the month long study period, eczema improved dramatically in infants receiving probiotic supplementation. Also, the concentration of fecal TNF-α decreased substantially in the *Lactobacillus*-treated children. (TNF-α is sometimes used as a marker of inflammation.) Overwhelmingly, the results of this study indicated that *Lactobacillus* GG reduced intestinal inflammation *and* allergies. By preventing intestinal inflammation, the barrier function of the gut is enhanced, thereby down regulating food allergy and accompanying eczema reactions (Majamaa and Isolauri, 1997). Likewise, in another small pilot study, *Lactobacillus* GG supplements significantly reduced the severity of eczema in infants with allergies to cow's milk (Kirjavainen et al., 2003).

After the first reports that probiotics reduced the severity of eczema in infants, investigators turned their attention to *adults* with allergies to try to figure out just *how* probiotics might alter immune activities.

> In a double-blind, **cross-over** study using adults with milk allergies, researchers found that milk-allergic adults experienced an increase in the activity of phagocytosis (increased expression of four different phagocytosis receptors) after drinking milk. Increased phagocytosis can cause inflammation. In the intestine, such inflammation was apparent as abdominal pain and diarrhea.
>
> These same individuals were then given probiotics. In milk-allergic folks, *Lactobacillus* GG *prevented* inflammation by down-regulating phagocytic activities (Pelto et al., 1998). Equally important, the probiotic reduced gastrointestinal discomfort. Thus, *Lactobacillus* GG normalized a gut that was previously damaged by increased intestinal permeability. Interestingly, in healthy folks who don't have allergies, *Lactobacillus* GG *stimulates* phagocytosis — thus, the same probiotic can have dual immune effects triggering different responses in healthy versus allergic individuals (Pelto et al., 1998).

How else might probiotic bacteria be anti-allergenic? In addition to altering phagocytosis, probiotic bacteria also aid in the digestion of milk proteins, breaking them into small particles that don't stimulate allergic responses (Apostolou et al., 2001). Alternatively, probiotic bacteria promote anti-allergenicity by altering IgA antibody and cytokine production.

In a small study, *Lactobacillus* GG-digested casein caused a shift in cytokine production in allergic individuals — a shift away from allergic IL-4 — indicating that intestinal bacteria degrade dietary antigens *and* modify their original allergenic properties (Sutas et al., 1996).

Modulation of another specific cytokine, may also play a substantial role in the ability of *Lactobacillus* GG to decrease allergic responses. *Lactobacillus* GG supplements were given for four weeks to children aged 7-42 months who had been previously diagnosed with eczema and food allergies. The probiotic supplement stimulated a transient increase in IL-10 levels in all individuals studied (Pessi et al., 2000). Why is this significant? IL-10 is important because it is a cytokine that "turns off" allergic pro-inflammatory components. Essentially, IL-10 prevents sensitivity reactions to substances that would otherwise be allergenic.

Some patients with allergic diseases like asthma are known to have deficiencies in IL-10 production. In these folks, probiotics may lessen allergy symptoms by blocking synthesis of the inflammatory and allergic chemical mediators responsible for their allergy symptoms (Pessi et al., 2000). Support for this comes from knowing that parasitic infections that stimulate IL-10 production provide protection against allergies (Das, 2002). In allergy settings, it is often desirable to increase levels of IL-10, in order to reduce inflammation. However, in those with allergies, it may be even more desirable to increase IL-12. Experimental studies in mice have found *Lactobacillus plantarum* — even when killed by heat prior to administration — stimulates production of IL-12. [Many gram-positive probiotic bacteria stimulate cytokine release from human immune cells even when the bacteria are dead. It is interesting to note that probiotic bacteria may not even need to be viable to mediate effects on the immune system, suggesting that certain components of their cell walls interact with gut-associated immune tissues in a way that mediates these beneficial actions (Cross et al., 2001).] In fact, at least three other strains of lactobacilli — *Lactobacillus lactis*, *Lactobacillus casei*, and *Lactobacillus* GG also stimulate production of IL-12 and IFN-γ (Pochard et al., 2002).

Indeed, most gram-positive bacteria stimulate high levels of IL-12, while gram-negative strains are not only poor inducers of IL-12 (Karlsson et al., 2002), but also may stimulate release of IL-10, which may suppress IL-12 from being secreted. Why is all of this significant? First, IL-12 directly suppresses production of the pro-allergic cytokine IL-4 and indirectly suppresses production of pro-allergic IgE allergic antibodies (See figure 7-3) (Murosaki et al., 1998). Additionally, IL-12 is known to be an important stimulus for Th-1 cells to produce IFN-γ (Cross, 2001). IFN-γ, in turn, plays its own role in directing the immune system *away* from pro-allergic activities. Thus, the bottom line is: IL-12 is a "good" cytokine when it comes to allergies! Any stimulus that increases release of IL-12 "programs" the immune system *away* from allergic tendencies!

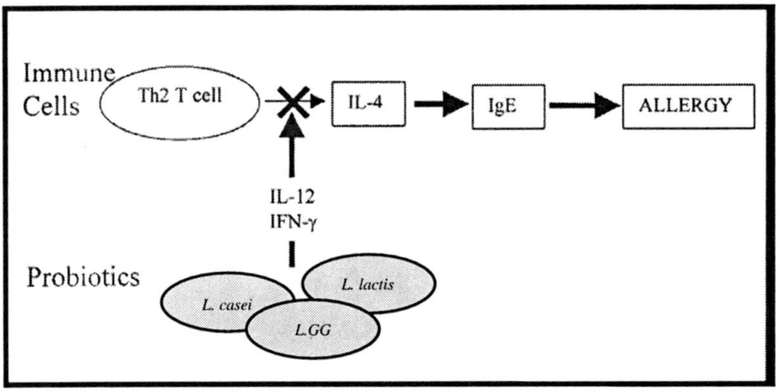

Figure 7-3. Probiotic bacteria like *Lactobacillus casei, Lactobacillus lactis*, and *Lactobacillus* GG stimulate release of IL-12 and IFN-γ, cytokines that inhibit allergic responses.

Certainly many strains of bacteria have been shown to modify the immune system, but not all of them direct the immune system *away* from allergies. In fact, some bacteria stimulate release of pro-inflammatory cytokines which cause other immunological difficulties. How can these seemingly opposite effects by similar strains of bacteria be explained? Well, the answer probably depends upon the *amounts* of specific cytokines that are stimulated. Therefore, different strains of probiotics regulate the immune system in different ways. There are strain-dependent differences in the ability of probiotics to stimulate immunoregulatory cytokines like IL-10 and IL-12. For example, it was recently demonstrated that *Lactobacillus paracasei* induced 4-7 times more IL-12 than IL-10, while *Lactobacillus rhamnosus* did just the opposite. *L. rhamnosus* stimulated 4-fold more IL-10. Therefore, not all probiotics will be effective at promoting anti-allergic responses. As we currently understand, the strains that are potent inducers of IL-12, like *Lactobacillus casei* and *Lactobacillus plantarum* are probably the lactobacilli with the best bets for down-regulating allergic responses (Cross et al., 2001).

What other cytokines might probiotics regulate in a beneficial manner? To answer this question, researchers assessed the effects of *Lactobacillus* GG on production of TGF-β. TGF-β is considered a key cytokine for promoting both IgA secretion and oral tolerance mechanisms (Das, 2002). In infancy, TGF-β production in the gut is not sufficient to protect against dietary antigens. However, there is a strong correlation between TGF-β concentrations in mother's breast milk and a newborn's ability to make specific IgA antibodies and avoid allergies (Rautava et al., 2002). In fact, for infants with a tendency toward developing allergic diseases, breast feeding is recommended as potentially beneficial, in part because of benefits provided by TGF-β. Investigators wanted to determine if *Lactobacillus* GG could stimulate production of TGF-β, and whether this would have beneficial effects on children at high risk for allergies.

> In a double-blind, placebo-controlled trial using 159 pregnant women with a family history of allergic diseases, half the women received *Lactobacillus* GG while the others took placebo pills. The women began using supplements four weeks before giving birth and continued the supplements while breast feeding until the infants were 3 months of age. In mothers who took the probiotic, TGF-β was significantly more concentrated in breast milk compared to mothers that took placebo.
>
> Some of the children born to the women who took part in this study were followed for two years. Maternal use of probiotics reduced the prevalence of eczema in these children. By the time the children were two years of age, only 15% of the infants born to mothers who received probiotics developed eczema, compared to 46% of children whose mothers were given placebo (Rautava et al., 2002).

This study is significant for two major reasons. First, it illustrates that maternal use of probiotics during pregnancy and lactation is a safe and effective way to prevent eczema in infants. Second, this study suggests that infants with allergic disease may have defective production of TGF-β, which could be improved by the use of probiotics (Rautava et al., 2002).

Bifidobacteria

Bifidobacteria have also been studied for their role in quelling allergies, since they are the predominant species found in the digestive tract of infants — reaching levels as high as 99% of total fecal flora within in the first week of life.

> One group of investigators specifically evaluated differences in bifidobacterial strains found in feces of healthy infants versus allergic infants. Several interesting things were observed. First, in allergic infants, *Bifidobacterium adolescentis* was the most common species found compared to *Bifidobacterium bifidum* which was the most prevalent species isolated from healthy infant specimens. This is important since the number of intestinal bifidobacteria have been found to be significantly decreased in a variety of medical conditions, including allergies (He et al., 2001).
>
> Second, since gut bacteria stimulate and modify the immune system, adhesive properties of the isolated bifidobacterial strains were compared. Adhesion of fecal bifidobacteria to human mucus was significantly greater in the bifidobacterial species identified from healthy infants than from allergic infants. This suggests that it may not be enough just to be colonized with the right species. Rather, to exert positive influences on the immune system, the bacteria must possess a critical level of adhesive properties in order to "normalize" the immune system.
>
> To study this further, two common probiotic strains, *Lactobacillus* GG and *Bifidobacterium lactis* were included in this study for comparison to the bifidobacteria identified in the infants' stools. Remarkably, the common probiotics had even greater adhesive abilities than the bifidobacterial species isolated from human specimens. These results illustrate that these commercially available probiotics possess some of the properties necessary to modify an "imbalanced" immune system.

Since lactobacilli and bifidobacteria have both been shown to play important roles in modifying the immune system, it is no surprise that two strains from these genera were combined head-to-head for anti-allergic effects. In a double-blind, placebo controlled clinical trial, infants with eczema were given supplements of either *Lactobacillus* GG, *Bifidobacterium lactis,* or placebo for two months. After two months, the infants receiving either strain of probiotic experienced a significant improvement – and, in many cases, complete clearing — of eczema. Consistent with the resolution of eczema, markers of inflammation and allergies in the blood and urine were also substantially educed in infants that received probiotic supplements (Isolauri et al., 2000).

Most of the clinical trials have involved children. However, probiotics can be just as effective in resolving eczema in adults. Take a look at the following story of one woman from California.

> N.N. spent much of her life battling eczema. She was covered from head to toe; 98% of her body was affected. In public, parents pulled their staring children away from her because of her appearance.
>
> N.N. had seen specialists for advice, but standard medical treatments were not working. She was at the point where the only thing conventional medicine could offer her was skin grafting. Figuring she had nothing to lose by "trying" one more thing, N.N. began taking three strains of probiotics three times a day: *Bifidobacterium bifidum*, *Lactobacillus acidophilus* NAS strain, and *Lactobacillus bulgaricus.*
>
> Within 48 hours of initiating probiotic therapy, N.N.'s skin was 50% clear of eczema. After using the probiotics for 7 days, her eczema had completely resolved. After only one week, the only evidence of her long struggle with eczema were the scars caused by years of scratching. N.N. has continued taking the probiotics and has done well ever since.

So, we've seen that probiotics can successfully *treat* allergic diseases, probably by modifying immune responses. But, can we actually *prevent* allergies in the first place? That is the avenue some researchers are exploring.

> In another recent double-blind, randomized, placebo-controlled clinical trial, *Lactobacillus* GG or placebo was given to pregnant women for two to four weeks before giving birth.

> After delivery, probiotic supplements were either continued by breast-feeding moms or given directly to the infants for six more months. All the women included in the study were chosen because they had a family history of allergic diseases such as eczema, hayfever, or asthma. Children born to these women were evaluated for eczema at ages 3,6,12,18, 24 and 48 months. *At both two and four years of age , the frequency of eczema was reduced by approximately 50% in infants given probiotics* versus those who received placebo (Kalliomaki et al., 2001b; Kalliomaki et al., 2003)!

This result (and other similar results, see Rautava et al., 2002 also) is astounding because it demonstrates that probiotics can actually *prevent* allergies! In this study, *Lactobacillus* GG correctly "programmed" immune systems that otherwise would have been prone to err on the side of being hypersensitive. Certainly, all the mechanisms that we've talked about may be responsible for this: probiotics (1) enhance gut-specific IgA responses which are often defective in children with food allergies, (2) enhance gut barrier functions by restoring normal gut flora, (3) modify impaired intestinal permeability, and (3) stimulate cytokines production, shifting the balance away from Th2 hypersensitivity.

Inhaled Allergies, Asthma, Food Allergies, Anaphylaxis

So far in this chapter, we've spent a great deal of time talking about how probiotics are beneficial in treating and preventing eczema in children. Now, we are going to consider data for using probiotics as treatment tools in management of other allergic conditions. Admittedly not much is known, and in some cases there isn't much support at all for using probiotics, but these are areas under active investigation. Results of ongoing studies are expected to be published in the near future.

One of the first studies in this area examined whether or not long-term yogurt consumption had any health benefits on young versus old adults. Study participants were followed for a year. At the end of the study, it was apparent that those who had consumed yogurt for a year had fewer allergy symptoms, less itching, and showed a trend toward decreased gastrointestinal upset, fewer colds, less coughing, and a reduction in wheezing. Specifically, elderly adults who had eaten yogurt daily for a year, had significantly fewer allergic IgE antibodies in their blood stream (Van de Water et al., 1999). Since many researchers are currently spending great amounts of time and money designing experimental drugs that lower allergic IgE antibodies, it would be great if something as simple and benign as daily yogurt were the answer for which they've been searching.

Allergic rhinitis

The prevalence of allergic rhinitis is increasing in the United States and around the world, affecting 40% of children younger than 6 years of age and 20% of adults. Symptoms include nasal congestion, runny nose, itchy eyes, sneezing, and fatigue. To my knowledge, there is only one study so far that has evaluated the effects of probiotics in patients with allergies, specifically birch pollen allergies.

> In a small, double-blind, placebo-controlled study, 38 adult patients consumed *Lactobacillus* GG or placebo for almost 6 months. In this study, *Lactobacillus* GG did not improve allergy symptoms to birch pollen any more than placebo did (Helin et al., 2002).

It could be argued that the treatment period was too short to see any benefits of the probiotic. It is possible also that *Lactobacillus* GG may take longer than 6 months to alter immune responses, or that another probiotic strain might prove more effective for treating this allergic condition. Additionally, you may recall that in animal models of allergy, probiotics are only effective at inducing oral tolerance during neonatal stages of immune development (Sudo et al., 1997). As a result, it is entirely possible that beneficial probiotic effects will be evident in humans *only* during infancy and, as such, probiotics may not be beneficial in treating allergies later in life.

On the other hand, it is reported, that regular dietary consumption of yogurt containing other strains of bacteria, namely *Lactobacillus bulgaricus* and *Streptococcus thermophilus,* improves eczema in individuals with allergic rhinitis. Data from experimental mice suggest that this may be due to the bacteria's ability to break down and degrade foods into smaller, less allergenic fragments. In a clinical trial that examined the effects of *Lactobacillus* on allergy symptoms, there were no significant improvements noted in clinical symptoms. However, after a year of eating yogurt supplemented with *Lactobacillus acidophilus*, there was a trend toward improved IFN-γ levels, indicating the therapy may have just been beginning to alter the immune system (Wheeler et al., 1997).

Asthma

Asthma is a chronic airway disorder characterized by inflammation, varying degrees of airway obstruction, and airway hyperresponsiveness. Patients with asthma may suffer from chronic coughing, wheezing, or shortness of breath. More than 15 million Americans including 5 million children suffer from asthma. In fact, asthma is the most common disease in children and is a leading cause of disability.

Recently, a double-blind crossover study examined the effects of yogurt containing *Lactobacillus acidophilus* in 15 adult asthmatic patients over two 1-month periods. Although no benefits were found in pulmonary function parameters during this short trial, there were trends in immune parameters which indicated a shift *away* from allergic responsiveness with probiotic-supplemented yogurt (Wheeler et al., 1997). While it is entirely likely that probiotics may not have beneficial results in asthma, other explanations for lack of effects in this study are likely. For example, it probably takes longer than one month for effects on the immune system and on the respiratory system to be observed. Additionally, perhaps the dosage of the probiotic used in this study was too low for immunomodulation to occur in the lungs, or perhaps another probiotic strain would have greater effects.

Dietary interventions for asthma?

While most published literature on asthma deals with *reducing symptoms* and *eliminating the frequency of attacks*, there is increasing interest in *preventing* asthma from occurring in the first place in children that are genetically "at risk" because of allergic disorders in close family members. While it would be great if probiotics were the answer to *preventing* asthma, the studies that address this question are still ongoing and have not yet been conducted for a sufficient period of time for a final assessment of the data (Kalliomaki et al., 2003). A question researchers have begun exploring is, can we prevent asthma with dietary manipulation?

Truth be told, the answer to that question isn't clear. In lieu of being able to tackle this question with data about probiotics, here's what we do know about diet, immunomodulation, and asthma based upon published literature. We know that exclusive breast feeding for a minimum of 3 months results in a 30% overall reduction in those who go on to develop childhood asthma — and this increases to a 50% reduction in children with a family history of allergic disorders. So breastfeeding offers valid and important protection against asthma (Mellis, 2002). These protective effects are probably attributed, at least in part, to immunomodulatory components of breast milk.

Anyone who has ever seen human breast milk probably will recall its high fat content. Breast milk is rich in long chain polyunsaturated fatty acids (LCPUFAs). LCPUFAs enhance Th1 responses and suppress Th-2 immune activities — both of which favor anti-allergenicity. Additionally, some LCPUFAs have antimicrobial effects and anti-inflammatory actions and enhance adhesive actions of lactobacilli. Thus, LCPUFAs found in human breast milk coupled with probiotics have activities that actually potentiate each other to ensure appropriate development of gut-associated lymph tissues to maintain an appropriate balance between Th-1 and Th-2 responses (Das, 2002).

Other dietary interventions that may have merit in preventing asthma involve eliminating certain allergenic foods (peanuts, cow's milk, eggs, soy) from mothers' diets while breast feeding and avoiding these foods completely in children less than one year of age (Mellis, 2002). However, on the other hand, some will argue that elimination diets don't *prevent* the allergic response, but rather these diets just *delay* the inevitable (Laiho et al., 2000).

Additionally, some studies have also found that soy-based formulas have less of a tendency to promote allergies than cow's milk-based supplements, once breast feeding stops (Mellis, 2002). Recently, some data also indicated allergic diseases are more common in infants whose mothers have a low dietary intake of saturated fatty acids while breastfeeding, or that young people who have a low vitamin C intake are at a greater risk of developing asthma (Laiho et al., 2000).

There are also ongoing clinical trials evaluating dietary supplements with specific antioxidants or fatty acids, like omega-3 fatty acids, for asthma interventions (Mellis, 2002; Laiho et al., 2000). Western diets tend to have high levels of n-6 fatty acids, obtained from meat and vegetable oil, but are low in n-3 fatty acids obtained from nuts, seeds, legumes, and fish. This fatty acid profile — high n-6 and low n-3 fatty acids — promotes IgE production, setting the stage for allergies and inflammation. Recently, two studies found that eating high levels of fatty fish improved lung function in both adult smokers and children (Jaber, 2002). On the other hand, an Australian study found than high levels of omega-6 polyunsaturated fatty acid significantly increased the risk of developing asthma (Jaber, 2002). Additionally, in the International Study of Asthma and Allergies in Childhood there was a clear correlation between intake of trans-fatty acids (found in margarine, hydrogenated vegetable oils in crackers, breads, cakes, and chips) and the prevalence of asthma, hayfever, and eczema. Although at this point, there are no official recommendations that people with asthma take fish oil or other n-3 fatty acid supplements to improve asthma symptoms, there is also no evidence of risks or adverse effects from doing so. Only time will tell whether there is merit to these dietary interventions.

At this point, I would be completely remiss if I didn't share with you a dietary change that our family made which completely eliminated asthma in my son and my husband. My son was diagnosed with asthma at 11 months of age and my husband has had asthma since he was two years old. I share this anecdotal scenario with you because it falls under the "can't hurt, might help" category, but please remember, no clinical trials have been done to validate what I am about to share with you. The closest thing to a scientific study to back up what I am about to tell you is the study referred to at the beginning of this chapter describing the anthroposophic lifestyles (Alm et al., 1999).

When my son was 28 months old, he was diagnosed with chronic, persistent *C. difficile* diarrhea. Five months after his diagnosis, we learned that the reason he couldn't get rid of this infection was because of inappropriate oral tolerance. His immune system had failed to learn that *C. difficile* and its toxins should be seen as "foreign", hence he did not make any antibodies against the microorganism or its toxins. In a manner of speaking, he had a specific, focal immune deficiency.

Of course, once this immune deficit was identified by the doctors, it sparked a battery of other immunological tests. While awaiting all test results, my husband and I decided that if our son suffered from an immune deficiency, we would do everything we possibly could do to boost his immune system. Mostly what we decided to do was change our diet. We didn't alter the types of foods we ate. We still ate the same meals and cooked from the same recipes, but we purchased only organic, natural ingredients. We made it a point to buy organic fruits, vegetables, beef, and poultry. Any product that we couldn't find organically was at least free of added colors, artificial flavors, and preservatives.

The most amazing thing happened! No, the diet didn't cure the *C. difficile* infection (which is what we were hoping for). Rather, within three weeks on the new diet, both my son and my husband were free of asthma! As I write this, it has been over one year since our dietary change and *it has been over one year since my son had a single asthmatic cough or wheeze* — this is a child who had been on *daily* maintenance medication for asthma during the previous 2 years! Some might say that he simply "grew out of it", which I might be tempted to believe if it weren't for the fact that my 38-year old husband also "grew out of it" at the same time! Clearly, there was some ingredient(s) — maybe a preservative in the processed foods we were eating or a pesticide residue on our vegetables — that my son and husband were allergic to. When that ingredient was removed from their diets, whatever the ingredient was, no more asthma...!

Like I said earlier, eating organic foods to prevent or treat asthma isn't scientifically proven. In fact, to my knowledge, the closest that clinical trials have come to evaluating this is the study published by Alm et al. (1999) in which it was demonstrated that children who eat organically have significantly fewer allergic illnesses than other children. However, if you are willing to shop differently for a finite period of time — give yourself 3 months of eating exclusively organically — maybe you'll be pleasantly surprised with the outcome! And if it works, please write and let me know!

Food Allergies and Anaphylaxis

Unfortunately, I haven't seen any literature describing whether probiotics have any benefits in human beings with food allergy anaphylaxis. **Anaphylaxis** is a life-threatening allergic reaction where airways in the lungs swell and close, making breathing impossible. Additionally, the heart can fail and death may occur. This is the type of reactions some people have to bee stings and peanuts. We found out — the hard way — in our family that some children (like my son) — develop anaphylactic food allergies to eggs.

This is another area that is just beginning to be explored and research is still in the "experimental animal" stage. However, animal studies do look promising for probiotics. A specific type of lactobacillus, *Lactobacillus casei* strain Shirota (LcS), is widely used in fermented milk products. This strain is known to suppress IgE — the antibodies that produce allergic and anaphylactic responses. LcS stimulates release of IL-12 from macrophages, which shifts cytokine production away from Th2-type and towards Th1-type responses.

Through genetic engineering, scientists have developed mice that experience anaphylaxis when exposed to eggs, just like people with allergies do. Excitingly, in these experimental mice, *Lactobacillus casei* Shirota strain prevents anaphylaxis when the mice are fed egg whites (Shida et al., 2002)!

Allergies and the Pancreas

For just a moment, let's take a break from talking purely about probiotics in allergic diseases, and consider the role of the pancreas. To be perfectly frank, the idea of allergic illness arising from pancreatic insufficiency is a rather new area that is only just beginning to be explored. Very few papers have been published on the subject. In addition to describing what has been published, I am also going to share the experiences of a friend, Dr. Michael McCann, a retired pediatric allergist and clinical immunologist who formerly practiced in the Cleveland, Ohio, area. Dr. McCann is a firm believer that pancreatic enzyme supplements and probiotics can work hand-in-hand to treat allergies. Dr. McCann has helped many individuals with severe food allergies lead a normal life again and his findings have been presented at several conferences (McCann, 1999; 2000).

As you may recall from chapter 1, the pancreas secretes enzymes that aid in food digestion. Physicians have noted that individuals with food allergies often experience relief from diarrhea, abdominal pain, gas, and bloating when they take pancreatic enzyme supplements. Likewise, patients with deficient pancreatic function experience adverse food reactions when they eat fatty foods, meats, or milk products. If the pancreas doesn't produce enough enzymes, foods won't be degraded as completely as they should be. As we've already discussed, when large food proteins are absorbed into the blood stream, the immune system responds to these "large" foreign invaders as if they are harmful by mounting an allergic response against them. Thus, insufficient secretion of pancreatic enzymes may contribute to the development of food allergies. It is important to note that pancreatic activity is deficient in children, especially low birth weight infants. Since there is an association between large amounts of undigested proteins and food allergies

(McNeish, 1984), could pancreatic enzymes be a new type of anti-allergy drug? This is what new studies are trying to figure out.

> A small double-blind placebo-controlled trial was undertaken in 10 individuals with confirmed food allergies. When pancreatic enzyme supplements were given along with foods to which these individuals were sensitive, there was a marked reduction in adverse symptoms and significantly less allergic inflammation in all 10 patients. This study, published in 2002, clearly demonstrates that pancreatic enzymes may have a beneficial effect, reducing intestinal allergic inflammation (Raithel et al., 2002).

Thanks to the generosity of Dr. McCann, I can also share with you some of his experiences during the past two decades using pancreatic enzymes to treat food allergic patients. Dr. McCann, knowing that I was diligently working on getting all of this information compiled, has graciously given me access to some of his own data concerning the use of pancreatic enzymes to treat allergic patients.

Since 1990, Dr. McCann has had more than 65 patients referred to him by other physicians who were unable to help these individuals. These patients all had severe allergies, including a lifetime of entire body eczema, asthma, food allergies, allergic rhinitis, anaphylaxis, and gastrointestinal symptoms of diarrhea or abdominal pain. In some cases, allergy skin testing revealed allergies to almost every food that was eaten. In addition to common food allergies like milk, eggs, wheat, or soy, some of these individuals had allergies to foods like corn, beans, rice, pork, bananas, potatoes, and peas. For many of these individuals, Dr. McCann simply recommended pancreatic enzymes and probiotics. Pancreatic enzymes can be obtained from a pharmacy with a prescription. Additionally, some health food stores may sell plant-derived pancreatic supplements. In Dr. McCann's studies, his patients enjoyed dramatic improvements in their health. Some patients saw their eczema and asthma completely resolve. Many were able to discontinue all other drug therapies, including antihistamines and steroids.

Overall, Dr. McCann found that for patients with multiple food allergies, it is sometimes impractical or impossible to avoid *all* the foods to which one is allergic. In this particular group of patients, pancreatic enzyme supplements may be the answer. Pancreatic supplements help to digest foods, eliminating their pro-allergenic properties. Pancreatic supplements were effective not only in preventing symptoms of allergy, but more importantly, in alleviating physical signs of allergy like asthma, gastrointestinal discomfort (including diarrhea), hives, anaphylactic-type reactions, and chronic eczema. Here are the stories of a few of his patients.

> J.M. was a 61 year old man who had suffered from total body eczema since he was a teenager. In attempt to control his allergies, he used high doses of steroids, antihistamines, and biweekly allergy shots.
>
> His skin was so severely covered in eczema that skin testing had to be performed on his buttocks. Skin testing revealed that he was allergic to 43 of 59 foods including carrots, peas, tomatoes, eggs, peanuts, milk, and cabbage. After eliminating from his diet 13 foods to which he was most allergic, J.M. began taking pancreas enzyme supplements with every meal and each snack.
>
> Over the next 3 months, his skin cleared up, but he suffered relapses. When *Lactobacillus acidophilus* DDS-1 strain was added to J.M.'s diet, the eczema cleared completely and did not recur for 3 years. Although he experienced a relapse, J.M.'s skin again cleared up with the combination of pancreas enzymes and probiotics and he enjoyed complete remission from symptoms and was able to stop all asthma/eczema/allergy medications for the next 5 years.
>
> Use of probiotics also reduced objective signs of allergy in J.M. While using probiotics, levels of allergic IgE antibodies decreased.

> A.K. was an 18 month old girl that suffered repeated episodes of severe asthma. Her mother also noticed hives and diarrhea in response to certain foods, especially peanuts. Skin testing confirmed a severe peanut allergy and also identified significant allergies to eggs, potatoes, beans, and peas. The patient recovered completely on a diet free of peanuts and eggs, *Lactobacillus acidophilus*, and pancreas enzymes.
>
> During the next five years, the child had no further episodes of asthma, hives, or diarrhea. She ate a regular diet, but avoided peanuts. Although she continued to take probiotics regularly, pancreatic supplements were given only when she ate eggs.

These cases illustrate that pancreas enzymes can degrade most food proteins in the stomach, rendering them less antigenic, before they reach the small intestines. However, pancreas enzymes don't address the underlying problem — that of a leaky gut. Gut leakiness is probably most often caused by an imbalance of gut normal flora and can be corrected by replacing disturbed gastrointestinal flora with probiotics.

While using pancreas enzyme supplements for allergies may sound like a new idea, as long ago as the 1930s it was reported that food allergic patients were deficient in pancreatic enzymes. Most importantly, several physicians independently found pancreatic enzyme replacement corrected allergic deficiencies — in particular, corrected food allergies — in more than 90% of allergic patients (roughly 380 allergic individuals were studied all together) (Oelgoetz et al., 1936). This initial discovery was published approximately 70 years ago. With these kinds of positive results, it is mind-boggling that no further studies have been published in this area for almost a century!

While pancreatic enzymes were effective in clearing up eczema in many of Dr. McCann's patients, a few individuals experienced regular relapses. Interestingly, when probiotics were added to their diets, the eczema cleared permanently. It seems that pancreas supplements plus probiotics work synergistically. Both pancreatic enzymes and probiotic bacteria may break down proteins to small sizes that are less allergenic. Additionally, we know that probiotics also modify the immune system in various ways to "program" it in a less allergenic fashion. Consistent with this approach, Dr. McCann's current working theory is that pancreas enzymes can be useful as initial treatments for folks that have multiple food allergies but it is probiotics that correct the underlying "leaky gut" problem and help these folks remain in remission.

Conclusion

Allergic illnesses, especially eczema and food allergies, are reflected by increased production of Th-2 allergic cytokines, and allergies arise when gut permeability is increased. Probiotic bacteria, can counteract allergic tendencies. Certain strains of lactobacilli and bifidobacteria have dramatic immunomodulatory actions in the immune system and, as such, these probiotics may be quite beneficial in restoring normalcy to a dysregulated gut and hyperactive immune system.

Notes

Notes

References

Alm JS, Swartz J, Lilja G, et al. Atopy in children of families with an anthroposophic lifestyle. Lancet. 1999;353:1485-1488.

Apostolou E, Pelto L, Kirjavainen PV, et al. Differences in the gut bacterial flora of healthy and milk-hypersensitive adults, as measured by fluorescence in situ hybridization. FEMS Immunol Med Microbiol. 2001;30:217-221.

Arvola R, Isolauri E, Rantal I, et al. Increased *in vitro* intestinal permeability in suckling rats exposed to cow milk during lactation. J Ped Gastroenterol Nutr. 1993;16:294-300.

Arvola T, Rantala I, Marttinen A, et al. Early dietary antigens delay the development of gut mucosal barrier in preweaning rats. Ped Res. 1992;32:301-305.

Bjorksten B, Naaber O, Sepp E, et al. The intestinal microflora in allergic Estonian and Swedish 2-year-old children. Clin Exp Allergy. 1999;29:342-346.

Bjorksten B, Sepp E, Julge K, et al. Allergy development and the intestinal microflora during the first year of life. J Allergy Clin Immunol. 2001:108:516-520.

Boedeker, EC. Adherent Bacteria: Breaching the mucosal barrier? Gastroenterol. 1994;106:255-257.

Cross ML, Stevenson LM, and Gill HS. Anti-allergy properties of fermented foods: an important immunoregulatory mechanism of lactic acid bacteria? Int Immunopharmacol 2001;1:891-901.

Das UN. Essential fatty acids as possible enhancers of the beneficial actions of probiotics. Nutrition. 2002;18:786-789.

Dunne C, Murphy L, Flynn S, et al. Probiotics: From myth to reality. Demonstration of functionality in animal models of disease and in human clinical trials. Antonie van Leeuwenhoek. 1999;76:279-292.

He F, Ouwehand AC, Isolauri E, et al. Comparison of mucosal adhesion and species identification of bifidobacteria isolated from healthy and allergic infants. FEMA Immunol Med Microbiol. 2001;30:43-47.

Helin T, Haahtela S, and Haahtela T. No effect of oral treatment with an intestinal bacterial strain, *Lactobacillus rhamnosus* (ATCC 53103), on birch-pollen allergy: A placebo-controlled double-blind study. Allergy. 2002.57:243-246.

Heyman M and Dexjeux JF. Cytokine-induced alteration of the epithelial barrier to food antigens in disease. Annal New York Acad Sci. 2000;915:304-311.

Isolarui E, Arvola T, Sutas Y, et al. Probiotics in the management of atopic eczema. Clin Exp Allergy. 2000;30:1604-1610.

Isolauri E, Kaila M, Arvola T, et al. Diet during rotavirus enteritis affects jejunal permeability to macromolecules in suckling rats. Ped Res. 1993;33:548-553.

Isolauri E, Majamaa H, Arvola T, et al. *Lactobacillus casei* strain GG reverses increased intestinal permeability induced by cow milk in suckling rats. Gastroenterol. 1993;105:1643-1650.

Jaber R. Respiratory and allergic disease: From upper respiratory tract infections to asthma. Prim Care Clin Office Pract. Prim Care. 2002;29:231-261.

Karlsson H, Hessle C, and Rudin A. Innate immune responses of human neonatal cells to bacteria from the normal gastrointestinal flora. Infect Immunity. 2002;70:6688-6696.

Kalliomaki M, Kirjavainen P, Eerola E, et al. Distinct patterns of neonatal gut microflora in infants in whom atopy was and was not developing. J Allergy Clin Immunol. 2001a;102:129-134.

Kalliomaki M, Salminen S, Arvilommi H, et al. Probiotics in primary prevention of atopic disease: A randomised placebo-controlled trial. Lancet. 2001b;357:1076-1079.

Kalliomaki M, Salminen S, Poussa T, et al. Probiotics and prevention of atopic disease: 4-year follow-up of a randomised placebo-controlled trial. Lancet. 2003;361:1869-1871.

Kirjavainen PV, Apostolou E, Arvola T, et al. Characterizing the composition of intestinal microflora as a prospective treatment target in infant allergic disease. FEMS Immunol Med Microbiol. 2001;32:1-7.

Kirjavainen PV, Arvola T, and Salminen SJ. Aberrant composition of gut microbiota of allergic infants: A target of bifidobacterial therapy at weaning? Gut. 2002;51:51-55.

Kirjavainen PV, Salminen SJ, Isolauri E, et al. Probiotic Bacteria in the Management of Atopic Disease: Underscoring the importance of viability. J Ped Gastrenterol Nutr. 2003;36:223-227.

Kruisselbrink A, Heijne Den Bak-Glashouwer M-J, Havenith CEG, et al. Recombinant *Lactobacillus plantarum* inhibits house dust mite-specific T-cell responses. Clin Exp Immunol. 2001;126:2-8.

Laiho K, Ouwehand A, Salminen S, et al. Inventing probiotic functional foods for patients with allergic disease. Ann Allergy Asthma Immunol. 2002;89 (Suppl):75-82.

Linneburg A, Ostergaard C, Tvede M, et al. IgG antibodies against microorganisms and atopic disease in Danish adults: The Copenhagen allergy study. J Allergy Clin Immunol. 2003;111:847-853.

Majamaa H and Isolauri E. Probiotics: A novel approach in the management of food allergy. J Allergy Clin Immunol. 1997;99:179-185.

McCann ML. Probiotics: Recent scientific applications of an ancient medical practice. Anti-Aging Conference, Las Vegas, NV, Dec. 17, 2000.

McCann ML. Treatment and possible prevention of food allergies with pancreatic enzyme supplements and probiotics. Presented to Conference on ADD/ADHD; Georgetown University, Arlington, VA, May 1999.

McNeish AS. Enzymatic maturation of the gastrointestinal tract and its relevance to food allergy and intolerance in infancy. Ann Allergy. 1984;53:643-648.

Mellis, CM. Is asthma prevention possible with dietary manipulation? Med J Australia. 2002;177:S78-S80.

Murosaki S, Yamamoto Y, Ito K, et al. Heat-killed *Lactobacillus plantarum* L-137 suppresses naturally fed antigen-specific IgE production by stimulation of IL-12 production in mice. J Allergy Clin Immunol. 1998;102:57-64.

Oelgoetz AW, Oelgoetz P, and Wittekind J. The treatment of food allergy and indigestion of pancreatic origin with pancreatic enzymes. Am J Digesti Dis. 1935;2:422-426.

Olhagen B and Mansson I. Intestinal *Clostridium perfringes* in rheumatoid arthritis and other collagen diseases. Acta Med Scand. 1968;184:395-402.

Pelto L, Isolauri E, Lilius E-M, et al. Probiotic bacteria down-regulate the milk-induced inflammatory response in milk-hypersensitive subjects but have an immunostimulatory effect in healthy subjects. Clin Exp Allergy. 1998;28:1474-1479.

Pessi T, Sutas Y, Hurme M, et al. Interleukin-10 generation in atopic children following oral *Lactobacillus rhamnosus* GG. Clin Exp Allergy. 2000;30:1804-1808.

Pochard P, Gosset P, Grangette C, et al. Lactic acid bacteria inhibit Th2 cytokine production by mononuclear cells from allergic patients. J Allergy Clin Immunol. 2002;110:617-623.

Raithel M, Weidenhiller M, Schwab D, et al. Pancreatic enzymes: A new group of antiallergic drugs? Inflamm Res. 2002;51: S13-S14.

Rautava S, Kalliomaki M, and Isolauri E. Probiotics during pregnancy and breast-feeding might confer immunomodulatory protection against atopic disease in the infant. J Allergy Clin Immunol. 2002;109:119-121.

Sepp E, Julge K, Vasar M, et al. Intestinal microflora of Estonian and Swedish infants. Acta Pediatrica; 1997;86:956-61.

Shida K, Makino K, Morishita A, et al. *Lactobacillus casei* inhibits antigen-induced IgE secretion through regulation of cytokine production in murine splenocyte cultures. Int Arch Allergy Immunol. 1998;115:278-287.

Shida K, Takahashi R, Iwadate E, et al. *Lactobacillus casei* strain Shirota suppresses serum immunoglobulin E and immunoglobulin G1 responses and systemic anaphylaxis in a food allergy model. Clin Exp Allergy. 2002;32:563-570.

Spitz J, Hecht G, Taveras M, et al. The effect of dexamethasone administration on rat intestinal permeability: The role of bacterial adherence. Gastroenterol. 1994;106:35-41.

Sudo N, Sawamura A, Tanaka K, et al. The requirement of intestinal bacterial flora for the development of an IgE production system fully susceptible to oral tolerance induction. J Immunol. 1997;159:1739-1745.

Sutas Y, Hurme M, and Isolauri E. Down-regulation of anti-CD3 antibody-induced IL-4 production by bovine caseins hydrolysed with *Lactobacillus* GG-derived enzymes. Scand J Immunol. 1996;43:687-689.

Van de Water J, Keen CL, and Gershwin ME. The influence of chronic yogurt consumption on immunity. J Nutr. 1999;129:S1492-S1495.

Wheeler JG, Shema SJ, Bogle ML, et al. Immune and clinical impact of *Lactobacillus acidophilus* on asthma. Ann Allergy Asthma Immunol. 1997;79:229-233.

Wold AE. The hygiene hypothesis revisited: Is the rising frequency of allergy due to changes in the intestinal flora? Allergy. 1998;53 (Suppl 46):20-25.

Chapter 8

Problems in Private Places Probiotics and Urogenital Infections

Many women suffer from periodic vaginal discomfort and urinary tract infections. Of course, on TV, we see advertisements for topical creams and oral pills, but how do probiotics fare in treating these conditions, or more importantly *preventing* them? This is what we will explore in the present chapter.

Every year, 1 billion women around the world suffer from nonsexually transmitted urogenital infections (Reid and Bruce, 2001a). These infections include bacterial vaginosis, yeast vaginitis, and urinary tract infections. In the United States these infections are *the most common reasons* women visit their primary care physicians and urologists. Even with treatment, many experience recurring symptoms. Serious complications can occur from these infections — especially during pregnancy — when premature labor is a big concern.

It's not uncommon for physicians to recommend yogurt to women suffering from recurrent urogenital infections. And there are plenty of anecdotal stories from women, supporting the use of yogurt for these conditions. However, there have only been a handful of clinical trials appropriately designed to truly determine how useful probiotics are in treating and preventing these infections. The majority of these studies offer encouraging results. Specific probiotic strains play a beneficial role in maintaining urogenital health.

Urogenital Flora

Where do urogenital flora come from? Bacteria that live in the **urogenital tract** (defined as bladder, kidneys, urethra, periurethra, vagina, and cervix) originated in the intestines. These bacteria passed out of the body with fecal matter and migrated to the vaginal and urethral areas. More than 50 different bacterial species are known to live in healthy female urogenital tracts, with the most common microorganisms being lactobacilli — at least in pre-menopausal women.

Numerous factors alter the bacterial composition of the vagina and urinary tract: availability of essential nutrients, antibiotics (can wipe out normal flora for 1-2 months after treatment has finished), oral hormonal contraceptives, steroid therapies, spermicides like nonoxynol-9 (kill beneficial hydrogen peroxide-producing lactobacilli strains) (Reid and Bruce, 2001a), immunosuppression, diabetes mellitus, and normal cyclic hormonal variations.

Amazingly, and for reasons we don't understand, the bacterial flora in the vagina changes constantly. Lactobacilli are the predominant species found in healthy women, yet at any given time, only 22% of women have a normal lactobacillus-dominated flora, even in the absence of obvious symptoms. Cyclic hormonal fluctuations are partially responsible for the floral fluctuations. For example, on the days when estrogen levels are highest during a woman's monthly cycle, lactobacilli are able to adhere to the urogenital wall and colonize more efficiently. Likewise, postmenopausal women using estrogen therapies typically have sufficient lactobacilli colonization and a low incidence of recurrent urogenital infections (Raz and Stamm, 1993).

Depletion of vaginal lactobacilli can have serious consequences since lactobacilli strains protect against infections from bacteria like *Neisseria gonorrhoeae*, *Trichomonas vaginalis*, *Gardnerella vaginalis*, HIV, urinary tract infections, bacterial vaginosis, and yeast infections (Gardiner et al., 2002; Reid and Burton, 2002). Additionally, in pregnancy, lack of vaginal lactobacilli can increase the risk of premature labor.

Lactobacilli protect from infection in several different ways. Lactobacilli attach to epithelial cells in the vagina and the urinary tract, preventing disease-causing microorganisms from adhering. Lactobacilli deplete nutrients that would otherwise be available for disease-causing microorganisms. Lactobacilli heighten immune responses so the risk of infection is reduced (Reid and Burton, 2003). Additionally, lactobacilli produce chemicals like acids, hydrogen peroxide, and surfactants that are toxic to other strains of bacteria. Although there is considerable variation in the mechanisms by which different strains of lactobacilli prevent invasion and infection by disease-causing microorganisms, these factors are probably interdependent allowing for a balanced vaginal flora (Osset et al., 2001; Velraeds et al., 1996). Three particular strains of *Lactobacillus* (*L. jensenii*, *L. acidophilus*, and *L. casei*) colonize the vagina in almost 97% of healthy, non-pregnant, pre-menopausal women. There is definitely a correlation between *loss* of these microbes (through antibiotic or spermicide use) and *increased susceptibility to urogenital infections.*

One way that women lose beneficial hydrogen peroxide-producing lactobacilli from their urogenital tracts is by using spermicides, like nonoxynol-9. "Healthy" hydrogen peroxide-producing lactobacilli strains are more susceptible to death by nonoxynol-9 than non-peroxide producing lactobacilli. This observation suggests that vaginal flora may become depleted of "healthy" lactobacilli in women who use spermicides, thus placing these women at an increasing risk of developing urogenital infections (McGroarty et al., 1992).

Recently 42 healthy women were asked to take one of several different probiotic regimens by mouth for 28 days. Before and after the study, vaginal flora was examined. Not all probiotic strains were good colonizers, but two strains stood out from the rest. These two strains, *Lactobacillus rhamnosus* GR-1 and *Lactobacillus fermentum* RC-14, resulted in healthy vaginal flora for 90% of patients. Results from this study indicate that taking specific strains of *Lactobacillus* — even taking them by mouth at doses of at least 100 million bacteria per day — can restore and maintain a normal urogenital flora (Reid et al., 2001a). These strains of bacteria, *Lactobacillus rhamnosus* GR-1 and *Lactobacillus fermentum* RC-14 were originally isolated from a healthy urogenital tract. Both of these bacteria adhere well to urogenital epithelial cells and inhibit growth as well as adhesion of disease-causing bacteria. *Lactobacillus rhamnosus* GR-1 possesses the additional property of being resistant to nonoxynol-9 and *Lactobacillus fermentum* RC-14 produces hydrogen peroxide (Gardiner et al., 2002) and a biosurfactant that prevents a broad range of disease-causing microorganisms from adhering to the urogenital tract including: *Escherichia coli, Enterococcus faecalis, Klebsiella pneumoniae, Pseudomonas aeruginosa*, Group B streptococci, *Providencia stuartii, Staphylococcus epidermis, Gardnerella vaginalis*, and *Candida albicans* (Reid and Bruce, 2001b).

Bacterial Vaginosis

Bacterial vaginosis, also referred to as nonspecific vaginitis, is the most common cause of urogenital symptoms in women. While 100 thousand to 1 million bacteria are found in each gram of vaginal secretions taken from healthy women, there is a marked increase in bacteria (1-100 trillion per gram of vaginal secretions) in those with bacterial vaginosis. Bacterial vaginosis is characterized by loss of *Lactobacillus*-predominant vaginal flora and replacement with *Gardnerella vaginalis*, *Escherichia coli*, anaerobic bacteria, or *Mycoplasma hominis*.

Almost 50% of women with bacterial vaginosis, have no obvious symptoms of infection. However, when symptoms do occur, they include a fishy odor that worsens after intercourse or menses, a thick gray vaginal discharge, or vaginal itching (13% of the time). Bacterial vaginosis is diagnosed by physicians based on the presence of at least three of the following four characteristics: the foul fishy odor, an alkaline (less acidic than normal) vaginal environment, the presence of at least 20% "clue cells" (vaginal cells with a striped appearance due to adherent bacteria), and a milky vaginal discharge. Alternatively, (1) loss of lactobacilli coupled with (2) an increase in *Gardnerella* and *Bacteroides* species and (3) an alkaline vaginal environment also suggest to medical personnel that a diagnosis of bacterial vaginosis is likely.

Bacterial vaginosis, even in the absence of obvious symptoms, has been associated with an increased risk of pelvic inflammatory disease, urinary tract infections, endometriosis, and infections after gynecologic surgeries (Reid and Bruce, 2001a). Bacterial vaginosis can cause complications during pregnancy including premature rupturing of membranes (breaking water), premature labor and delivery, and even death of the fetus or newborn. Use of intrauterine devices (IUDs) is a major risk factor for developing bacteria vaginosis. Other factors that correlate with an increased tendency for bacterial vaginosis are cigarette smoking, multiple sexual partners, use of a diaphragm, rape, and a history of abnormal Pap smears.

Common therapies for bacterial vaginosis are inadequate, since as few as 61% of women remain "cured" one month after treatment is completed (Schmitt et al., 1992). Antibiotic vaginal creams and suppositories, such as metronidazole (Flagyl®) and clindamycin (Cleocin®,) are the most common therapies to treat bacterial vaginitis.

Sometimes, these antibiotics are prescribed orally as well. In fact, some physicians report a higher cure rate with oral rather than vaginal formulations. However, side effects limit the use of these drugs when they are prescribed orally. Women taking oral metronidazole must completely abstain from alcohol. Additionally, a nasty metallic taste in the mouth often occurs with this drug. Oral clindamycin, on the other hand, can cause severe, even life-threatening disruptions in the gastrointestinal flora. A microorganism known as *Clostridium difficile* can overgrow in the gastrointestinal tract (occurs in approximately 10 out of every 100 patients) causing a situation known as **pseudomembranous colitis** (see chapter 5 for more details). Regardless of whether these two drugs are used orally or vaginally, side effects are possible, antimicrobial resistance can develop, and *Escherichia coli* or *Enterococcus* may overgrow in the vagina (Hillier et al., 1990).

Reoccurrence of bacterial vaginosis — even right after antibiotic treatment — is a serious problem. Recurrence may be related to: reinfection from male partners, persistence of an unidentified factor that makes women susceptible to infection, microorganisms that are inhibited but not killed during antibiotic therapy, or the failure to reestablish protective *Lactobacillus*-predominant flora after therapy.

Different strains of lactobacilli have been used successfully to treat vaginitis. In one study, 28 women who suffered from recurrent vaginitis (more than five infections each year) were given suppositories containing *Lactobacillus GG* and asked to insert the suppositories vaginally twice daily for seven days. The patients returned for assessment 7 days after completing the therapy. All women self-reported improvement in symptoms like itching, and physicians reported a decrease in redness, irritation, and abnormal vaginal discharge following *Lactobacillus* therapy (Hilton et al., 1995).

In another small study, 32 women diagnosed with *Lactobacillus*-deficient bacterial vaginitis were enrolled in a clinical trial. In this study, 17 women received treatment with estrogen and *Lactobacillus acidophilus* — either one or two tablets inserted vaginally each night at bedtime while 15 other women were given placebo. Treatment continued for a total of 6 days. Overall, the results from this study found that two weeks after beginning therapy there was a 77% cure rate in the estrogen/probiotic group compared to a 25% cure rate in the placebo group. The benefits were even more substantial four weeks after initiating treatment, when 88% of those receiving estrogen and lactobacilli were "cured" versus 22% of the women taking placebo (Parent et al., 1996).

In another clinical trial, women with bacterial vaginosis were entered into a study where *Lactobacillus acidophilus* vaginal suppositories were given to 28 women and placebo was administered to 29 women. All women were colonized vaginally by *Bacteroides* prior to beginning the study. Immediately after completing the study, 16 of the 28 women treated with lactobacilli had normal vaginal smears and 12 of the 16 had no detectable *Bacteroides* present. These results were compared to those receiving placebo in which none of the 29 women had normal vaginal smears. However, after the next menstrual cycle, benefits of the probiotic were almost entirely lost. Only 3 of the women who had received *Lactobacillus* were still free of bacterial vaginosis (Hallen et al., 1992). Although results from this study were initially promising, the benefits of probiotic therapy were not maintained for extended periods of time. This is because probiotics do not colonize for extended periods of time. Thus, for continued benefit, periodic re-treatment or continuous maintenance treatment with probiotics is necessary.

Several other clinical trials evaluated whether administering lactobacilli by mouth would reduce the signs and symptoms of recurrent bacterial vaginosis and vaginal yeast infections. Although one study was well designed initially, the results were complicated by a high drop-out rate of study participants. However, it was concluded that eating yogurt containing *Lactobacillus acidophilus* is associated with larger numbers of live *Lactobacillus acidophilus* colonizing the rectum and vagina and this could, in turn, lead to fewer episodes of bacterial vaginosis (Shalev et al., 1996).

More recently, oral use of probiotics was evaluated again by another group of investigators. Of 10 women treated with probiotics for 14 days due to recurrent urogenital infections, 6 had complete resolution of symptoms within one week of beginning therapy with *Lactobacillus rhamnosus* GR-1 and *Lactobacillus fermentum* RC-14 when these supplements were taken by mouth, suspended in skim milk (Reid et al., 2001b). Prior to therapy, most patients in this study had constant pelvic pain, urinary frequency, pain during urination, or vaginal irritation. Patients remained healthy for many months following probiotic use after the study had concluded.

Additionally, a group of 64 healthy women was recruited to participate in a 60 day, randomized, double-blind clinical trial in which half were given daily *oral* capsules of either *Lactobacillus rhamnosus* GR-1 and *Lactobacillus fermentum* RC-14, while the other half of the women received placebo. Interestingly, prior to initiation of the study, none of the women reported any vaginal symptoms, although 16 of 64 (25%) had evidence of bacterial vaginosis, defined as low levels of lactobacilli and the presence of disease-causing bacteria. Half-way through the study and/or again at the end of the study, there was a substantial increase in vaginal lactobacilli, a substantial reduction in vaginal yeast, and a significant reduction of disease-causing bacteria in the vagina of women that received probiotics, but not in women prescribed placebo (Reid and Bruce, 2001a; Reid and Burton, 2002; Reid et al., 2003). This study represents the first in which an oral probiotic combination was definitively shown to reduce vaginal colonization by disease-causing bacteria and yeast.

Bacterial vaginosis in pregnancy

Bacterial vaginosis should always be treated in pregnant women, even when no symptoms are present. However, experts also recommend that the antibiotics used to treat bacterial vaginosis should be avoided in pregnancy, due to possible risks to the unborn child. How should clinicians handle these opposing guidelines? Probiotics! Probiotics may be especially useful for pregnant women. A clinical trial was conducted in 84 women with bacterial vaginosis who received either no treatment, vaginal treatment with yogurt containing *Lactobacillus acidophilus*, or vaginally-applied acetic acid tampons during their first trimester of pregnancy. Treatments were given as two doses daily for 7 days and repeated one week later. One month after therapy began, symptomatic improvements were most dramatic in those receiving yogurt therapy (Neri et al., 1993).

According to one report, *Lactobacillus* therapy is routinely used in one European clinic for pregnant women who are considered to be at high risk for delivering prematurely when warning signs of bacterial vaginitis are present. When women actively participate in their therapy, by monitoring vaginal acidity levels twice a week and by taking probiotics to restore their normal vaginal flora, there is only a 0.3% rate of very early premature births compared to a 4.1% rate in patients who do not participate in self-care regimens of self-monitoring and probiotic therapy. These results support active participation and early intervention by women who are at risk for having low-birth weight, premature children (Saling et al., 2001). Thus, probiotics may be a very favorable therapeutic option for treating bacterial vaginosis during pregnancy.

Although many studies have successfully used probiotics to treat women with bacterial vaginosis, there are some reports in the medical literature that have not found probiotics to be beneficial (Fredricsson, 1989). The reason for the discrepancies are unclear, but may be related to the specific strain of bacteria used or the method by which the bacteria were administered into the vagina. For example, in a study where *Lactobacillus* did not improve bacterial vaginitis, the probiotic was administered as a vaginal milk douche (Fredricsson, 1989). It is possible that bacteria did not remain in the vagina long enough to exert positive health benefits when given in this manner.

Yeast Vaginitis

Yeast infections in the vagina (also referred to as moniliasis or candidiasis) occur frequently in women. Yeast infections are the second most common form of vaginitis in the United States. Roughly 75% of women will have at least one yeast infection and 45% will have a second attack at some point during life. However, approximately 5% of females suffer from chronic, persistent or recurrent episodes. A survey conducted in 2000 American women older than 18 years of age found more than 17% of black women and 6% of white women had at least one yeast infection during the previous two months. Additionally, 8% of women reported four or more episodes during the previous year (Foxman et al., 2000) and 5% of those surveyed suffer from recurrent, frequent infections that no longer respond to regular medical treatments. Vaginal yeast infections are considered to be "recurrent" when a woman experiences four or more infections within a twelve month period.

Yeast vaginitis is defined as inflammation of the vagina or vulva due to invasion by *Candida* species. Although *Candida albicans* is responsible for 85-90% of vaginal yeast infections, two other species, *Candida glabrata* and *Candida tropicalis*, also cause vaginitis and are more difficult to eliminate than *Candida albicans*. Unfortunately, recurrent infections are probably caused by drug-resistance among non-*Candida albicans* species.

Common symptoms of vaginal yeast infections include intense vaginal or vulvar itching, a cottage-cheese-like vaginal discharge, and redness or swelling of the labia. Sometimes, rash-like lesions are also present and some women complain of vaginal soreness, vulvar burning, and pain during sexual intercourse when they have a yeast infection. On the other hand, up to 20% of women are colonized by *Candida* without ever experiencing any symptoms.

In order for yeast to cause infections, they must adhere to and penetrate into epithelial tissues. Invasion of the epithelium leads to redness and increased vaginal discharge. In acidic environments — when lactobacilli are present — yeast have difficulty attaching to the vagina. However, in more alkaline environments — as when lactobacilli are absent — *Candida* species adhere tightly to vaginal cells.

Risk factors for yeast vaginitis include pregnancy, diabetes, high estrogen-containing oral contraceptives, spermicides, and antibiotic use. High blood sugar levels (associated with diabetes) make it easier for *Candida albicans* to bind tightly to vaginal cells; however, for those with diabetes, this can be minimized with tight control over blood sugar. Estrogenic components of oral contraceptives and increased levels of estrogen during pregnancy are also believed to increase adhesive properties of yeast and speed yeast growth rates. On the other hand, low estrogen levels — prior to the onset of menses and after menopause — are associated with a greatly reduced incidence of vaginal yeast infections. Spermicides such as nonoxynol-9 may also increase adhesive properties of *Candida,* allowing yeast cells to adhere to the urogenital tract more easily (McGroarty et al., 1990). It is not a surprise that antibiotics disturb vaginal normal flora and allow yeast to grow. In fact, many women are automatically given a prescription for an antifungal agent each time they are given a prescription for an antibiotic, since they know they are likely to experience a vaginal yeast superinfection as a consequence of taking oral antibiotics.

Treatment regimens often consist of antifungal agents that are used in the vagina as creams or suppositories. Common over-the-counter (available without a prescription) vaginal treatment regimens use the drugs butoconazole (Femstat®), clotrimazole (Mycelex®), miconazole (Monistat®), or tioconazole (Vagistat®). The antifungal cream terconazole (Terazol®) is also available with a prescription. There are some drawbacks to these treatments. For example, vaginal creams and suppositories are messy, they must be used just prior to bedtime for maximal benefits, and depending upon the product selected, up to seven nights of continuous use may be required for a cure.

Alternatives to vaginal antifungals, are the antifungal drugs diflucan (Fluconazole®) and ketoconazole (Nizoral®) which are available as tablets taken by mouth. For most yeast infections, one tablet is usually curative. For chronic infections, sometimes low doses must be used continuously to prevent subsequent re-infections. When yeast infections occur chronically there may be an underlying immune deficiency. Low levels of IgA antibodies often correlate with recurrent vaginal yeast infections. Additionally, in some women, high levels of IgE (allergic) antibodies have been observed, suggesting that some women may suffer an allergic-type response when colonized by yeast.

Lactobacilli are the most important barriers to vaginal yeast infections. This is because lactobacilli compete with *Candida* for essential nutrients, lactobacilli block adhesive properties of *Candida*, and lactobacilli produce substances that interfere with yeast growth. Although there are few formal studies evaluating probiotics as therapies for vaginal yeast infections, the data does suggest benefits, particularly in *prevention* of infections (as opposed to treatment). In fact, experts believe it is unlikely probiotics will *cure* a yeast infection, since yeast can coexist with lactobacilli. On the other hand, probiotics may *prevent recurrences* by restoring normal flora *after* antifungal treatments, before disease-causing bacteria and yeast grow back and dominate the vagina (Reid, 2002a). Clinical trials seem to support this.

In one study 13 women with recurrent vaginal yeast infections were evaluated for at least 1 year, during which time they ate yogurt containing *Lactobacillus acidophilus* for 6 months and did not eat yogurt during the other 6 month period. During the period when patients were eating yogurt containing probiotics, there was a three-fold decrease in the number of vaginal yeast infections. Additionally, in this study, there was a correlation between the presence of *Lactobacillus acidophilus* in the rectum and in the vagina. When *Lactobacillus acidophilus* was present in their stools, the probability that the bacterium would colonize the vagina was nearly 55%. In contrast, when *Lactobacillus acidophilus* was absent from the stools, there was only a

15.5% probability that it would be found in the vagina. These results suggest daily consumption of *Lactobacillus*-enriched yogurt increases the chance of *Lactobacillus* colonization in the urogenital region and decreases the risk of vaginal yeast infections (Hilton et al., 1992).

Another study also evaluated *Lactobacillus casei* variant GG in women with recurrent yeast infections. The probiotic therapy, used vaginally twice daily for 7 days, improved vaginal symptoms in all women in this study. These results suggest that use of probiotics *after* antifungal therapy may restore normal flora in women with recurrent yeast infections (Hilton et al., 1995).

Another blinded, placebo-controlled clinical trial studied the safety and efficacy of *Lactobacillus acidophilus* strain NAS vaginal suppositories (Gynatren®) alone or in combination with an oral probiotic preparation containing *Lactobacillus acidophilus* NAS strain, *Bifidobacterium bifidum* Malyoth strain, and *Lactobacillus bulgaricus* strain LB-51 (Healthy Trinity®) in 27 college women with recurrent candidal infections. The women took oral capsules daily and used vaginal suppositories three times weekly. These women participated in the study for an average of 3.3 months. During this time, there were dramatically fewer recurrent yeast infections in women using vaginal *Lactobacillus acidophilus* strain NAS (with or without oral probiotics) compared to women given placebo. These findings demonstrate the efficacy of vaginal suppositories in directly delivering hydrogen peroxide-producing lactobacilli to the urogenital area (Metts et al., 2000; Metts et al., 2003).

Vaginal candidiasis is a common problem for women living with HIV infections due to their immunocompromise. With use of current antiviral drugs, women with HIV are living longer, and yeast infections have a dramatic impact on their quality of life. In a double-blind placebo-controlled study, 164 HIV-infected women were instructed to insert either *Lactobacillus acidophilus* (Healthy Trinity®), clotrimazole (an antifungal), or placebo capsules vaginally once a week. These women were followed for an average of 21 months. During the study, the likelihood of having a yeast infection was decreased by about 50% for women taking either the probiotic or the antifungal, compared to women given the placebo (Williams et al., 2001).

Although there are only a few clinical trials that have actively studied the use of probiotics to prevent recurrent vaginal yeast infections, there is a great deal of word-of-mouth support of probiotics for this use. In fact, reports of various yogurt products being effective treatments for recurrent yeast infections span the medical literature — as far as 25 years back (Sandler, 1979; Will, 1979; Bach, 1992). Eating yogurt is a simple and tasty way for women to self-medicate and take control of their health and well being. (As an interesting side note, one of the first published observations describing the utility of yogurt for preventing vaginal yeast infections also mentioned that when yogurt was prescribed to three women, not only did their yeast infections clear up, but life-long eczema also went away. Interestingly, when these women stopped eating yogurt, the eczema returned. See chapter 8 for more about probiotics and eczema.)

Urinary Tract Infections (UTI)

Hundreds of millions of women experience urinary tract infections each year (Reid and Bruce, 2001a). The term UTI refers to any situation in which there are more than 100 to 10,000 bacteria present in each milliliter of urine (obtained by mid-stream, clean catch method) and symptoms suggestive of a UTI are also present. Although symptoms are not always consistent, some individuals complain of urinary frequency or urgency, pain when urinating, incontinence, pain in the abdomen or back, or blood in the urine when experiencing a UTI. When UTIs become complicated and the infection spreads to involve the kidneys, symptoms are more severe and include fever, chills, fatigue, back pain, and diarrhea.

The first time an individual has a UTI, it tends to resolve quickly with treatment and complications are unlikely. Recurring UTIs may be due to several factors. Unresolved *bacteriuria* (bacteria in the urine) describes a situation in which, despite appropriate treatment, bacteria persist in the urinary tract. This occurs when bacteria are resistant to antibiotics or when patients have been non-compliant and have not taken the complete antibiotic therapy as prescribed. On the other hand, *bacterial persistence* occurs when urine cultures originally become sterile during antibiotic therapy, but reinfection — by the same microorganism — occurs due to an infection high within the urinary tract. Upper urinary tract infections can be due to an infected prostate gland (men), infected cysts, or infected kidney stones. Additionally, a *reinfection* can occur at any time with new microorganisms after a previous infection has cleared up.

Up to 85% of the time, UTIs in non-hospitalized women are caused by *Escherichia coli*, followed by *Staphylococcus saprophyticus*, and enterococci (Reid and Bruce, 2001a). Risk factors for developing a UTI include sexual intercourse with multiple partners or use of spermicidal agents like nonoxynol-9. As mentioned previously, spermicides have a harmful effect on vaginal flora, killing lactobacilli which causes a loss of acidity. An alkaline (less acidic) environment promotes growth of disease-causing gram-negative bacteria (Reid et al., 1990). Postmenopausal women are also at risk for UTIs due to loss of estrogen. Additionally, previous urogenital surgeries and bladder dysfunction are also risk factors for UTIs.

Common medical therapy relies upon various antibiotics, given for one to seven days, to treat uncomplicated UTIs. Symptoms usually subside within three days. However, those with recurrent episodes must stay on long-term low maintenance doses of antibiotics. Continuous low dose antibiotic treatment is recommended for women who experience two or more UTIs in a six month period — OR — three or more episodes per year. Complicated infections that involve the kidneys usually require hospitalization and intravenous antibiotics. During pregnancy, up to 40% of women with bacteria in their urine — even if no symptoms are present — go on to develop a complicated UTI affecting their kidneys. Because this often leads to premature labor and delivery of a low-birth weight infant, all pregnant women with evidence of bacteria in their urine require treatment. Unfortunately, antibiotic therapy may be associated with serious side effects. An additional concern with antibiotics is the increasing incidence of bacterial resistance to many drugs.

Although it is not uncommon to find disease-causing bacteria in the urinary tract of healthy women, studies indicate that lactobacilli should, by far, be the predominate bacteria present. This suggests that lactobacilli maintain a balance in the normal flora of the urinary tract, preventing infection. It is clear that in order to persist in an environment of continuous urinary flow, disease-causing bacteria must be able to attach strongly to the urinary tract mucosal surface.

Not much is known about the mechanisms by which the urinary tract defends itself against disease-causing bacteria, but it is believed that antibodies and normal lactobacilli are the key players. Lactobacilli prevent urinary tract infections by interfering with the ability of disease-causing bacteria to bind to the epithelial cells that line the urinary tract (Reid et al., 1987). Lactobacilli also produce substances that are toxic to harmful bacteria, such as hydrogen peroxide, thereby suppressing growth of bacteria that are harmful to the urinary tract, including *Escherichia coli.*

Escherichia coli is the microorganism most commonly associated with recurrent UTIs. For most women, hydrogen peroxide-producing lactobacilli inhibit growth of this microorganism. However, in women prone to recurrent UTIs, there is a marked absence of hydrogen peroxide-producing strains of lactobacilli in the vagina, and therefore, a higher likelihood of vaginal colonization by *Escherichia coli.* This suggests that a lack of hydrogen peroxide-producing lactobacilli in the vagina is an important feature that permits *Escherichia coli* colonization in the urinary tract (Gupta et al., 1998). As a result of this observation, several studies have used *Lactobacillus* supplementation to treat women with recurrent urinary tract infections.

In the late 1980s, 5 women who suffered from recurrent UTIs were treated twice a week with a specific strain of lactobacillus, *Lactobacillus casei* var *rhamnosus* GR-1, which was administered directly into their vaginas. Following use of this probiotic, each patient enjoyed an infection-free period ranging from 4 weeks to 6 months. This study, although limited, was the first to demonstrate potential utility of lactobacilli to prevent recurring urinary tract infections in women (Bruce and Reid, 1988).

A few years later, 41 women with recurrent UTIs entered another clinical trial to compare the effects of vaginal *Lactobacillus* suppositories to placebo. There was a 21% recurrence rate of UTI among women receiving probiotic therapy versus 47% UTI recurrence in the placebo group, again suggesting *Lactobacillus* is a safe and effective treatment for reducing UTI recurrence (Reid et al., 1992).

In another example, a 33 year old female with a history of recurrent UTIs and multiple vaginal infections was administered *Lactobacillus casei* var *rhamnosus* GR-1, three times over the course of six months. During the 6 month treatment period, the patient was symptom-free. Prior to beginning treatment, no lactobacilli were found in the vagina of this patient. However, seven weeks after the first dose of the probiotic, *L. casei* var *rhamnosus* GR-1 was recovered from the vagina suggesting that this organism is capable of surviving in the vagina for long periods of time after being introduced (Reid et al., 1994).

In another study involving 55 women, two lactobacilli strains,

Lactobacillus casei GR-1 and *Lactobacillus fermentum* B-54, were administered twice a week vaginally for a year. The incidence of UTI was 79% *less* while using the probiotic combination than the incidence during the previous year, prior to starting probiotic therapy (Reid and Bruce, 2001a).

See below for the story of one child with recurrent urinary tract infections excerpted from an article submitted for publication by a Ukrainian physician and scientist, Gerasimov (2003).

> A.M., a 6 year old girl, complained of burning when she urinated and it was determined that she had a urinary tract infection. An ultrasound was performed but found no abnormalities with her kidneys or bladder. However, *Escherichia coli* and white blood cells were present in her urine. She was treated with cephalexin and her symptoms resolved.
>
> One month later, she experienced pain while urinating, plus back pain and fever. Again, a large number of *Escherichia coli* were detected in her urine. This time her infection was treated with intravenous ampicillin and gentamicin. Again, all of her symptoms improved.
>
> However, once again, about a month later, she complained of fever, fatigue, and back pain, as well as pain and frequency of urination. This time, the child was pale, with signs of systemic toxicity. Laboratory studies noted a moderately elevated white blood cell count in her blood and urine, and *Escherichia coli* (serotype 07) was found in both urine and fecal specimens. The microorganism was susceptible to ceftriaxone and cefadroxil, but was resistant to ampicillin and gentamicin.
>
> This child was then treated with intravenous ceftriaxone for 3 days, followed by oral cefadroxil for 18 days. After 7 days on antibiotic therapy, her urine was free of *Escherichia coli*, but serotype 07 was still found in her stools.
>
> After completion of antibiotics, *Lactobacillus acidophilus* DDS-1 (Megadophilus Dairy Capsules®) was given to the little girl twice daily for one month, then continued just once daily. Her physician selected this strain because the bacterium inhibited the growth of *Escherichia coli* serotype O7 in his preliminary laboratory tests.
>
> After two months of probiotic therapy, *Escherichia coli*, serotype 07 was no longer found in the little girl's stools. During the 5 months that this child was followed and continued to take the probiotic, the child did not experience any further reoccurrences of urinary tract infections.

However, not all studies have yielded such encouraging results. In one trial of women with recurrent UTIs, twice-weekly use of *L. casei* var *rhamnosus* did not prevent recurrent infections during the 6 month time period that these women were followed by physicians (Baerheim et al., 1994). Discrepancies between this study and the many positive results obtained by others may be due to many factors, including the particular bacterial strain that was used, the dosage prescribed, or the formulation of the product.

This next patient case illustrates probiotics are definitely helpful, but not necessarily magic bullets for all women.

> Eight years ago, Jane Boucher, an internationally-known speaker and author in her mid 40s was literally at death's door. Her career came to a screeching halt when she developed symptoms of a bladder infection.
>
> Unfortunately, her symptoms continued to worsen despite antibiotic therapy. She was terribly weak and lost a great deal of weight, until her 5 foot, 7 inch frame weighed only 100 pounds. One doctor told her that she just had "honeymoon cystitis." Another physician told her that she needed to see a psychiatrist. After all, his reasoning went, if the physical symptoms couldn't be cured by his medical treatment they must all be in her head. During this time, she also developed symptoms of irritable bowel syndrome. She was suffering from terrible bladder and bowel troubles. At times she was so bloated and her abdomen so distended she appeared to be several months pregnant. There were times she wanted to die.
>
> For years she traveled all over North America, from Mexico to Canada, Cleveland to Los Angeles. She saw numerous physicians and spent thousands of dollars. Meanwhile, all this time, her urine cultures contained enterococci. Although one would think identifying the cause of her symptoms would be the first step towards solving the problem, this was easier said than done in Jane's case. The microorganism Jane Boucher carries in her body is resistant to all known antibiotics. When microorganisms are resistant to antibiotics, what do you do? You treat them with probiotics, of course!
>
> For the past several years, Jane has taken *Lactobacillus* supplements and used Chinese herbs. She indicated, "Probiotics really helped, but haven't gotten rid of the bacteria completely. I still test positive for *Enterococcus*." At the present time, Jane is back on the lecture circuit and is about 80-90% well. Ms. Boucher has the utmost respect for probiotic researchers and is optimistic that she may still find a probiotic that will cure her infection 100%. (Jane asked me to include her full name and she encourages women to contact her though her website.)

Other

Certainly, probiotics are not all created equally. As already mentioned, two strains in particular, *Lactobacillus rhamnosus* GR-1 and *Lactobacillus fermentum* RC-14, possess many desirable qualities when it comes to treating urogenital infections. These two strains adhere well to urogenital epithelial cells as well as inhibit growth and adhesion of disease-causing bacteria. Additionally, *Lactobacillus rhamnosus* GR-1 is resistant to nonoxynol-9, and *Lactobacillus fermentum* RC-14 produces hydrogen peroxide and surfactants which kill disease-causing bacteria (Reid and Bruce, 2001a). The properties of these two strains complement each other well when they are combined. These two strains seem to colonize and remain in the vagina longer than other probiotics. So far, it seems that probiotics aren't capable of displacing indigenous flora to become the dominant microbes. At best, probiotics stick around for only a few days or weeks (Reid, 2002b). A recent study found that when these two probiotics were inserted vaginally in capsule form, *Lactobacillus rhamnosus* GR-1 persisted in the vaginal tract for up to 19 days and *Lactobacillus fermentum* RC-14 was detectable for 5 days after vaginal instillation (Gardiner et al., 2002).

Additionally, these two strains of probiotic bacteria may possess antiviral properties. A recent study in healthy women compared the effects of a probiotic vaginal capsule containing *Lactobacillus rhamnosus* GR-1 and *Lactobacillus fermentum* RC-14 with commercially-available capsules containing *Lactobacillus rhamnosus* GG. The majority of women (73%) who received the GR-1/RC-14 capsules still had these organisms present vaginally two weeks after stopping the product — compared to only 3 women (21%) who received *Lactobacillus* GG. The probiotic bacteria recovered by vaginal swabs from these women were then further tested for ability to inhibit yeast and several different viral strains. Both GR-1 and RC-14 strains consistently inhibited growth of *Candida* and killed two different viruses within 10 minutes. These results clearly indicate that probiotics — even those that are closely related — don't behave similarly. The potent antiviral activity of strains GR-1 and RC-14 may have broad implications, perhaps even suggesting that women colonized by these lactobacilli may be at less risk of acquiring sexually transmitted diseases. (Cadieux et al., 2002). Definitely, more studies are needed in this area. Since vaginal flora may become disturbed at any point during the menstrual cycle, restoration of the flora by use of self-care products may be helpful to many women.

While *Lactobacillus rhamnosus* GR-1 and *Lactobacillus fermentum* RC-14 appear to have some amazing properties and could be very beneficial to many women, at the present time, these specific strains are, unfortunately, not commercially available.

Conclusion

As we already know, different lactobacilli strains possess properties that suppress activities of disease-causing bacteria and yeast. Most likely, various properties of different lactobacilli strains are necessary for maintaining a healthy urogenital environment. Although the lactobacilli strains that seem to best colonize the vagina such as *Lactobacillus casei* GR-1 and *Lactobacillus fermentum* RC-14 are not commercially available at this time, it is envisioned that in the future women may be able to use products containing these strains *vaginally* once daily for three days to *treat* bacterial vaginosis and *orally* once daily to maintain a healthy vaginal environment (Reid and Bruce, 2001a; Reid, 2002b).

Another lactobacilli strain, *Lactobacillus crispatus* CTV-05, is also being investigated for use as a probiotic. At the present time, not much is known about *Lactobacillus crispatus* CTV-05 other than that it is a potent hydrogen peroxide producer (Reid, 2002a; Reid and Bruce, 2001b). Since this strain is still in the early experimental stages for use as a probiotic, there are no products containing this microorganism commercially available right now. This microorganism has not yet even been evaluated in clinical trials to determine whether it is effective for treating urogenital infections in women.

Right now, there is some evidence that indicates *Lactobacillus acidophilus* may provide some benefits to some women with urogenital ailments. Since this product is widely available, *Lactobacillus acidophilus* may be an alternative until *Lactobacillus casei* GR-1 and *Lactobacillus fermentum* RC-14 become commercially available. Nearly all women have abnormal vaginal flora at some point in any given monthly cycle and probiotic consumption may be a natural way for women to restore and maintain a healthy vaginal environment. Probiotics can help to prevent infections, permitting women to rely on therapies other than antibiotics and antifungals. This is desirable since antibiotics and antifungals have adverse effects, disrupt normal flora, and increase antibiotic resistance among microorganisms (Reid, 2002b).

Note: In this chapter, emphasis was placed on studies conducted within the past 15 years. However, benefits of probiotics in this area date back to the 1920s. For a complete review of early studies conducted between 1920 and the early 1980s, please refer to an article published in the International Dairy Journal (Sieber and Dietz, 1998).

Notes

Notes

References

Bach C. Reader identifies yogurt containing culture effective in relieving candidal vaginitis. Nurse Practitioner. 1992:17:9.

Baerheim A, Larsen E, and Digranes A. Vaginal application of lactobacilli in the prophylaxis of recurrent lower urinary tract infection in women. Scand J Prim Health Care. 1994;12:239-243.

Bruce AW and Reid G. Intravaginal instillation of lactobacilli for prevention of recurrent urinary tract infections. Can J Microbiol. 1988;34:339-343.

Cadieux P, Burton J, Gardiner G, et al. *Lactobacillus* strains and vaginal ecology. JAMA. 2002;287:1940-1941.

Fredricsson B, Englund K, Weintraub L, et al. Bacterial vaginosis is not a simple ecological disorder. Gynecol Obstet Invest. 1989;28:156-160.

Foxman B, Barlow R, D'Arcy H, et al. Candida vaginitis: Self-reported incidence and associated costs. Sex Transm Dis. 2000;27:230-235.

Gardiner GE, Heinemann C, Bruce AW, et al. Persistence of *Lactobacillus fermentum* RC-14 and *Lactobacillus rhamnosus* GR-1 but not *Lactobacillus rhamnosus* GG in the human vagina as demonstrated by randomly amplified polymorphic DNA. Clin Diag Lab Immunol. 2002;9:92-96.

Gerasimov SV. Probiotic prophylaxis in pediatric recurrent urinary tract infections (UTI). 2003; Clin Pediatr. In press.

Gupta K, Stapleton AE, Hooton TM, et al. Inverse association of H_2O_2-producng lactobacilli and vaginal *Escherichia coli* colonization in women with recurrent urinary tract infections. J Infect Dis. 1998;178:446-470.

Hallen A, Jarstrand C, and Pahlson C. Treatment of bacterial vaginosis with lactobacilli. Sex Trans Dis. 1992;19:146-148.

Hillier S, Krohn MA, Watts DH, et al. Microbiologic efficacy of vaginal clindamycin cream for the treatment of bacterial vaginosis. Obstet Gynecol. 1990;76(3 Pt 1):407-413.

Hilton E, Isenberg HD, Alperstein P, et al. Ingestion of yogurt containing *Lactobacillus acidophilus* as prophylaxis for candidal vaginitis. Ann Int Med. 1992;116:353-357.

Hilton E, Rindos P, and Isenberg H. *Lactobacillus GG* vaginal suppositories and vaginitis. J Clin Microbiol. 1995;33:1433.

McGroarty JA, Soboh F, Bruce AW, et al. The spermicidal compound nonoxynol-9 increases adhesion of Candida species to human epithelial cells *in vitro*. Infect Immun. 1990;58:2005-2007.

McGroarty JA, Tomeczek L, Pond DG, et al. Hydrogen peroxide production by *Lactobacillus* species: Correlation with susceptibility to the spermicidal compound nonoxynol-9. J Infect Dis. 1992;165:1142-1144.

Metts J, Famula TR, and Clemens RA. *Lactobacillus acidophilus*, strain NAS (H_20_2 positive) in reduction of recurrent candidal vulvovaginitis. Presented at American Academy of Family Physicians Annual Scientific Assembly, Atlanta, GA, October 5, 2000.

Metts J, Famula TR, Trenev N, et al. *Lactobacillus acidophilus*, strain NAS (H_20_2 positive) in reduction of recurrent candidal vulvovaginitis. Nutrition Res. 2003, submitted.

Neri A, Sabah G, and Samra Z. Bacterial vaginosis in pregnancy treated with yogurt. Acta Obstet Gynecol Scand. 1993;72:17-19.

Osset J, Bartolome RM, and Garcia E. Assessment of the capacity of *Lactobacillus* to inhibit the growth of uropathogens and block their adhesion to vaginal epithelial cells. J Infect Dis. 2001;183:485-491.

Parent D, Bossens M, Bayot D, et al. Therapy of bacterial vaginosis using exogenously-applied Lactobacilli acidophili and a low dose of estriol: A placebo controlled multicentric clinical trial. Arzneim-Forsch. Drug Res 1996;46:68-73.

Raz R and Stamm WE. A controlled trial of intravaginal estriol in postmenopausal women with recurrent urinary tract infections. N Engl J Med 1993 Sep 9;329:753-756.

Reid G, Beuerman D, Heinemann C, et al. Probiotic *Lactobacillus* dose required to restore and maintain a normal vaginal flora. FEMS Immunol Med Microbiol. 2001a;32:37-41.

Reid G and Bruce AW. Could probiotics be an option for treating and preventing urogenital infections? Medscape Women's Health. 2001a;6:9.

Reid G and Bruce AW. Selection of *Lactobacillus* strains for urogenital probiotic applications. J Infect Dis. 2001b;183:S77-S80.

Reid G, Bruce AW, Fraser N, et al. Oral probiotics can resolve urogenital infections. FEMS Immunol Med Microbiol. 2001b;30:49-52.

Reid G, Bruce AW, McGroarty JA, et al. Is there a role for lactobacilli in prevention of urogenital and intestinal infections? Clin Microbiol Rev. 1990;3:335-344.

Reid G, Bruce AW, and Taylor M. Influence of three-day antimicrobial therapy and *Lactobacillus* vaginal suppositories on recurrence of urinary tract infections. Clin Ther. 1992;14:11-16.

Reid G and Burton J. Use of *Lactobacillus* to prevent infection by pathogenic bacteria. Microb Infect. 2002;4:319-324.

Reid G, Charbonneau D, Erb J, et al. Oral use of *Lactobacillus rhamnosus* GR-1 and *L. fermentum* RC-14 significantly alters vaginal flora: Randomized, placebo-controlled trial in 64 healthy women. FEMA Immunol Med Microbiol. 2003;35:131-134.

Reid G, Cook RL, and Bruce AW. Examination of strains of lactobacilli for properties that may influence bacterial interference in the urinary tract. J Urol. 1987;138:330-335.

Reid G, Millsap K, and Bruce AW. Implantation of *Lactobacillus casei* var *rhamnosus* into vagina. Lancet. 1994;344:1229.

Reid G. Probiotics for urogenital health. Nutr Clin Care. 2002a;5:3-8.

Reid G. The potential role of probiotics in pediatric urology. J Urol. 2002b;168:1512-1517.

Saling E, Schrieber M, al-Taie T. A simple, efficient and inexpensive program for preventing prematurity. J Perinatal Med. 2001;29:199-211.

Sandler B. Lactobacillus for vulvovaginitis. Lancet. 1979;2:791-792.

Schmitt C, Sobel JD, and Meriwether C. Bacterial vaginosis: Treatment with clindamycin cream versus oral metronidazole. Obstet Gynecol. 1992;79:1020-1023.

Shalev E, Battino S, Weiner E, et al. Ingestion of yogurt containing *Lactobacillus acidophilus* compared with pasteurized yogurt as prophylaxis for recurrent candidal vaginitis and bacterial vaginosis. Arch Fam Med. 1996;5:593-596.

Sieber R and Dietz U-T. *Lactobacillus acidophilus* and yogurt in the prevention and therapy of bacterial vaginosis. Int Dairy J. 1988;8:599-607.

Velraeds MMMC, Van der Mei HC, Reid G, et al. Inhibition of initial adhesion of uropathogenic *Enterococcus faecalis* by biosurfactants from *Lactobacillus* isolates. Appl Environ Microbiol. 1996;62:1958-1963.

Will TE. *Lactobacillus* overgrowth for treatment of monilliary vulvovaginitis. Lancet. 1979;2:482.

Chapter 9

So Many Choices, So Little Advice
Selecting a Probiotic

"Okay," you say. "I'm convinced! I really want to try probiotics to treat my symptoms, but how do I choose one? Which one will work for *me*?"

I'm often asked this question. Unfortunately, there's no simple answer. One reason it's tough to answer is that some medical conditions respond better to one probiotic than another. Another fact that makes this difficult is that we simply don't all respond the same way. This isn't unique to probiotics. Even prescription drugs are this way. Think about it. If a single drug were the answer for treating everyone with high blood pressure, we wouldn't have a need for the more than 50 different high-blood-pressure medications on the market today. In essence, what works for me, may not work for you. It is naïve to assume that a single probiotic strain will be the cure-all for everyone — or even in the same individual at different stages of a disease. There is no probiotic that is a magic bullet. A single microorganism can't be all things to all people. The intention of this chapter is not to recommend any one product over another. The selection of strains will depend upon the intended medical use as well as safety and biological considerations. Rather, it is my desire to communicate to you why all probiotics are not created equally, and to provide you — the consumer — with the information you need to select a quality product.

Probiotics are purchased over-the-counter. They are not prescription items. You might ask, "Well, then how can they be any good if they don't require a prescription?" In order for me to answer that question, you have to understand what is required to bring a prescription drug product to market — in short — money! The big drug companies spend billions of dollars conducting large clinical trials and race against the clock in order to get their products to market before the patent runs out (typically 17 years from the date the patent is filed) so that they can have market exclusivity and be able to reap profits before generic manufacturers grab a piece of the market share. Unfortunately, the problem for probiotics and the pharmaceutical industry is this: a naturally occurring microorganism cannot be patented. From the pharmaceutical industry's perspective, without patent protection, there is little incentive to spend billions of dollars on clinical trials, when the "guy down the street" can mass produce and sell the product, too.

On one hand, purchasing probiotics over-the-counter translates into increased convenience for you; on the other hand, this means that your health insurance won't pay for them. You, the consumer, must pay the full amount out of your own pocket for probiotics. Since these costs can add up and be quite pricey, you want to make certain that the product you select is a good, quality probiotic.

Before we proceed, it is essential to have a clear definition of what a probiotic is in the first place. The definition I use for the term "probiotic" is the following: *A preparation or a product containing a sufficient number of live microorganisms to alter the flora of the host and bring about beneficial health effects.* This definition is based upon a similar one proposed by Schrezenmeir and de Vrese (2001). By this definition, a probiotic may be found in a food like yogurt, or may be a product that is independently sold and labeled as a probiotic substance, whether that be a tablet, capsule, powder, suppository, or douche. Most probiotics are marketed as either a food or a drug. According to a recent *USA Today* news story, the yogurt maker, Dannon©, recently launched a probiotic drink called Actimel® in the United States. This fermented milk beverage has been sold in Europe for years and packs 10 billion *Lactobacillus casei* into each 3.3 ounce serving (Rubin, 2003). On the other hand, probiotic "pills" — tablets and capsules — are readily available over the internet and through health food stores.

Our definition of "probiotic" also indicates that microorganisms must be alive and present in large enough quantities to alter and improve properties of the normal flora in order for positive health benefits to occur. To fulfill the last part of this definition, probiotics need to live up to some high manufacturing standards. Unfortunately, however, since manufacturers of probiotics are not regulated by governmental agencies, there is a great deal left to chance when it comes to selecting a good quality probiotic.

Because probiotics aren't subjected to regulation by any governing body, manufacturers are under no obligation to perform *any* type of quality assurance testing to verify either the purity of the product or to assure the viability of the bacteria by the time the product reaches the consumer. Worse, yet, probiotic manufacturers are free to claim any health benefits they want in order to sell their products. Obviously, these issues are problematic. Unfortunately, some products don't even contain the microbial species stated on the label, and many products don't contain the declared amounts of bacteria in each dose. Recently, some researchers investigated claims made by manufacturers of yogurt-type milk products. According to product labels, these yogurts contained live and active cultures. In this study, it was noted that the bacterial species *actually* contained in the products often differed from those stated by the manufacturer. Additionally, the number of live bacteria varied greatly among different brands tested (Holzapfel et al., 2001) and even between different lots produced by the same manufacturer (Majamaa et al., 1995). In fact, in one of twelve brands of yogurt evaluated, *no* live bacteria were found at all (Holzapfel et al., 2001)! According to Rita Rubin, a health and science reporter for *USA Today*, the FDA proposed more stringent regulation of dietary supplements in March 2003 when the agency realized that 8 of 25 probiotic supplements tested contained fewer than 1% of the number of live bacteria consumers expected them to have (Rubin, 2003).

These problems are all too common. Often the probiotic strain listed by the manufacturer as the "active ingredient" is *not* truly the strain that is in the product. To illustrate this point, let me share with you what a group of investigators recently discovered about one of the products they were using in clinical trials. The clinical trial was conducted with a product that was supposed to contain *Lactobacillus acidophilus*, 1.0×10^9 microorganisms per dose. However, upon closer examination, the product actually contained *Lactobacillus casei*, but only 4.4×10^7 bacteria per dose — two orders of magnitude fewer bacteria and an entirely different species than what the manufacturer had claimed (Majamaa et al., 1995).

Manufacturers of probiotics often use misleading or false advertising to sell their products. For example, just last week, a friend sent me a web address advertising a new probiotic and asked me for my opinion. I was told the product is sold by a company that I'll refer to as Company X and the new probiotic contains several different strains of bacteria. When I visited Company X's website, I noticed numerous references from the medical literature which this company insinuated were evidence of health benefits from their product. However, I had never heard nor seen Company X's product mentioned anywhere in the medical literature, so I took a closer look at those references. Not a single clinical trial in any of those references had actually been conducted using Company X's product. Company X cited clinical trial data that had used different products, in fact, different strains of bacteria altogether than those found in their own product. Clearly, if there were any governmental regulation in the industry, this false advertising would be halted and lawsuits would be filed.

The next time you visit the supermarket, check out the labels on the yogurts. The ones that indicate their products contain "live and active cultures" are subtly proposing that their product contains beneficial healthy bacterial. Likewise the next time you visit a health food store, take a look at the probiotic supplements or, better yet, search the internet for the keyword "probiotic". You will no doubt find hundreds if not thousands of probiotics on the market, promoted as beneficial for one disease or another. *Most times those health claims have never been substantiated.* No quality, reliable clinical trials have ever been conducted for *most* probiotic products promoted for health purposes. In fact, it always scares me when I hear a health food store clerk giving out medical advice to unsuspecting consumers in an area that he/she clearly knows nothing about, ie. "You just take 2 of these pills a day for good gastrointestinal health..." But, with an industry that has no obligation to live up to any type of standards, how can a consumer possibly separate the good from the bad, the beneficial from the harmful? How do you avoid purchasing snake oil?

Discuss the Use of Probiotics with Your Health Care Provider

To select the correct probiotic, the appropriate first step is to consult a knowledgeable physician, and whenever possible, a physician who specializes in the field in which you hope to find the use of probiotics beneficial. For example, if you are considering using probiotics in your three year old child who has a history of asthma, eczema, and food allergies, the best place to start searching for information on an appropriate probiotic would be with your child's allergist. On the other hand, if you have had intolerable diarrhea and abdominal cramps and are thinking of trying a probiotic to restore normal digestive functions, it is wise for you to discuss this with your gastroenterologist.

The reasons for physician involvement are several-fold. First, although probiotics are remarkably safe, there are some individuals who should not take probiotics or should do so only under close medical supervision. Such people are those who could, in theory, be at risk for developing an infection from the bacteria in the probiotic. Probiotics are best avoided by folks with severe immunosuppressive illnesses like HIV/AIDs or cancer. Additionally, there are some drugs that weaken the immune system and could, theoretically, lead to a greater tendency for infections to occur when taking probiotics. Steroids and some "immunomodulator" medicines used for rheumatoid arthritis are two examples of such drugs. As with any other medicine or supplement, it is a good idea if you discuss your intentions with a physician who can help you to decide if probiotics are right for you.

With that disclaimer stated, probiotics are remarkably safe. Bifidobacteria and lactic acid bacteria have rarely caused disease. Their safety track record in fermented milk, vegetables, and cereals is superb. According to one expert who reviewed 143 human clinical trials between 1961 and 1999, during almost 30 years of use, there were *no* adverse effects reported in any of the 7526 people who participated in probiotic clinical trials (Madsen, 2001).

Occasionally, however, there have been reports of blood infections (sepsis) or heart infections (endocarditis) from *Lactobacillus*, but in most of these cases, the source of the infection was *not* probiotics but rather normal gastrointestinal flora (Griffiths et al., 1992; Antony et al., 1996; Horwitch et al., 1995; Patel et al., 1994). These situations are rare and usually only occur when the immune system is severely weakened by cancer, organ transplantation, diabetes, HIV, recent surgery, tissue injury, or drug-induced immune problems (Chomarat et al., 1991; Schlegel et al., 1998). There has been speculation that probiotic bacteria could become resistant to antibiotics; however, while natural antibiotic resistance of bifidobacteria and lactobacilli has been occasionally reported (Matteuzzi et al., 1983; Ishibashi and Yamazaki, 2001; Gupta, 1995), it is not usually a concern for most patients using probiotics.

Reports of fungal infections in the blood as a result of using *Saccharomyces boulardii* are also very rare (Niault et al., 1999). Again, the likelihood of this yeast exiting the intestinal tract and entering the blood stream is typically only a concern in situations of major immunocompromise such as cancer chemotherapy or severe intestinal injury (Cesaro et al., 2000; Pletincx et al., 1995).

Like any medical therapy, using probiotics does involve a small risk, however, the safety of probiotics has been confirmed through centuries of experience. In fact, just to give an idea of how long probiotic bacteria have been used successfully in foodstuffs with beneficial effects: one Persian translation of the Bible credits Abraham's longevity to consumption of sour milk (in other words, the milk was fermented by bacteria). Additionally, in 76 BC, the Roman historian Plinius recommended fermented milk products for treating gastrointestinal infections (Schrezenmeir and de Vrese, 2001). It is comforting to know that despite thousands of years of experience with probiotics, secondary infections caused by probiotic bacteria are extremely rare. In fact, the most common complaint during the first 1-2 weeks of probiotic therapy is flatulence or gas, but even this subsides within a few days.

Another reason to include your physician specialist in a discussion of probiotics is to determine if the physician recommends one product over another, either from personal experience or from reading about benefits in the medical literature. We know that all probiotics are not created equally. For example, although a *Lactobacillus*-deficiency is known to contribute to urogenital infections in women, only a few specific strains of lactobacilli have demonstrated beneficial effects in treating these types of infections. In this circumstance, it would not make sense to take supplements containing bifidobacteria for urogenital infections when it hasn't been thoroughly tested nor found beneficial. Keep in mind, the success of one bacterial species used in a certain application <u>*does not*</u> suggest all related strains will produce a comparable response. In fact, often probiotic products don't indicate to consumers the specific strain of bacteria contained in the product, and quite frankly, even the medical literature doesn't always tell us exactly which strain was tested in clinical trials. A physician can help you determine whether or not there is evidence in peer-reviewed medical journals supporting use of a particular probiotic product, or bacterial strain, for the medical use that you intend it. Likewise, a physician may be able to help you acquire probiotics, even ones that aren't commercially available for sale to the general public. Keep in mind that while probiotic manufacturers often cite clinical trials in their literature or on their websites, *rarely* was the clinical trial actually conducted with the specific product that the manufacturer is selling. A physician can help you to determine if there is evidence published in peer reviewed scientific journals describing the mechanism by which the probiotic may be effective. If there is no basis in the literature for a probiotic to be effective for a particular medical use, then chances are good, the product won't be effective!

A physician can also help determine an appropriate dose for you. Probiotic products often say, "Take one or two capsules a day for intestinal health." These products never clarify what they mean by "intestinal health." Are they claiming that is the dose necessary to cure a gastrointestinal ailment? Or is this the dose needed to maintain homeostasis?

With close inspection of any given product, you may notice each individual probiotic capsule contains a few million bacteria. At first, that sounds like a HUGE amount. However, if you search the medical literature, you'll find clinical trials use much larger doses — on the orders of hundreds of billions or even trillions of bacteria — each day to bring about gastrointestinal healing. For many probiotic products marketed, you'd have to take 30 or more capsules every day to even come close to taking the dosage that's really necessary. Unless you consult with your physician or read the literature yourself, you won't really know what dose is right for you.

Recently, it was suggested by several prominent investigators, not only do you need a certain *number* of microorganisms to have beneficial effects on digestive tract flora, but also *simultaneous* use of *several different strains* of bacteria probably has a greater impact than a single strain. This makes sense. After all, there are 450-500 different strains of microorganisms normally living in our gastrointestinal tracts at any given time, accounting for up 100 trillion bacteria in every gram of our feces. Greater health benefits are likely when several different species of bacteria are introduced into the gut simultaneously. In fact, this has been the rationale, in recent years, for new probiotics that combine two, three, five, and even eight different bacterial strains into one commercially available product. By including your physician in the decision-making process, you can find out what the clinician has seen effective in his/her own practice and ask which species of bacteria or which commercially available product he/she has read about most often in the medical literature.

Although discussing probiotics with your physician sounds like a reasonable and straightforward approach, you may be surprised at how little physicians in the Western world know about the topic — and you can use this opportunity to educate them and get them thinking. Our society, during the last 100 years, has been much more focused on eliminating microorganisms from our environment and from our bodies, than studying the symbiotic relationships that we, as humans, share with the trillions of "bugs" that live in us. This is why many physicians are skeptical about probiotics. Few medical schools promote the use of probiotics, or even mention them during the years of medical training. This was clearly evidenced by a recent survey of family physicians. Although the survey was conducted by a high school student, the results of the survey were startling and were reported in the *Canadian Medical Association Journal* (Edmunds et al., 2001). The student, knowing that antibiotic treatment destroys beneficial intestinal flora and often results in diarrhea, mailed a brief questionnaire to 100 physicians inquiring about their probiotic prescribing practices. Although all responding physicians indicated that they prescribe ***antibiotics*** on a regular basis, only 10% indicated that they often or always recommend probiotics with antibiotic prescriptions. *Even more shocking was that only 18% of physicians were even aware that there was any research on probiotics!* If your physician is wary of probiotics or claims there is no data to support their usefulness, you may take the opportunity to gently and kindly educate your doctor. Through no fault of their own, many clinicians have simply not been exposed to prescribing practices of probiotics. Remember, it has only been within the last 15 years that the probiotic field has even *existed* in Western literature and it has only been within the last 5 years that our knowledge has literally exploded. Prior to 1990, only 22 articles in the Medline database were found on the topic of probiotics. However, more than 1000 articles have been published between 1992 and 2002. In fact, there were more than 200 articles published in the first six months of 2002 alone (Marteau et al., 2002)! A good doctor is willing to listen, be educated, and brought up to speed with current medical literature. If a physician is unwilling to listen and learn, red warning flags should go up in your mind. In fact, Fergus Shanahan, a gastroenterologist at the University of Cork in Ireland expressed these same sentiments when he indicated in an interview with *USA Today* that while probiotics are not magic bullets, they should not be dismissed (Rubin, 2003).

What if you discuss probiotics with your doctor, and you find him/her open and willing to let you try a probiotic approach, but he/she simply lacks the experience to make a recommendation...how do you select a product? You do the homework! With the internet, information is literally at our fingertips — only a click away. However, be certain that the information you are getting is accurate. Stay away from anecdotal stories on probiotic manufacturer's web sites. Remember, there is no regulation in the industry so these folks can claim whatever they want. Instead, take a close look at what is reported in the medical literature. The National Library of Medicine has a web site available free to the public, called PubMed. This database summarizes thousands of medical journals that are accessed easily and does so for free — there is no charge to use this service! The web address is: http://www.nlm.nih.gov

If you must do your own homework, start out at PubMed by typing some key words. For example, "probiotic" and "allergy." Summaries of articles published by physicians and scientists will pop up and can be easily read. You can read summaries or abstracts of articles on the web site for free. Many full-length articles are also available for free, directly from the PubMed web site, although other articles may be purchased for a small fee. Additionally, articles can also be obtained through a local university library at minimal cost, too. When skimming through the text of these articles, make note of the specific strain of bacteria used — whether treatment was beneficial or not — and note the name and location of the product's manufacturer. <u>It is important to use the same exact product mentioned in the literature</u>, whenever possible. You need to use the same product, at the same dosages as cited in clinical trials. Remember, even closely related bacterial species don't always behave the same. Don't forget, this is an area where there is no governmental regulation. Unlike the pharmaceutical industry, probiotic manufacturers do not need to prove their products are safe or effective in order to sell and market them.

Whenever there is difficulty ascertaining which strain of bacteria was used in an article or the name and location of the probiotic's manufacturer, your physician or a librarian may be able to assist you. Think how impressed your physician will be if you bring an article from the medical literature to your next appointment to discuss with him/her. The age of information and technology has come such a long way in a few decades to where patients are able to be proactive in caring for themselves! When searching for a probiotic, those most likely to benefit humans by improving intestinal microbial balance are organisms within the genus *Lactobacillus* and *Bifidobacterium;* however, other species will also turn up on your literature searches — like *Saccharomyces* (yeast) or *Escherichia.*

As I mentioned, lactobacilli strains will no doubt pop up when you search the literature. As you already are aware from reading this book, lactobacilli promote vitamin production and food digestion. They also rely mainly on sugars for digestion and produce short chain fatty acids like lactic acid. Short chain fatty acids are an important source of energy for the epithelial cells lining the intestine. Lactobacilli also produce hydrogen peroxide and toxins — both of which suppress growth of other gut bacteria. Likewise, bifidobacteria are also lactic acid producers. These species are needed for manufacturing B vitamins and may also reduce cholesterol levels (Mombelli and Gismondo, 2000). There are some studies that suggest reduced levels of bifidobacterial species in the gut may be the reason that children develop eczema (Laiho et al., 2002). Additionally, both lactobacilli and bifidobacteria may have antioxidant properties which may be beneficial for management of asthma (Laiho et al., 2002). In general, lactobacilli and bifidobacteria are all around "good guys". But your job will be to identify a product with the correct species and strain for the ailment you are interested in treating.

Once you have identified a particular species, with medical evidence of its usefulness, it is relatively easy, using the internet, to contact the company and find out how you can purchase the product. Some companies will only ship their products directly to you, while other companies routinely sell their products to supermarkets or health foods stores but will ship directly to you if you cannot find a local store that sells it. What if, however, you have not been able to identify a specific brand or company in the literature...Then what? How does one know whether a probiotic is truly of good quality, whether the product contains the bacterial species it claims, or if there are sufficient numbers of microorganisms — still alive — by the time it reaches your door to exert the desired medical effect? While these questions are a bit more difficult to answer definitively, it is still possible to do a bit of homework on your own by telephoning the manufacturer and asking a few questions about their manufacturing and quality assurance practices. If you are told there is no one available to answer your questions, then there probably are few, if any, quality assurance tests in place. This may not be a product worth purchasing. I have telephoned companies like that.

For example, I recently attempted to contact three different companies with questions about their probiotic preparations. I won't mention any company names, but will instead refer to these three companies as company #1, #2, and #3. Company #1 is a very well-known multi-level-marketing manufacturer of vitamins and alternative medicines. Company #2 is a little-known manufacturer of kefir — a yogurt-like beverage available in supermarkets and health food stores. Company #3 is a small pharmaceutical manufacturer that, in addition to FDA-approved medicines, also manufactures a non-FDA approved probiotic powder.

When I called to inquire about quality control procedures, I was told by company #1 that they did not answer technical questions by telephone. I was informed that I had to e-mail or fax my questions to the company. At company #2, the receptionist was unable to answer my questions, but I received a phone call several hours later *from the president of the company.* According to "the president", even though there are no governmental regulations and therefore no obligation to perform certain quality control procedures, this company routinely tests not only the products that they manufacture, but also competitor's products, to see how many live microorganisms survive the manufacturing process. Additionally, I was specifically informed which particular product — of the many products this company sells — contains the most microorganisms per cup (by virtue of the quality assurance tests conducted). I was also informed how their product compares head-to-head with various competitors' products (several orders of magnitude more probiotic organisms). Additionally, I received a bit of education and found out that "plain" kefir/yogurt products contain roughly 20% more live microorganisms than flavored products because bacteria survive better without addition of sugars associated with fruit flavorings. Unlike the "brush off" that I got from company #1, the answers to my questions far exceeded my expectations with company # 2.

My experience with company #3 was similar to that of company #2. Although the receptionist was unable to answer my questions, I received a telephone call from *the director of marketing*. Again, not only was I satisfied with the answers to my questions, but I also learned other things that I had not known. For example, this company has so much faith in their probiotic powder when treating gastrointestinal disorders such as pouchitis, inflammatory bowel disease, or diarrhea, that in conjunction with a physician's request, this company was shipping a FREE thirty days supply of their product directly to patients in order to get them started on probiotic therapy. I also found out that company #3 has sales representatives making stops at physician's offices to educate them about their product. What this tells me is: company #3 wants to work with physicians to treat patients and they have a great deal of faith in their product because they have clinical trial data to back up their claims. As a result of my interaction with these companies, I purchased company #2's kefir and company #3's probiotic powder, but I avoided any products from company #1. On a related note, several weeks after my initial inquiries, a representative from company #3 telephoned me — just to follow up — and asked whether or not their product had worked. How many times have you been called by a pharmaceutical company, after taking their product, just to see how you are feeling? Company #3 is selling a quality product, without a doubt.

Questions to Ask

When speaking with manufacturers of probiotic products, some "quality assurance" types of questions to ask or consider are the following:

What medical treatment(s) has your product been successfully used to treat and where is this information published? Be certain that a reputable manufacturer makes a product containing the microorganism(s) of interest and make sure that this product has already been *proven* effective for the medical ailment you are hoping to treat. It is essential to know whether or not a properly designed clinical trial — for treating a clearly defined medical condition — has been conducted if you plan to use the product for a specific medical condition. It is important to rely only on products with a documented history of success in the medical literature and NOT the company's own personal "success" stories. If the company directs you to medical literature citing a success with a particular strain of bacteria — be certain that the clinical trial actually used the precise product manufactured by this company in the studies, and not a competitor's product. This is very important because there are numerous differences in manufacturing and shipping processes — from one company to another — and these differences dramatically affect the final number of live microorganisms, overall product stability, and possible health benefits to you.

What types of quality control tests do you perform? Although the scientific details may not be important, what is important is that there are, in fact, routine procedures in place to assure the product contains the microorganism that they claim as the "active ingredient" and that their product is free of contaminants that could be harmful. Ideally, the company should be manufacturing the product using good manufacturing practices approved by the Food and Drug Administration. Quality control checks should be in place to assess the stability of the product over time, as well as evaluate functional properties of the bacteria to be certain that health benefits are still likely (ie. after being grown in laboratories, do bacteria still adhere to epithelial cells of the gut? of the urogenital tract?).

Although not a scientist or a physician, Natasha Trenev, founder and president of Natren, Inc.©, has worked with probiotic bacteria for 30 years. According to Trenev, many probiotic manufacturers fail to consider the growth medium in which they culture their bacteria. Trenev says, "Scientists shouldn't separate bacteria from their natural fermentation media." For example, one of Trenev's strains of *Lactobacillus acidophilus* grows best in milk and it needs calcium to adhere to epithelial cells. For optimal probiotic performance, researchers and probiotic manufacturers should grow their probiotics in the "preferred" environments.

Trenev also explained how bacteria don't waste energy. They don't produce byproducts unless stimulated to do so. According to Trenev, probiotic manufacturers often lose the beneficial effects that the probiotics demonstrated in small laboratory settings when they scale up production. When production is scaled up and the bacteria are grown in "foreign" environments, according to Trenev, "The bacteria are now honed for survival and they don't produce beneficial bacteriocins and other byproducts." Trenev gave an example, "Probiotic bacteria don't produce lactase unless grown in a lactose-containing (milk) medium." She continued, "Bacteria are really quite intelligent. They don't produce these substances [hydrogen peroxide, lactase, bacteriocins, glycoproteins for attaching to epithelial cells, etc.] for our sakes. They do it for their own survival, and they won't do it unless stimulated" — stimulated by appropriate growth conditions.

Probiotics are often used in fermented foods such as yogurts and other milk products, as well as fermented meats and vegetables like fresh sausages and sauerkraut. During the fermentation process, several bacterial by-products such as acetic acid, lactic acid, and bacterial toxins are produced — thus making the final product more acidic. Such changes may affect the stability and longevity of the product and may alter the bacteria's functional properties.

Not only must probiotics be able to withstand the acidity of yogurts and fermented milks, but they must also be resistant to lysozyme — an enzyme in saliva that kills gram-positive bacteria. They must survive stomach and bile acids. As a result, tolerance to harsh conditions imposed by the gut is one of the first criteria that must be established for a probiotic to be a successful therapeutic agent. Long-term industrial processing and storage conditions also influence the functional properties of probiotic agents. Thus, it is necessary to use a probiotic product from a manufacturer that periodically performs quality-assurance testing on its product to assess the viability and activities of the microorganisms. For example, one well-known gastroenterologist claims to have had great success using a particular strain of *Lactobacillus* in the early 1990s in patients with gastrointestinal-related disorders. This was when this strain was obtained directly from the laboratory of the gentleman who initially isolated it. However, now that the product has been produced industrially for more than a decade and is commercially available, the probiotic seems to have lost its effectiveness due to the very nature of the manufacturing process itself. Now, the bacteria lack certain adhesive properties that they possessed when they were originally isolated.

Intestinal adhesion of bacteria correlates with health benefits. So, prerequisites for probiotic activity are (1) survival during transit through the digestive tract and (2) adhesion to the gastrointestinal tract. Some strains of probiotics adhere better to the small intestines, while others bind preferentially within the large intestines (Isolauri et al., 2002). Adhesion may also depend upon the age and the immune status of the host. It is also possible that some strains adhere better to damaged areas of the intestinal tract as opposed to healthy tissues. Because adhering to the intestinal wall is absolutely necessary for colonization and since adherence is also necessary for stimulating the immune system, probiotics should be tested regularly by their manufacturers to assess their binding capacity for intestinal cells. It comes as no surprise that different strains of bacteria exhibit various adhesion properties. Additionally, the industrialization process itself has been associated with a reduction in adhesion ability of bacteria. If adhesion properties are modified over time, the probiotic health benefits will also be reduced. Thus, even the same product produced in the same manufacturing facility may vary in its potency between batches, especially as more and more time passes from when the original bacterial isolate was collected (Tuomola et al., 2001).

How many live and active microorganisms are in each dose of your product? Part of our definition of "probiotic" indicates that bacteria must be present in large enough numbers to alter the normal flora. Even though many probiotics indicate on their label that each capsule, teaspoonful, or cup contains a specified number of live bacteria, that may not be an adequate reflection of the number of bacteria remaining alive by the time the product reaches your doorstep. The number of organisms many manufacturers state on their product refers to the viable bacteria when the product is first manufactured, but there may be considerably less — or even no — live microorganisms remaining by the time the product reaches you unless it is shipped and stored appropriately.

What is the expiration date for this product? How many microorganisms are still alive and active through the expiration date? How should this product be stored and how is it shipped to maximize longevity and stability? Unfortunately, many probiotic products do not contain an expiration date at all. In these circumstances, it is impossible to know how long the product has been sitting around. Ideally, expiration dates should be set such that the number of live microorganisms stated on the product are still viable through that date. To achieve this, the manufacturer actually needs to put extra microorganisms in the product initially, since it is reasonable to expect a 10% loss of viable organisms by the expiration date, even when stored appropriately. This is the acceptable limit for loss of potency within the pharmaceutical industry for FDA-approved drugs.

Probiotic products must stay cool and refrigerated for optimal activity. Products that are not shipped on ice may sit in hot warehouses or unrefrigerated delivery trucks. These products won't provide health benefits if the microorganisms have not survived transit (Heller, 2001). The probiotic manufactured by company #3 (discussed above) is shipped direct to the consumer on ice via second day air. Additionally, the product possesses an expiration date, through which the manufacture guarantees 450 billion microorganisms will be alive in each packet, as long as the product is kept refrigerated.

The storage process alone causes a significant decline in numbers of live probiotic bacteria, even when stored appropriately. In one study, it was demonstrated that after five weeks of storage, some yogurt products contained no live *Bifidobacteria bifidum* at all (Shah et al., 1995). Additionally, because the intestinal tract is the normal environment for bacteria, the oxygen content and water activity during shipping and storage must be considered by the manufacturer when ensuring stability of the products. One manufacturer of probiotics has spent a great deal of time developing delivery systems to enhance bacterial viability. Some of their probiotics are put into an oil matrix, inside a two-piece hard gel capsule. Then all water and air are removed from the oil to lengthen the product's half-life. Finally, they weld the capsule back together.

Another factor influencing the stability of products has to do with interactions between two or more probiotics in a single product. For example, beneficial interactions occur when the two species *Streptococcus thermophilus* and *Lactobacillus bulgaricus* are stored together When these two species are combined in yogurt, organisms rapidly multiply because of cross-feeding of both microorganisms. In contrast, some bacterial species have antagonistic effects towards each other when combined due to production of bacterial toxins, hydrogen peroxide, or lactic acid (Heller, 2001). In these situations, even if the product is stored properly, there will still be a detrimental loss of microorganisms by the time the product reaches the consumer.

As a result of all of the above mentioned "manufacturing" criteria necessary for good quality probiotics, whenever possible, probiotics should be purchased from top-notch pharmaceutical companies who perform regular quality control evaluations.

What You Can Do to Maximize Probiotic Activity

Once you have purchased a quality probiotic product, there are several things you can do to increase the activity of the microorganisms. The probiotic should be stored in the refrigerator to ensure the longevity of the product. Heat, even just prolonged room temperature, reduces the number of live and active bacteria.

Once ingested, the amount of probiotic bacteria that survive transit through the gastrointestinal tract depends upon many factors including: degree of stomach acidity, length of time exposed to gastric acids, concentration of and length of time exposed to bile acids, and level of bile acid enzyme activity. Some strains of bacteria are hardy and able to withstand acidic conditions better than others. Other strains survive harsh conditions when exposed to bile salts (Berrada et al., 1991; Lankaputhra et al., 1995; Noh et al., 1993;). Because probiotics are susceptible to acidic conditions, it may be beneficial to take probiotics on an empty stomach. Ingesting probiotics one hour before food, or two to three hours after eating, ensures that the production of stomach acid and bile salts is at low levels. For this reason, it is also recommended that probiotics are taken with plain yogurt or milk — since these foods do not stimulate acid production in the intestinal tract.

Due to the complex and hostile environment of the gastrointestinal tract, it is unlikely that a single probiotic bacterial strain is capable of significantly altering the microbial environment of the host. Many experts recommend combinations of strains to change and positively influence the host's gastrointestinal tract (Dunne et al., 1999). Certainly, a portion of probiotic bacteria survive passage through the gastrointestinal tract (Pahwa et al., 1987; Langhendries et al., 1995; Benno et al., 1992; Ling et al., 1994; Pochart et al., 1992). In fact, up to 25% of probiotics may be recovered in the feces. However, the bacteria do not implant, grow, multiply, and stick around in the gastrointestinal tract for any appreciable length of time. Within a few days — 7 days to 3 weeks — of stopping bacterial supplements, the number of probiotic bacteria recovered in feces declines to zero. In fact, usually within two weeks of stopping a probiotic, there are no more probiotic bacteria present in feces. These results indicate that any benefits derived from taking probiotics quickly disappear when the products are stopped. For this reason, it is important to keep taking probiotics once they have been initiated.

Some researchers have identified *Lactobacillus plantarum*, and to a lesser extent, *Lactobacillus rhamnosus* as having the best ability to colonize the intestine (Bengmark, 1998). These microorganisms tolerate more acidic conditions than most other bacteria. *Lactobacillus plantarum* is the most common bacteria found in naturally fermented foods. It has a unique ability to inhibit growth of disease-causing bacteria and is used by the food industry to increase product shelf-lives.

Desirable Properties for Probiotics	
Resistance to digestive enzymes, acids, bile	***-Survives passage through gastrointestinal tract*** ***-Modulates immune system*** ***-Excludes disease-causing bacteria*** ***-Speeds healing of damaged intestinal lining***
Derived from human origin	***-Species-specific interactions with host***
Documented health benefits	***-Proposed health benefits are "true"***
Safe	***-Minimal risk to consumer*** ***-Cannot transfer antibiotic resistance***
Other	***-Viable product; good shelf life***

Table 9-1. Desirable properties for probiotics (adapted from Laiho et al., 2002)

Dosing Issues

Unfortunately, since there is no formal regulatory agency governing the use of probiotics, there are no clear guidelines for dosing them, either. Most clinical trials have relied upon a minimum of 100 billion microorganisms given daily. While that may sound like a lot, in fact, that number is probably on the low-end of the range of microorganisms needed to bring about changes in the complex intestinal environment. Many probiotic products sold actually contain several fold fewer microorganisms than that per dose. For example, a rather well-known *Lactobacillus* preparation contains only a fraction of that amount in each dose, requiring many capsules daily, to get even a fraction of the number of microorganisms that might have a therapeutic benefit.

On the other hand, VSL#3®, a probiotic combination product that contains 4 different strains of *Lactobacillus* (*L. casei, L. plantarum, L. acidophilus, L. bulgaricus*), 3 strains of *Bifidobacterium* (*B. longum, B. breve, B. infantis*), and 1 strain of *Streptococcus* (*S. thermophilus*), comes in 6-gram dose-packets. Each packet contains 450 billion LIVE microorganisms at the time of manufacture, and when kept refrigerated, is guaranteed to still contain 450 billion LIVE bacteria through the product's expiration date. I happen to be particularly fond of this product for several reasons. First, I know from first hand experience that this product can bring about major, beneficial changes within the gastrointestinal tract. Secondly, this product is manufactured by a well-known pharmaceutical company. Thirdly, the product is shipped direct to the user ON ICE by 2nd-day air to make sure the bacteria remain viable. Fourth, as far as I am aware, the product contains the greatest number of live bacteria per dose than any other product. And fifth, the product contains 8 different strains of probiotics, whose actions complement one another. While I happen to like this product, I know there are other probiotics on the market that are just as good. Other products have helped thousands of people, and I certainly don't want to downplay the others.

When taking probiotics to treat a medical condition, the key is large doses initially. Lower maintenance doses may work once the condition has stabilized . Again, I'll use VSL#3®, purely as an example, since it has been widely reported beneficial for gastrointestinal inflammation in recent clinical trials. In adults, dosages have ranged anywhere from 1-4 packets (6-24 grams) of bacteria per day initially in clinical trials (see http://www.questcor.com for details). In small children, 6 grams (1 packet) of VSL#3® each day might be sufficient as an initial dose. In fact, once the condition has stabilized and the bowel has been populated with "good bacteria", say after 3 months or so, it may be permissible to lower the dosage to a fraction of the original dose if the probiotic is continued as a maintenance therapy.

Certainly, the most common way for probiotics to be administered is via the mouth, but I would be negligent if I didn't also mention that some probiotics have been administered rectally by enemas for various types of colorectal inflammation. Additionally, vaginal probiotic delivery has also been used successfully to treat recurrent urinary tract or vaginal infections, and probiotics have also been infused directly into the bladder when treating chronic urinary tract infections (Mombelli and Gismondo, 2000).

Conclusion

Hopefully, it is now evident that not all probiotics are created equally. While there are some quality probiotics on the market that meet our broad definition, there are probably many companies that manufacture products that do not meet all the criteria — especially in regards to supplying live bacteria in large enough numbers to alter the normal flora and bring about health benefits. This is one of many reasons why it is recommended that a physician be included in the decision-making process, since clinicians are likely to have experience with quality products. I have been careful throughout this book to NOT make a habit of describing products by brand name or manufacturer. Likewise, I have rarely included specific dosages used in clinical trials for treating different conditions. I left this information out intentionally, because I want you to use probiotics only with the knowledge and consent of your physician, at the doses he/she prescribes.

By selecting quality products, using appropriate storage conditions, and ingesting probiotics on an empty stomach, you can obtain maximal benefits from taking probiotics. Note: More information about selecting *quality* probiotics and a few examples of specific products available in the United States are available on line at: http://www.usprobiotics.org

Notes

Notes

References

Antony SJ, Stratton CW, Dummer JS. *Lactobacillus* bacteremia, description of the clinical course in adult patients without endocarditis. Clin Infect Dis. 1996;23:773-778.

Bengmark S. Immunonutrition: Role of biosurfactants, fiber, and probiotic bacteria. Nutrition. 1998;14:585-594.

Benno Y, Mitsuoka T. Impact of *Bifidobacterium longum* on human fecal microflora. Microbiol Immunol. 1992;36:683-694.

Berrada N, Lemeland J-E, Laroche G, et al. *Bifidobacterium* from fermented milks: Survival during gastric transit. J Dairy Sci; 1991;74:409-413.

Cesaro S, Chinello P, Rossi L, et al. *Saccharomyces cerevisiae* fungemia in a neutropenic patient treated with *Saccharomyes boulardii*. Support Care Cancer. 2000;8:504-505.

Chomarat M, Espinouse D. *Lactobacillus rhamnosus* septicemia in patients with prolonged aplasia receiving ceftazadime-vancomycin. Euro J Clin Microbiol and Infect Dis. 1991;10:44.

Dunne C, Murphy L, Flynn S, et al. Probiotics: From myth to reality. Demonstration of functionality in animal models of disease and in human clinical trials. Antonie van Leeuwenhoek. 1999;76:27-292.

Edmunds L. The underuse of probiotics by family physicians. CMAJ. 2001;164:1577.

Gupta PK, Mital BK, Gupta S. Antibiotic sensitivity pattern of various *Lactobacillus acidophilus* strains. Indian J Exp Biol. 1995;33:620-621.

Griffiths JK, Daly JS, Dodge RA. Two cases of endocarditis due to *Lactobacillus* species, microbial susceptibility, review, and discussion of therapy. Clin Infect Dis. 1992;15:250-255.

Heller KJ. Probiotic bacteria in fermented foods: Product characteristics and starter organisms. Am J Clin Nutr. 2001;73:374S-379S.

Holzapfel WH, Haberer P, Geisen R., et al. Taxonomy and important features of probiotic microorganisms in food and nutrition. Am J Clin Nutr. 2001;73:365S-373S.

Horwitch CA, Fureth A, Larson AM, et al. Lactobacillemia in three patients with AIDS. Clin Infect Dis. 1995;21:1460-1462.

Ishibashi N, Yamazaki S. Probiotics and safety. Am J Clin Nutr. 2001;73:465S-470S.

Isolauri E, Kirjavainen PV, Salminen S. Probiotics: A role in the treatment of intestinal infection and inflammation? Gut. 2002;50:iii54-iii59.

Laiho K, Ouwehand A, Salminen A, et al, Inventing probiotic functional foods for patients with allergic disease. Ann Allergy Asthma Immunol. 2002;89(Suppl):75-82.

Langhendries JP, Detry J, Van Hees J, et al. Effect of a fermented infant formula containing viable bifidobacteria on the fecal flora composition and pH of healthy full-term infants. J Pediatr Gastroenterol Nutr. 1995;21:177-181.

Lankaputhra WEV, Shah NP. Survival of *Lactobacillus acidophilus* and Bifidobacterium sp. in the presence of acid and bile salts. Cult Dairy Prod J. 1995;30:2-7

Ling WH, Korpela R, Mykkanen H et al. Lactobacillus strain GG supplementation decreases colonic hydrolytic and reductive enzyme activities in healthy female adults. J Nutr 1994;124:18-23.

Madsen KL. The use of probiotics in gastrointestinal disease. Can J Gastroenterol. 2001;15:817-822.

Majamaa H, Isolauri E, Saxelin M et al. Lactic acid bacteria in the treatment of acute rotavirus gastronenteritis. J Ped Gastrenterol Nutr. 1995;20:333-338.

Marteau P, Seksik P, Jian R. Priobiotics and health: New facts and ideas. Curr Opin Biotechnol. 2002;13:486-489.

Matteuzi D, Crociani F, Bridigi P. Antimicrobial susceptibility of Bifidobacterium. Ann Microbio (Paris)l. 1983;134A:339-349.

Mombelli B, Gismondo MR. The use of probiotics in medical practice. Int J Antimicrobiol Agents. 2000;16:531-536.

Niault M, Thomas F, Prost J, et al. Fungemia due to *Saccharomyces* species in a patient treated with enteral *Saccharomyces boulardii*. Clin Infect Dis. 1999;28:930.

Noh DO, Gilliland SE. Influence of bile on cellular integrity and beta-galactosidase activity of *Lactobacillus acidophilus*. J Dairy Sci. 1993;76:1253-1259.

Pahwa A, Mathur BN. Assessment of a bifidus containing infant formula. Part II. Implantation of *Bifidobacterium bifidum*. Indian J Dairy Sci. 1987;40:364-367.

Patel R, Cockerill FR, Porayko MK, et al. Lactobacillemia in liver transplant patients. Clin Infect Dis. 1994;18:207-212.

Pletincx M, Legein J, Vandenplas Y. Fungemia with *Saccharomyces boulardii* in a 1-year-old girl with protracted diarrhea. J Pediatr Gastroenterol. Nutr. 1995;21:113-115.

Pochart P, Marteau P, Bouchnik Y. Survival of bifidobacteria ingested via fermented milk during their passage through the human small intestine: An *in vivo* study using intestinal perfusion. Am J Clin Nutr. 1992;55:78-80.

Schlegel L, Lemerle S, Geslin P. *Lactobacillus* species as opportunistic pathogens in immunocompromised patients. Eur J Clin Microbiol Infect Dis. 1998;17:887-888.

Schrezenmeir J, de Vrese M. Probiotics, prebiotics, and synbiotics — approaching a definition. Am J Clin Nutr. 2001:361S-364S.

Shah NP, Lankaputhra WEV, Britz KL. Survival of *L. acidophilus* and *Bifidobacterium bifidum* in commercial yogurt during refrigerated storage. Int Dairy J. 1995;5:515-521.

Tuomola E, Crittenden R, Playne M, et al., Quality assurance criteria for probiotic bacteria. Am J Clin Nutr. 2001;73:393S-398S.

Chapter 10

It's Not A Typo
What are Prebiotics?

No, that's not a typo in the title of this chapter. I really meant to say *pre*biotics instead of *pro*biotics. What's the difference? That's what we are going to explore next.

Since diet is the main factor determining which bacteria live in our guts, it makes sense that the composition of gut normal flora can be modified through food — by changing our diet. Most intestinal bacteria get their energy from our left-overs. By that I mean, bacteria survive by metabolizing the sugars (carbohydrates) in our gastrointestinal tracts that we haven't used. These sugars come from undigested food residues and gastrointestinal mucus secretions. The quality and type of sugars available for bacterial use depend mostly upon the extent that the sugars don't get absorbed or used by upper portions of our own digestive tracts. Any unabsorbed and undigested sugars that reach the bacteria living in the lower portions of our intestines, are available to be metabolized and broken down by bacteria in a process called **fermentation**. Once sugars are broken down, the resulting products are primarily short chain fatty acids and gases, namely hydrogen and carbon dioxide.

What is a Prebiotic?

Specifically, a prebiotic is a non-digestible food ingredient that beneficially affects the host (us) by selectively stimulating growth and activity of specific bacteria in the intestinal tract. In other words, prebiotics are foods not for us, but for bacteria. Prebiotics stimulate growth of "good" bacteria in our digestive tracts.

By promoting growth of one or more species of "healthy" bacteria, the environment of the gastrointestinal tract naturally benefits.

Typically, bifidobacteria and lactobacilli are the genera that grow best when prebiotic foods are ingested. The selective growth advantage of these "healthy" bacteria can be deleterious to "harmful" bacteria like bacteroides and clostridia.

At the present time, several small sugars are under investigation for their roles as prebiotics. Although many sugars are considered "candidate" prebiotics for human use (See table 10-1), the two that have been most widely studied are inulin and fructooligosaccharides.

Possibly Useful Prebiotics	
Arabinogalactose	Palatinose
Fructooligosaccharides	Polydextrose
Inulin	Pyrodextrin
Isomatlooligosaccharides	Raftiline
Lacitol	Sorbitol
Lactulose	Soybean oligosaccharide
Manitol	Xylooligosaccharides/Xylitol
Oligomate	

Table 10-1. Compounds that may be useful as prebiotics. Of this list, inulin and fructooligosaccharides (FOS) have been most widely studied.

Criteria for a Prebiotic

Indigestible

In order for prebiotics to be effective, they must not be digested, not be broken down, in the harsh conditions of the digestive tract. This means prebiotics must reach the intestines — where the majority of bacteria reside — still intact. Therefore, prebiotics must be resistant to stomach acids, pancreatic enzymes, and digestive juices in the upper portions of the gastrointestinal tract.

Fermentation

Once prebiotics reach the large intestines, the sugars are fermented by bacteria (or broken down by chemical reactions) into relatively simple substances that serve as energy sources for bacterial growth. Interestingly, bacterial species differ in the types of sugars required for rapid growth. For example, early studies found that bifidobacteria grew well on fructose-type sugars, while lactobacilli, *Escherichia coli*, and *Clostridium perfringes* grew poorly on these sugars (Cummings et al., 2001).

It is now widely accepted that the sugars oligofructose and inulin selectively stimulate growth of bifidobacteria (Wang and Gibson., 1993). (By the way, the word in the previous sentence was *inulin*, not insulin. Insulin, is the hormone that lowers blood sugar. *Inulin* is a type of sugar that stimulates growth of friendly bacteria in the gut. Although the two words are spelled similarly, they are totally unrelated and have absolutely nothing to do with each other!) In turn, bifidobacteria inhibit growth of *Escherichia coli* and *Clostridium perfringes* — two potentially disease-causing microorganisms (Gibson et al., 1995; Wang and Gibson, 1993). Additionally, we now know that a naturally occurring sugar called raffinose stimulates growth of lactobacilli (Tortuero et al., 1997). From reading earlier chapters of this book, we recall that lactobacilli suppress growth of numerous disease-causing microorganisms by producing acids, peroxide, and specific bacteriocins.

The chemical structures of sugars are probably important determinants of whether or not different bacteria can use them as energy sources, but very few studies have addressed this yet. So far, only one study has extensively looked at the impact that different types of sugars — with different chemical structures — have on different strains of bacteria. From this analysis, it was determined that sugars with straight chemical structures were broken down by bacteria more easily than sugars with branched structures. Moreover, fructans were extensively fermented by most bacteria, but not by clostridial species (Cummings et al., 2001). What does this mean in practical terms? A person suffering from *Clostridium difficile* diarrhea would possibly benefit from large doses of fructose-based sugars, since these sugars act as a growth stimulus for "good" bacteria while simultaneously suppressing the growth and activities of "bad" bacteria. Clearly, though, more experimentation in this area is needed before any health claims can be promoted for fructose-based foods.

When sugars are digested by bacteria, the major products of this metabolism are short chain fatty acids and gases. As we learned in earlier chapters, specific short chain fatty acids such as acetic acid, propionic acid, and butyric acid have beneficial effects in the gut, specifically in controlling growth of unwanted disease-causing bacteria. Ingestion of prebiotics definitely increases acidic conditions in feces, which suppresses growth of harmful bacteria. Of the sugars examined so far, starch consistently produces the most butyric acid, while oligofructose and inulin are the lowest producers of butyric acid. Arabinogalatan and polydextrose produce propionic acid, while oligofructose produces mostly acetic acid (Cummings, 1995). So far, no distinguishing features have become evident, yet, to match a specific prebiotic with changes in short chain fatty acid production that yield particular health benefits. However, this avenue of research is only just beginning to be explored.

Unwanted Side Effects

Unfortunately, hydrogen and carbon dioxide, major byproducts of sugar fermentation, may also cause irritating side effects when prebiotics are ingested. These gases can cause abdominal pain, flatulence, belching, and bloating (Stone-Dorshow and Levitt, 1987; Pedersen et al., 1997).

Typically when sugars reach the large intestines in a non-digested form, a laxative effect is seen. However, evidence for this in human studies of prebiotics has been unclear. The few human studies carried out so far have not reported significant laxative effects. In fact, the majority of studies have not reported significant changes in stool habits at all (Bouchnik et al., 1997; Gibson et al,. 1995; Alles et al., 1996). However, in theory, since prebiotics stimulate microbial growth, stimulate peristaltic movements of the gut, and increase the amount of fecal matter passed, prebiotics are probably beneficial for folks that have difficulty with constipation (Marteau and Boutron-Ruault, 2002). However, the likelihood of an outright laxative effect from prebiotics is probably extremely small and not a problem for most people.

Clinical Trials

Hepatic encephalopathy

Prebiotics like lactulose are widely used already in the medical community and are superior to placebo for treating hepatic encephalopathy. Hepatic encephalopathy is a term that describes detrimental effects that liver failure has on the brain and central nervous system. Symptoms of hepatic encephalopathy can range from mild confusion to complete unresponsiveness or coma. This condition occurs when there are high levels of ammonia in the blood, a complication that develops as a consequence of liver failure. Ammonia is produced in the gastrointestinal tract by intestinal bacteria. Usually, it is the liver's job to detoxify ammonia from the blood stream. However, in folks with liver failure, toxic levels of ammonia build up in the blood.

Lactulose is a common prescription drug for folks with liver failure. Lactulose stimulates growth of "good" bacteria which produce short chain fatty acids. Acidic conditions in the colon tend to draw ammonia out of the bloodstream and into the colon, where ammonia is then converted into a more readily excretable form. Signs and symptoms of hepatic encephalopathy improve when the prescription prebiotic lactulose is used (Marteau and Boutron-Ruault et al., 2002).

Mineral absorption

Although not widely studied yet, there is limited scientific evidence that suggests prebiotics enhance absorption of calcium, and possibly magnesium, iron, and zinc (Scholz-Ahrens et al., 2001; For a more thorough review of animal and human studies, see Teitelbaum and Walker, 2002). Although the exact significance of this isn't clear at this time, enhanced vitamin and mineral absorption could be relevant for folks that have osteoporosis or anemia. Further studies are under way to determine whether prebiotics can reduce the risk of osteoporosis. One of the major risk factors for developing osteoporosis (brittle bones that break easily) is insufficient intake of dietary calcium. Early studies suggest that oligofructose, inulin, or lactulose may aid in absorption of calcium and other minerals.

Cardiovascular effects

In experimental laboratory rats, numerous studies have found that prebiotics reduce high cholesterol levels — specifically high triglycerides and high low density lipoproteins (LDL). Elevated triglyceride and LDL cholesterol levels are risk factors for developing heart disease or clogged arteries.

Whether or not prebiotics are beneficial in humans with high cholesterol is presently unclear. However, inulin does lower triglycerides in healthy human volunteers (Jackson et al.,1999; Williams, 1999). For example, when 54 healthy, middle-age patients were given either 10 grams of inulin or placebo for 8 weeks, there was a trend toward lower triglyceride values in those receiving inulin compared to placebo at the end of the study (Jackson et al., 1999).

In patients with non-insulin dependent diabetes mellitus — a group of people noted for having elevated cholesterol levels — 8 grams of fructooligosaccharides or placebo was given to study participants daily for 14 days. After two weeks, individuals ingesting fructooligosaccharides had significant reductions in blood sugar levels, total cholesterol, and LDL cholesterol while participants that received placebo had no changes in these parameters (Yamashita et al., 1984). In another study that evaluated patients with mild-to-moderately high cholesterol levels, patients received 18 grams of inulin daily for 6 weeks and then the same participants received placebo for 6 weeks. During the inulin phase of the study, patients had significant reductions in total and LDL cholesterol levels, but had no change in triglyceride levels (Davidson et al., 1998).

High triglyceride or LDL cholesterol levels are typically treated with cholesterol-lowering drugs like gemfibrozil (Lopid®) or atorvastatin (Lipitor®). Although these drugs are widely used, there are some risks associated with their use including liver damage and muscle breakdown. Future studies will be needed to determine whether sufficient doses of prebiotics can be given to lower triglyceride or LDL levels without causing serious adverse effects. If so, prebiotics may become an alternative to conventional medicine for treating high cholesterol.

Cancer

Another area for further research involves the role of inulin-type sugars in reducing the incidence of cancer. It is widely known that during digestion, numerous substances are produced in the gut that are potentially harmful to the body. Studies have shown in both human and animal experiments that consumption of bifidobacteria and lactobacilli dramatically reduces the generation of these harmful chemicals (Hudson and Marsh, 1995). Likewise, it makes sense that similar reductions in harmful toxins would be evident if prebiotics were ingested, since growth of **endogenous** bifidobacteria and lactobacilli (those already existing in the body) would increase.

In experimental conditions, numerous studies conducted in laboratory rats have observed that prebiotics like inulin are associated with a reduced likelihood of pre-cancerous, microscopic changes that occur prior to the onset of colon cancer. For example, a recent study compared the protective effects of inulin and oligofructose in mice exposed to various disease-causing microorganisms and tumor-inducers. In these experiments, there was a dramatic reduction in pre-cancerous colon changes in the group of mice that was fed inulin and oligofructose compared to animals that received placebo. Additionally, the prebiotics protected the mice against infections caused by *Candida, Listeria*, and *Salmonella* (Buddington et al., 2002).

Interestingly, when it comes to protecting against colon cancer, a combination of prebiotics and probiotics seems to have greater protective effects than either prebiotics or probiotics used alone (Reddy et al., 1997; Rowland et al., 1998). For example, in laboratory experiments, administration of *Bifidobacterium longum* (a *pro*biotic) decreased the incidence of pre-cancerous changes in rats' intestines by 26%, inulin (a *pre*biotic) reduced the incidence by 41%, but the combination of *Bifidobacterium longum* with inulin reduced the incidence of these changes by 80% (Rowland et al., 1998). Also, for unknown reasons, inulin appears to have a greater protective effect against colon cancer than oligofructose (Reddy et al., 1997). Other studies also support anti-cancer effects of prebiotics. For example, the growth of experimental tumors was reduced in mice fed non-digestible carbohydrates (15% inulin, oligofructose, or pectin) compared with mice receiving placebo (starch) (Taper et al., 1997).

Although the reasons for protective effects of prebiotics are unknown, there are several theories. For example, inulin stimulates changes in gastrointestinal mucus — changes that exert protective effects and are associated with a reduced risk of colon cancer (Fontaine et al., 1996). It is also possible that prebiotics stimulate protective enzymes in the gut (Treptow-van Lishaut et al., 1990). Additionally, it is clear that when wheat bran and other starches are fermented by probiotic bacteria, there is increased production of butyric acid in the gut. Research has consistently shown butyrate directly stimulates cell growth in normal cells, while simultaneously inhibiting growth of cancerous cells. In fact, in cancerous cells, butyrate may even trigger a programmed cell death, to prevent growth and spread of tumors (Hague et al., 1995; Marchetti et al., 1997). Another way butyric acid protects against intestinal damage is by stimulating increased production of protective enzymes in the gastrointestinal tract (glutathione transferase π) (Treptow-van Lishaut et al., 1990). Indeed, butyric acid is an important energy source for colon cells and its presence also protects from damage caused by harmful cancer-causing chemicals (Abrahamse et al., 1999). (For a more in-depth look at animal and human studies in this area, see Teitelbaum and Walker, 2002.)

Other

Studies in animals and humans suggest that prebiotics may also play promising roles in inflammatory bowel disease, prevention of gallstones, and prevention of gastrointestinal infections (Marteau and Boutron-Ruault, 2002). Clearly, more clinical trials are needed to determine the precise roles for prebiotics in human diseases.

How to Obtain Prebiotics

Fructooligosaccharides

In theory, it is possible to ingest sufficient amounts of prebiotics through dietary means alone. Numerous fruits and vegetables contain prebiotic sugars. Examples that you may find in the produce department of your grocery store include onions, garlic, leeks, chicory, bananas, asparagus, and Jerusalem artichokes. You may also note fructooligosaccharides (often referred to as FOS) on ingredient labels of common foods. Fructooligosaccharides are used for their thickening properties in items like bread and dairy products. However, for most of us eating a typical Western diet, we probably only get about 2 grams of fructooligosaccharides in our diet each day, which is considerably less than optimal. Research indicates that at least 4-8 grams of fructooligosaccharides are needed to significantly change gut flora for the good. And most clinical trials have used 10-15 grams. This is quite a large amount. When you consider that most prescription drugs are in *milligram* or even *microgram* quantities, 4-15 grams is a huge amount. As a result, the best way to ingest enough fructooligosaccharides to positively benefit your normal flora is probably through FOS-containing supplements — capsules and powders that are widely available in most health food stores — and some common vitamin supplements.

Lactulose

Another prebiotic, lactulose, is a prescription item available only in pharmacies. It is used medically as a treatment for severe liver disease. Lactulose helps to rid the body of dangerously high ammonia levels in the blood and prevents further complications. Lactulose is also sometimes prescribed as a treatment for constipation since it is associated with mild laxative effects.

Unfortunately, lactulose comes as a thick, gooey liquid, but it can be mixed with fruit juice or milk to improve its taste. It is a good idea to avoid using laxatives while using lactulose. And when lactulose is used regularly, on a long term basis, periodic blood work should be done to check your electrolyte and carbon dioxide levels to be certain that they are within normal limits.

Other

Common foods like wheat germ and honey, as well as exotic man-made sugars, are also currently under investigation as prebiotics.

Synbiotics

In order to maximize benefits from prebiotics, we need a better understanding of what these sugars do to the bacteria in our bodies. We need to know which are the best sugars for stimulating growth of individual bacterial species, what prebiotic doses are needed, and what numbers of "healthy" bacteria are needed for optimal health. The term *synbiotic* has recently been coined to refer to products that contain both prebiotics and probiotics. *Synbiotic* is correctly used *only* when referring to a product that contains a prebiotic sugar that selectively stimulates growth of the particular strains of probiotic bacteria also contained in the product.

An example of a synbiotic product is kefir (a drinkable yogurt containing several species of "healthy" bacteria) that contains fructooligosaccharides. In this case, the fructooligosaccharides serve as selective "foods" for the probiotic yogurt-bacteria. Although relatively new in the United States, these types of products are widespread throughout parts of Europe and the Middle East. As our knowledge expands, it is likely that a great many more synbiotic products will regularly be available on our supermarket shelves.

Conclusion

The European Commission responsible for studying non-digestible oligosaccharides in 1999 summed up our knowledge about prebiotics well when they indicated:

- there is strong evidence for prebiotic effects in humans,
- there is strong evidence that prebiotics have beneficial effects on bowel habits in humans,
- there is promising evidence that inulin may increase calcium absorption in humans,
- there is preliminary evidence that inulin may have beneficial effects on lipid levels,
- and there is preliminary evidence in experimental animals that prebiotics have preventative effects on colon cancer (Van Loo et al., 1999).

Although the study of prebiotics is a relatively new field, it is an area of research that is rapidly expanding. With all the positive health benefits that can be derived from prebiotics and probiotics, it is only a matter of time before synbiotics are commonplace in our diets.

Notes

Notes

References

Abrahamse SL, Pool-Zobel BL, Rechkemmer G. Potential of short chain fatty acids to modulate the induction of DNA damage and changes in the intracellular calcium concentration in isolated rat colon cells. Carcinogenesis. 1999;20:629-634.

Alles MS, Hautvast JGAJ, Nagengast FM, et al. Fate of fructo-oligosaccharides in the human intestine. Br J Nutr. 1996;76:211-221.

Bouhnik Y, Flourie B, D'Agay-Abensour, et al. Administration of transgalacto-oligosaccharides increases fecal bifidobacteria and modifies colonic fermentation metabolism in healthy humans. J Nutr. 1997;127:444-448.

Buddington KK, Donahoo JB, Buddington RK. Dietary oligofructose and inulin protect mice from enteric and systemic pathogens and tumor inducers. J Nutr. 2002;132:472-277.

Cummings JH, Macfarlane GT, Englyst HN, et al. Prebiotic digestion and fermentation. Am J Clin Nutr. 2001;73:415S-420S.

Cummings JH. Short chain fatty acids. In: Gibson GR, Macfarlane GT, eds. Human colonic bacteria: Role in nutrition, physiology, and pathology. Boca Raton, FL: CRC Press, 1995:101-130.

Davidson MH, Synecki C, Maki KC, et al. Effects of dietary inulin in serum lipids in men and women with hypercholesterolemia. Nutr Res. 1998;18:503-517.

Fontaine N, Meslin JC, Lory S, et al. Intestinal mucin distribution in the germ-free rat and in the heteroxenic rat harbouring a human bacterial flora: Effect of inulin in the diet. Br J Nutr. 1996;75:881-892.

Gibson GR, Beatty ER, Wang X, et al. Selective stimulation of bifidobacteria in the human colon by oligofructose and inulin. Gastroenterology. 1995;108:975-982.

Hague A, Elder DJE, Hicks DJ. Apoptosis in colorectal tumour cells: Induction by the short chain fatty acids butyrate, propionate, and acetate and by the bile salt deoxycholate. Int J Cancer. 1995;60:400-406.

Hudson MJ, Marsh D. Carbohydrate metabolism in the colon. In: Gibson GR, Macfarlane GT, eds. Human colonic bacteria: Role in nutrition, physiology and pathology. CRC Press, Inc., Boca Raton, FL, 1995.

Jackson KG, Taylor RJ, Clohessy AM, et al. The effect of the daily intake of inulin on fasting lipid, insulin, and glucose concentrations in middle-aged men and women. Br J Nutr. 1999;82:23-30.

Marchetti C, Migliorate G, Moraca R, et al. Deosycholic acid and SCFA-induced apoptosis in the human tumor cell-line HT-29 and possible mechanisms. Cancer Lett. 1997;114:97-99.

Marteau PR and Bourton-Ruaulat MC. Nutritional advantages of probiotics and prebiotics. Br J Nutr. 2002;87:S153-S157.

Pedersen A, Sandstrom B, Van Amelsvoort JMM. The effect of ingestion of inulin on blood lipids and gastrointestinal symptoms in healthy females. Br J Nutr. 1997;78:215-222.

Reddy BS, Hamid R, Rao CV. Effect of oligofructose on colonic preneoplastic aberrant crypt foci inhibition. Carcinogenesis. 1997;18:1371-1374.

Rowland IR, Rumney CJ, Coutts JT, et al. Effect of *Bifidobacterium longum* and inulin on gut bacterial metabolism and carcinogen-induced aberrant crypt foci in rats. Carcinogenesis. 1998;19:281-285.

Scholz-Ahrens KE, Schaafsma G, van den Heuvel EGHM, et al. Effects of prebiotics on mineral metabolism. Am J Clin Nutr. 2001;73:459S-464S.

Stone-Dorshow T and Levitt MD. Gaseous response to ingestion of a poorly absorbed fructooligosaccharide sweetener. Am J Clin Nutr. 1987;46:61-65.

Taper HS, Delzenne NM, Roberfroid MB, et al. Growth inhibition of transplantable mouse tumors by non-digestible carbohydrates. Int J Cancer. 1997;71:1109-1112.

Teitelbaum JE and Walker WA. Nutritional impact of pre-and probiotics as protective gastrointestinal organisms. Annu Rev Nutr. 2002;22:107-138.

Tortuero F, Fernandez E, Ruperez P, et al. Raffinose and lactic acid bacteria influence caecal fermentation and serum cholesterol in rats. Nutr Res. 1997;17:41-49.

Treptow-van Lishaut S, Rechkemmer G, Rowland IR, et al. The carbohydrate crystalean and colonic microflora modulate expression of glutathione S-transferase subunits in colon of rats. Eur J Nutr. 1999;38:76-83.

Van Loo J, Cummings J, Delzenne N, et al. Functional food properties of non-digestible oligosaccharides: A consensus report from the ENDO project (DGXII AIRII-CT94-1095). Br J Nutr. 1999;81:121-132.

Wang X, Gibson GR. Effects of the *in vitro* fermentation of oligofructose and inulin by bacteria growing in the human large intestine. J Appl Bacteriol. 1993;75:373-380.

Williams CM. Effects of inulin on lipid parameters in humans. J Nutr. 1999; 129:1471S-1473S.

Yamashita K, Kawai K, Itakura M. Effects of fructo-oligosaccharides on blood glucose and serum lipids in diabetic subjects. Nutr Res. 1984;4:961-966.

Chapter 11

What Next? Future Directions for Probiotics

From a goat herder eating his home-made yogurt in a tent in Tibet thousands of years ago to a cure for chronic, debilitating diseases today, probiotics have come a long way. What might the future hold for probiotics?

As we've seen from earlier chapters, there are huge volumes of data from hundreds of human studies supporting probiotics for treating diarrhea, inflammatory bowel disease, allergic conditions, and urogenital infections. Clearly, probiotics aren't just for the gut any more! Since we now recognize that probiotics modify the entire systemic immune system, researchers are beginning to move beyond the gastrointestinal tract to investigate probiotic protection at other sites.

The purpose of this chapter is to highlight some other medical fields that are currently evaluating the role of probiotics. The following information is based upon the use of probiotics in experimental animal models, human volunteers, or small studies using only handfuls of patients. At this point, there is only a limited amount of data supporting probiotics for the following medical conditions. However, research is on-going in these areas. Only as we continue to do research and acquire more data will we fully comprehend the potential that probiotics offer for treating these and other medical conditions.

Cancer Prevention

Colon Cancer

In industrialized societies, colon cancer is the second most common cause of cancer death (lung cancer is most common). According to data that has been gathered through animal studies, probiotic bacteria seem to play important roles in colon cancer prevention, possibly due to effects on metabolism, the immune system, or other protective mechanisms. Human studies evaluating correlations between consumption of fermented milk products and the risk of colon cancer have been contradictory; therefore, at this point, it is only an educated guess that probiotics may reduce the risk of tumors in the human large intestines. There are three proposed ways that probiotics could protect us from colon cancer: (1) probiotics may inhibit bacteria that convert dietary pre-carcinogens into carcinogens, (2) probiotics may inhibit tumor formation, and/or (3) probiotics may bind/inactivate carcinogens.

Chemicals known to be **carcinogens** are often administered to animals to evaluate tumor formation in the colon. Several experimental scenarios using this type of model system have found probiotics prevent carcinogen-induced tumors in animals. For example, even though rats were exposed to a carcinogen, administration of *Bifidobacterium longum* prevented pre-cancerous changes in their colons. Interestingly, combining lactulose — a prebiotic that stimulates growth of bifidobacteria (prebiotics are covered in chapter 10) — with *B. longum* provided even greater protection against the carcinogen than either *B. longum* or lactulose alone (Challa et al., 1997). Similar results have also been reported in experimental rats fed *Lactobacillus acidophilus*. Dietary supplementation with *Lactobacillus acidophilus* delayed the incidence of chemically-induced colon cancer, suggesting that probiotics interfere with initial stages of intestinal tumor formation (Goldin and Gorbach, 1980; Goldin et al., 1996). The protection that this probiotic offered was not complete, but rather the probiotic *delayed* onset of tumor formation in animals that had been administered an intestinal carcinogen (Goldin and Gorbach, 1980).

In order for colon cancer to develop, certain things must occur. First, certain key **genes** must develop **mutations**. These mutations allow cells to grow and multiply uncontrollably. Studies suggest that various strains of *Lactobacillus*, *Streptococcus*, *Lactococcus*, and

Bifidobacterium are capable of *preventing* mutations in human genes. The exact mechanisms by which this occurs is unknown, but it has been speculated that probiotics produce antioxidants, or prevent pro-carcinogens from being metabolized into carcinogens, or secrete enzymes that inactivate carcinogens (Bodana and Roa, 1990). Protection from a carcinogen's mutagenic activity seems to depend upon the number of live probiotic organisms ingested (Pool-Zobel et al., 1993; Pool-Zobel et al., 1996; Hosoda et al., 1992). It appears that a certain "threshold" or critical number of probiotic bacteria must be present to protect against the types of mutations that lead to tumor formation.

Another possible theory to explain protective effects of probiotic bacteria involves the idea that probiotics may "scavenge" mutation-causing metabolic products. Several studies have shown probiotic bacteria may literally bind to carcinogens, decreasing absorption of carcinogens into the blood stream and promoting elimination of carcinogens in feces (Orrhage et al., 1994; Morotomi et al., 1986; Zhang et al., 1991). Eating fried meats is known to cause a rather high likelihood of DNA damage, presumably due to the production of toxic by-products called heterocyclic amines. These by-products simply occur naturally during the cooking process. In one study, consumption of *Lactobacillus acidophilus* with fried meat reduced DNA damage in humans by 28% (Wollowski et al., 2001). Additionally, in several different experimental situations where beef extract and nitrosated beef extract were used as **mutagens**, *Lactobacillus casei* quite effectively prevented mutagenic effects normally caused by heterocyclic amines (Renner and Munzer, 1991).

Still another school-of-thought to explain colon cancer prevention with probiotics suggests that probiotics decrease activities of enzymes that normally activate carcinogens. Harmful and "healthy" bacteria differ in their enzymatic activities. For example, harmful bacteria such as clostridia and enterobacteria have high β-glucuronidase, nitroreductase, and azoreductase activities; these enzymes convert pro-carcinogens into direct-acting carcinogens. These enzymes may also be responsible for prolonging the activities of harmful cancer-causing agents, by retaining harmful compounds in the body. Additionally, some species of bacteria produce large amounts of ammonia, which can also be harmful if the body cannot detoxify it properly. In experimental rats, ingestion of bifidobacteria significantly decreases the activity of β-glucuronidase. Likewise, in healthy human volunteers, *Lactobacillus* GG lowers levels of harmful enzyme activities 2 to 4-fold (Goldin et al., 1992; Goldin and Gorbach, 1984). Additionally, it is of interest to note, in five healthy human volunteers receiving *Bifidobacterium longum* supplements, significant decreases in several clostridial strains were observed, as well as significant reductions in fecal ammonia concentrations and β-glucuronidase activity. [Keep in mind, clostridial species make up a large proportion of fecal microflora in patients with colon cancer (Benno et al., 1992).] Thus, since *Lactobacillus* GG and bifidobacteria lower the activities of enzymes that may activate carcinogens, there is speculation that probiotics may lower the risk of colon cancer, in part, by inhibiting harmful enzymatic activities. This would promote elimination of carcinogens from the body, rather than allowing the body to recycle and reabsorb toxic compounds (Goldin et al., 1992).

It is also possible that probiotic anti-carcinogenic effects may be related to increased production of short chain fatty acids (SCFA). In laboratory experiments, butyrate potently inhibits growth of colon cancer cells. Furthermore, both butyrate and propionate stimulate activities of an enzyme that acts as a detoxification system for potentially mutagenic compounds (glutathione *S*-transferase-π) (Stein et al., 1996).

Although animal studies have shown promising results suggesting that probiotics may slow or prevent mutations from arising that lead to colon cancer, future research is needed to determine whether these results translate into a role for probiotics as a preventative for human colon cancer. (For a more thorough review of both animal and human studies that have been conducted to date in this exciting area, see Teitelbaum and Walker, 2002.)

Cervical Cancer

Although radiation is the first-line treatment for uterine cervical cancer, it has limitations. Ideally, another therapy, perhaps a probiotic, to modulate the immune system locally could be added to radiation therapy to prevent spread, recurrence, and metastasis of the cancer.

A randomized, placebo-controlled clinical trial involving 228 women with late stage cervical cancer was carried out to evaluate whether heat-killed *Lactobacillus casei*, injected intradermally (under the skin) offered any benefits over radiation therapy alone. Specifically, researchers were curious to see if the probiotic could shrink the tumor or prolong survival more than radiation therapy alone. While there were no differences in tumor size when *Lactobacillus casei* was added to the treatment regimen, the 4-year survival rate was significantly longer in those who received the probiotic (69% versus 46%). Unexpectedly, women who received *Lactobacillus casei* were also less likely to experience low white blood cell counts (this is a limiting side effect of radiation therapy) compared to women who had radiation alone. The incidence of leukopenia was 26% in women getting lactobacilli injections versus 48% in those who received only radiation. Likewise, only 4% of those who had lactobacilli added to their therapy suffered from neutropenia versus 17% of the other women (Okawa et al., 1993).

Although injections of *Lactobacillus casei* improved survival, lengthened the time women were in remission, and were associated with a lower incidence of leukopenia and neutropenia, the injections did cause some discomfort for women. A few women developed a short-lived fever, others reported discomfort, pain, or irritation of the skin near the injection site. Since *Lactobacillus casei* appears to be a useful immunomodulator, it will be interesting for researchers to determine if it is beneficial in other types of cancer.

Other tumors and cancers: lung, bladder, leukemia

We've known since the 1960s that certain microorganisms stimulate the immune system and these immunostimulating effects may fight against certain types of cancers. In the early 1980s, several investigators experimentally caused various types of cancer to occur in mice, including sarcomas and leukemia. Of 28 different strains of lactobacilli selected for study, *Lactobacillus casei* had significant anti-tumor effects and inhibited tumor growth in mice. Investigators injected the probiotic (after killing the bacteria with heat) into the intraperitoneal cavity of mice either before or after tumors became established. Mice that received heat-killed *Lactobacillus casei* survived longer and had smaller tumors than mice that were not exposed to the probiotic. In this case, anti-tumor activity of the probiotic was due to enhanced activation of macrophages (Kato et al., 1981).

Several years later, a different group of researchers studied the efficacy of *Lactobacillus casei* in another mouse model of cancer — lung cancer and its associated metastasis into the plural cavity, which is the area surrounding the lungs. First, these investigators found that administering heat-killed *Lactobacillus casei* into the pleural cavity inhibits metastasis of lung cancer (Matsuzaki and Yokokura, 1987). Second, they noted that intrapleural injections of heat-killed *Lactobacillus casei* prolongs survival of mice (Matsuzaki et al., 1988). Again, in these studies the beneficial effects of *Lactobacillus casei* seems to be related, at least in part, to increased activation of macrophages, with their enhanced phagocytic functions and activation of other lethal white blood cells called natural killer cells, which release potent chemicals that kill tumor cells and infectious microbes.

Using another mouse model to study effects of *Lactobacillus casei* in cancer metastasis, some researchers evaluated whether the probiotic had beneficial effects in preventing cancer if the microorganisms were given to mice by mouth. In this situation, oral administration of live *Lactobacillus casei*, but not heat-inactivated *Lactobacillus casei,* suppressed growth of tumors and enhanced activities of the immune system. Therefore, even when given orally, *Lactobacillus casei* stimulates immune responses and acts as an immunomodulator, protecting against cancer (Kato et al., 1994).

More recently, attention has turned to investigating *Lactobacillus casei* in recurring bladder tumors. Even after surgical removal, bladder tumors often return. Approximately 50-80% of affected individuals will experience tumor recurrence. To assess this, *Lactobacillus casei* was administered into the bladders of experimental mice for 10 days, beginning on the same day that a tumor was implanted. The probiotic continued to be delivered the same way for a total of 10 days. There was a significant delay in time until tumors appeared, and tumors were smaller in mice that had received probiotics. These beneficial effects were due to activation of macrophages and increased release of specific cytokines: IFN-γ, TNF-α, and IL-12 (Takahashi et al., 2001). Activated macrophages directly release TNF-α and IL-12. These two cytokines help activate other white blood cells (specifically helper T cells) to release other anti-tumor cytokines like IFN-γ. Additionally TNF-α (an acronym for **t**umor **n**ecrosis **f**actor-α) directly causes tumor cells to die.

With all of the positive effects of *Lactobacillus casei* in various types of experimental cancers in mice, the probiotic was finally evaluated for efficacy in humans with cancer. The product used in a clinical trial was a probiotic preparation widely available in Japan. The product is called BLP® and is manufactured by Yakult Honsha Co Ltd.©, in Tokyo, Japan. BLP® has been available in Japan for more than 20 years. In a double-blind, placebo controlled trial of 138 patients who had undergone surgery to remove bladder cancer, live *Lactobacillus casei*, was administered orally. The probiotic prolonged the time until tumor returned by about 1.8-fold. Additionally, when tumors returned, they were not as severe as they had been previously (Aso et al., 1995).

Enzyme Deficiencies

Lactose intolerance

Another area of investigation for probiotic bacteria is in the area of lactose intolerance. Lactose intolerance occurs when levels of *lactase*, the enzyme that normally breaks down and metabolizes the sugar lactose, are too low. In primary lactose malabsorption, lactase activity decreases in childhood or adolescence, and symptoms of lactose intolerance become apparent in adulthood. On the other hand, secondary lactase insufficiency may result as a consequence of gut inflammation, sprue disease, or bacterial or parasitic infections.

Symptoms of lactose intolerance occur any time folks that don't produce adequate amounts of lactase, consume milk or other lactose-containing products. While the condition is not serious, symptoms of diarrhea, abdominal cramping or pain, bloating, and gas occur within 30 minutes to 2 hours after eating or drinking food that contains lactose. These symptoms are often quite distressing to patients. Most lactose-intolerant individuals still produce *some* lactase. The varying amounts of lactase produced by different affected individuals explains why one person cannot drink even half a glass of milk without experiencing symptoms, while another person may drink one or two glasses, but not three.

Lactose intolerance is easily diagnosed in a doctor's office in several different ways. One diagnostic test monitors blood sugar levels. People with normal levels of lactase, break lactose down into the sugars glucose and galactose. The liver further breaks down galactose to glucose. Glucose is then absorbed into the blood stream, and under normal conditions, the amount of glucose in the blood stream rises. Blood glucose, of course, can be easily measured. On the other hand, those that don't produce sufficient amounts of lactase, have no increase in blood sugar levels after ingesting lactose since they are unable to metabolize the sugar.

Another diagnostic test used to identify lactose intolerance involves breath samples. When lactose is not broken down in the intestines by lactase, gut bacteria begin to metabolize the sugar. In the process of lactose fermentation, hydrogen is produced. Hydrogen is a gas that is detectable in the breath. Since, normal individuals do not have any hydrogen detected in their breath, the presence of hydrogen in breath samples is another way to diagnose lactose intolerance.

A third method to diagnose lactose intolerance involves collection of stool samples. Undigested lactose that is fermented by bacteria in the colon creates lactic acid and other short chain fatty acids as by-products. These metabolic break-down compounds can be identified in stool samples.

Typically, the advice given to lactose intolerant individuals focuses on avoiding food that contains lactose. However, this is easier said by the doctor than done by the patient. Although milk and milk-products are obvious sources of lactose, lactose is also found in processed breakfast cereals, instant potatoes and soups, margarine, lunch meats, salad dressings, candies, and boxed mixes for pancakes or cookies. Some "nondairy" products like coffee creamers also contain lactose. Additionally, most people don't realize that 20% of prescription drugs and 6% of over-the-counter medicines also contain lactose. So, without reading all the ingredients on every food or drug label, it is unlikely that lactose-intolerant individuals will be successful at sticking to a strict lactose-free diet.

For those who experience adverse effects to even very small amounts of lactose, lactase enzyme supplements are available to digest food more easily. Additionally, recent research shows that yogurt containing live and active bacterial cultures may be a good source of the lactase enzyme. Of course, this seems contradictory since yogurt is fairly high in lactose. However, evidence shows that bacterial cultures used to manufacture yogurt produce large amounts of lactase — the "missing" enzyme needed for appropriate lactose digestion.

Numerous studies in humans have found better lactose digestion and less hydrogen in the breath of lactose intolerant people after consuming yogurt versus milk (for a review of 13 more studies, please refer to de Vrese et al., 2001), but the reasons for this are not entirely clear. However, in theory, the probiotic bacteria in yogurt produce their own lactase enzyme and improve lactose digestion in this way (Marteau et al., 2001).

The effects of non-yogurt probiotic bacteria in lactose intolerance are not entirely clear, but at this point 10 studies (de Vrese et al., 2001) have examined the effects of various bacteria including *Streptococcus thermophilus, Lactobacillus bulgaricus, Bifidobacterium bifidum, Lactobacillus acidophilus, Lactobacillus casei, Lactobacillus lactis,* and *Bifidobacterium longum* in lactose digestion. Each of these bacterial strains improves lactose digestion more than milk (as evaluated by decreased hydrogen exhalation) but these probiotic supplements were not as effective as yogurt. While it is safe to say that probiotic bacteria *may* improve symptoms caused by undigested lactose, it is also necessary to point out that this is an area that has barely begun to be studied and is still in its infancy.

Sucrase-isomaltase deficiency

Sucrase-isomaltase deficiency is an inherited condition associated with certain genetic mutations, which impairs sucrose absorption. Accumulation of sucrose in the intestines causes diarrhea, abdominal cramps, and bloating. One study described the benefits of *Saccharomyces cerevisiae* (fresh baker's yeast) in eight children affected by this condition. It seems that this yeast strain may be capable of supplying the missing enzyme, thus preventing uncomfortable abdominal symptoms (Harms et al., 1987).

Gastrointestinal disorders

Short bowel syndrome

Another possible use for probiotics may be in management of short bowel syndrome. Short bowel syndrome occurs whenever the functions of the small bowel have been compromised, either by disease or by surgery. Unfortunately, short bowel syndrome is associated with many problems including weight loss, diarrhea, abdominal bloating, fatigue, and passage of intestinal bacteria to other parts of the body (bacterial translocation). The latter often causes infection and death and is probably due, in part, to lack of intestinal peristalsis, bacterial overgrowth in the intestines, loss of gut-associated lymph tissues, and degeneration of the mucosal layer of the intestines (Eizaguirre et al., 2002).

Experimentally, rats with 80% of their small intestines surgically removed, serve as model systems for studying short bowel syndrome. In rats lacking most of their small intestines, those that received probiotic supplementation with *Bifidobacterium lactis* fared better overall. The probiotic group of rats gained more weight; and fewer gut bacteria migrated out of the intestines to cause infection at other body sites (the probiotic reduced the risk of bacterial translocation by 43% and 1/3 avoided bacterial translocation all together) (Eizaguirre et al., 2002). This preliminary animal data suggests probiotics may significantly lower the risk of adverse effects in those affected by this condition.

Irritable bowel syndrome

Irritable bowel syndrome (IBS) is a chronic disorder in which bowel habits are altered. IBS occurs twice as often in women than men and is often associated with psychiatric disorders like anxiety. Some patients with irritable bowel syndrome suffer from constipation-predominant IBS, while others experience diarrhea-predominant IBS, and others alternate back and forth between the two extremes.

Those with constipation-predominant IBS complain of recurrent abdominal pain and cramping, bloating after meals, relief from abdominal symptoms after having a bowel movement, the sensation that there is still stool that needs to be passed immediately after a bowel movement, and sometimes mucus in their stools. On the other hand, diarrhea-predominant IBS is associated with cramping pain, diarrhea, bloating, explosive stools, incontinence, and rectal bleeding.

High fiber diets, exercise, and fluids are often recommended for treatment of IBS, despite that fact that these things rarely help. Sometimes, drugs that alleviate abdominal cramping, by slowing down gut motility, are prescribed by physicians for diarrhea-predominant IBS. In IBS, the problem is not lack of dietary fiber, inactivity, or lack of water. Quite frankly, fiber can worsen symptoms in some folks since it causes flatulence and can aggravate bloating.

Recently, bacterial infection and intestinal inflammation have been suggested as possible causes of IBS. Consistent with this notion are several facts: (1) antibiotics like metronidazole and vancomycin transiently suppress IBS symptoms, (2) IBS, especially constipation-predominant IBS, is often a hospital-acquired problem, (3) certain bacterial species (such as clostridia or enterobacteria) produce large volumes of gas and cause bloating, and (4) IBS symptoms can be reversed by using human probiotic infusions (Dr. Thomas Borody, personal communication; Andrews and Borody, 1993).

Intestinal colonization by strains like *Lactobacillus plantarum* has been associated with elimination of gas and eradication of gas-producing bacterial strains in healthy volunteers (Johansson et al., 1993). More and more, data is suggesting that those with irritable bowel syndrome may have an overgrowth of bacteria in their small intestines. Use of antibiotics (Pimentel et al., 2000) or better yet, probiotics (Nobaek et al., 2000; Niedzielin et al., 2001; Halpern et al., 1996) frequently alleviates abdominal discomfort and can even lead to a complete remission of symptoms for some folks with IBS.

According to Dr. Thomas Borody, director of the Centre for Digestive Diseases and the Probiotic Research Centre in Sydney, Australia, "Of 670 patients that we have treated with human probiotic infusions, more than 50% of them were IBS patients. IBS infection is due to some form of clostridia. How do we know this? Because they get well when they are treated with vancomycin, but IBS comes back as soon as the drug stops. Human probiotic infusions are *curative* more than 50% of the time."

Of course, what Dr. Borody refers to as a "human probiotic infusion" is replacement of the entire gastrointestinal flora by a series of fecal enemas from healthy donors. Typically, this process is carried out following a short course of antibiotics that reduce the amount of bacteria in the intestines. Remaining flora is then removed by potently flushing out the intestines (with drugs similar to those used prior to a colonoscopy), and bowel flora is replaced with a series of fecal enemas. The "healthy" new flora contains microorganisms that are capable of eliminating clostridial spores. This treatment has major advantages over other treatments, first of all, *because it is curative*! Additionally, this procedure alleviates motor dysfunction, fermentative disturbances, and peristaltic abnormalities (delayed gastric emptying), bloating, nausea, **dysphagia**, and even chronic fatigue (Probiotic Therapy Research Centre).

If you aren't quite ready for the human probiotic infusion approach, perhaps oral probiotics will work for you. However, Dr. Borody cautions you to be aware that commercially-available oral probiotics are not capable of implanting permanently in the gut because they lose their ability to adhere to epithelial cells through the culturing process in commercial laboratories. Only fresh human probiotics from another human being retain that capability and can implant long term. On the other hand, if you are prepared to continue taking oral probiotics on a long-term basis, then commercial probiotics may work just fine.

Here are summaries of some of the latest studies:

> In a double-blind, placebo-controlled study, a group of 60 patients with IBS were given either *Lactobacillus plantarum* 299v or placebo for 4 weeks. During the study, abdominal pain and gas cleared up significantly for those receiving the probiotic; furthermore, for up to a year after participating in this study, patients assigned to the probiotic group reported better overall gastrointestinal function than the placebo group (Nobaek et al., 2000).

> Another small human trial evaluated *Lactobacillus* or placebo in 29 patients with IBS over a period of 12 weeks. Criteria examined were abdominal pain, bloating or gas, daily number of stools, consistency of stools, mucus content of stools, and general physical state. Every patient received both *Lactobacillus acidophilus* for six weeks and placebo for six weeks. However, neither doctors nor patients knew which treatment was administered during either phase of the study. During the trial, patients were asked to keep track of their symptoms on a daily basis. When the data was analyzed, there was a significant therapeutic benefit — assessed by reduction of gastrointestinal symptoms — for 50% of patients while they received *Lactobacillus* compared to when they consumed placebo (Halpern et al., 1996).

> A recent randomized, double-blind placebo-controlled trial of 40 patients with IBS also reported symptomatic improvement in 95% of those receiving *Lactobacillus plantarum* versus 15% in the placebo group (Niedzielin et al., 2001). All patients receiving the probiotic reported improvement in abdominal pain and there was also a trend towards improvement in constipation.

> In another study, 19 women with IBS completed a double-blind cross-over trial in which they received supplements of *Lactobacillus casei* GG. Although there were no significant differences in abdominal pain or bloating when these women took the probiotic, there was a tendency towards less diarrhea, suggesting that this particular probiotic strain may be most beneficial for patients with diarrhea-predominant IBS (O'Sullivan and O'Morain, 2000).

Additionally, as I was writing this chapter, a press release was issued from The BioBalance Corporation©, regarding their probiotic which goes by the trade name of Probactrix®. Probactrix® contains *Escherichia coli* strain M17. The results of a recent randomized, double-blind, placebo-controlled clinical trial using Probactrix® in 20 IBS patients, who experienced severe symptoms of diarrhea and constipation for an average of 8 years, were reported. During the clinical trial, 10 patients who started the trial on placebo dropped out of the study because of continuing symptoms, as opposed to 10 patients who started the trial on *Escherichia coli* M17 and completed the study. Those that received the probiotic experienced substantial improvements in their bowel movements, had less mucus in their stools, and required less straining during defecation. This small pilot study provides compelling evidence for this probiotic that is already available in Israel and Russia.

Constipation

Since some studies report dramatic improvements in constipation and easier stool passage after antibiotic therapy (Celik et al., 1995; Borody et al., 1989) or probiotic therapy (Andrews et al., 1992; Mollenbrink and Bruckschen, 1994; Kasper, 1998; Andrews and Borody, 1993), it stands to reason that modification of gut flora may be of value in treating constipation if no obvious reasons for it can be identified. By altering gut flora, constipation has been alleviated in individuals of all ages, from children to geriatric patients (Borody et al, 1989; Kasper, 1998).

A few clinical trials have formally evaluated probiotics as treatments for constipation.

> One study, conducted more than a decade ago in constipated individuals, used fecal enemas to treat constipation. (For some participants in this study, constipation was related to

irritable bowel disease.) This somewhat "distasteful" therapy was used for 33 patients with chronic constipation. Twenty-five patients, or 76%, experienced significant improvement following therapy and none of them required further laxatives to treat constipation (Andrews and Borody, 1993).

Another study used *Escherichia coli* Nissle 1917 strain in 134 patients who had suffered from constipation for an average of 19 years. After 4 weeks of therapy, patients receiving the probiotic were passing almost 5 stools per week compared to less than 3 stools per week for the placebo group. By the 8th week of treatment, those receiving the probiotic were passing 6 stools per week while those taking placebo passed fewer than 2 stools per week (Mollenbrink and Bruckschen, 1994).

Positive results were also obtained from a double-blind crossover study in which 50 constipated patients received 3 grams (300 billion organisms) of *Lactobacillus casei* daily for 30 days. The overall response rate to probiotic therapy was 67% (Kasper, 1998).

Diverticulitis

Diverticulitis is inflammation of the diverticula, which are small pouches that form at weak spots in the intestinal tract. In these small sacs, bacteria often overgrow, causing infection and abdominal pain. Almost always, diverticulitis is associated with either diarrhea or constipation. Some folks with diverticulitis require almost constant therapy with antibiotics to suppress growth of bacteria within these inflamed pouches. Bacteria also frequently cause excessive gas production which causes bloating and enlarges the abdomen. The constant bloated feeling often causes folks to stop eating, which can, of course, lead to malnutrition. Additionally, just the overgrowth of bacteria robs the body of nutrients and contributes to malnutrition by causing malabsorption.

At the present time, there is only one study examining the efficacy of probiotics in treating diverticulitis. In 79 patients treated first with an antibiotic, followed by lactobacilli for 12 months, this regimen controlled gastrointestinal symptoms and prevented complications associated with diverticulitis, including bacterial infections in the blood. Thus, it is likely that probiotics may be effective, safe, and well-tolerated in those with diverticular disease (Giaccari et al., 1993).

Small bowel overgrowth

Bacteria can overgrow in the small intestines for many reasons, including motility disorders and diverticulitis. Unfortunately, symptoms associated with overgrowth are frequently chronic with numerous relapses. Preliminary studies suggest a possible role for *Lactobacillus plantarum* and *Lactobacillus* GG in individuals whose symptoms fail to resolve after typical antimicrobial measures (Vanderhoof et al., 1998).

Peptic ulcer disease

Within the past decade, it has become widely accepted that a bacterium called *Helicobacter pylori* (*H. pylori*) is the cause of gastric ulcers — nearly 100% of the time. Treatment of gastric ulcers commonly consists of a combination of 3-4 drugs — regimens that consist of both acid-suppressing drugs and several antibiotics. However, these regimens are not without problems including bloating, nausea, diarrhea, and taste disturbances.

Within the past few years, investigators have begun to focus their attention on probiotics as possible treatments for eliminating *H. pylori*. Because lactobacilli strains are among the few organisms that can survive high concentrations of acid, this genus has been the most widely studied. As early as 1996, scientific investigators realized that lactobacilli and bifidobacteria inhibit ulcer formation (Uejima et al., 1996). A few years later, it was also demonstrated that lactobacilli suppress *H. pylori* growth (Aiba et al., 1998).

It is suspected that production of large amounts of acetic acid may be responsible for lactobacilli's ability to suppress *H. pylori*. Investigators also compared 17 different strains of lactobacilli to see if any species could eliminate *H. pylori* entirely. One specific strain of *Lactobacillus acidophilus* — strain CRL639 — not only *inhibited* growth of *H. pylori*, but also out-right *killed* all *H. pylori* within 48 hours of exposure (Lorca et al., 2001). This effect was probably mediated by release of a specific toxin produced by strain CRL639. Similar results have been obtained by other investigators using various strains of *Lactobacillus*. Three different probiotics all obtained from Natren, Inc.©, *Lactobacillus delbruckii* subspecies *bulgaricus* strain LB-51, *Lactobacillus acidophilus* strain NAS, and *Lactobacillus acidophilus* strain DDS-1 were tested in a laboratory for their ability to inhibit growth of *H. pylori*. All three lactobacilli strains inhibited *H. pylori*, but the NAS strain inhibited it best (Rasic et al., 1995). As a result of these initial laboratory studies, 15 patients with *H. pylori* gastritis entered into a 2 month study in which they were given *Lactobacillus acidophilus* strain NAS. Of 14 patients who completed the study, *H. pylori* was completely eradicated in 6 of them (Mrda et al., 1998)!

Other researchers have also determined that some strains of *Lactobacillus reuteri* may inhibit *H. pylori* activities by preventing the ulcer-forming bacterium from binding to epithelial cells in the gut. Use of probiotics containing *Lactobacillus reuteri* may prevent or aid in elimination of *H. pylori* infection (Mukai et al., 2002).

So far, a study in 29 humans found consumption of the probiotic *Lactobacillus gasseri* (LG21) provided significant relief from colonization with *H. pylori* since it suppressed *H. pylori* growth and reduced gastric inflammation (Sakamoto et al., 2001). Additionally, several studies have demonstrated that combining probiotic therapy such as *Lactobacillus* GG with the usual multi-drug regimens for eliminating *H. pylori* infection resulted in a lower incidence of side effects — bloating, nausea, diarrhea, and taste disturbances (Cremonini et al., 2002). This is important because the side effects associated with multi-drug regimens can cause people to stop taking their drugs too soon, leading to ulcer reoccurrence. Furthermore, addition of *Lactobacillus* GG to multi-drug combinations also significantly increases the likelihood that *H. pylori* will be completely eliminated from the gut (Armuzzi et al., 2001a; Armuzzi et al., 2001b; Canducci et al., 2000; Sheu et al., 2002). (For a review, clinicians should see Marteau et al., 2002.)

Cardiovascular disease

Reduce risk of blood clotting and lower high cholesterol

Although cholesterol is essential for many different body functions, too much cholesterol contributes to clogged arteries and leads to **cardiovascular** diseases. Cholesterol is a precursor that is essential for production of hormones and bile acids. Our bodies either obtain cholesterol from dietary sources, or manufacture it in the liver. Although bile acids are made in the liver and stored in the gall bladder, these acids are ultimately dumped into the gastrointestinal tract, where they can be excreted in feces, or — if certain bacteria are present — gut flora chemically modifies bile acids, recycles them and converts the acids back into cholesterol.

Lactobacilli may modify metabolic pathways of cholesterol in the gut and reduce the risk of heart disease, by preventing blood clots and clogged arteries. In laboratory experiments, *Lactobacillus reuteri* and *Lactobacillus johnsonii* reduced blood cholesterol levels in mice, rats, and pigs (Mombelli and Gismondo, 2000). However, experiments in humans haven't been quite as convincing (for a complete review, see Teitelbaum and Walker, 2002).

The only positive study reported in humans so far involved a 6 week trial conducted in a group of Polish men with moderately elevated cholesterol levels. *Lactobacillus plantarum* 299v significantly reduced both LDL ("bad") cholesterol levels as well as fibrinogen — a protein suspected to increase the risk of blood clots (Bukowska et al., 1998). It is believed that enzymes produced by *Lactobacillus plantarum* prevent cholesterol precursors (bile salts) in the gut from being reabsorbed into the blood stream. This study is one of the first to indicate that probiotics may play a role in preventing coronary artery disease. However, these data should be considered very preliminary.

High blood pressure

High blood pressure, also known as hypertension, is a major risk factor for heart attacks and strokes. The big pharmaceutical companies manufacture hundreds of different drugs aimed at lowering blood pressure. These drugs, available by prescription only, are effective and work by many different ways to bring blood pressure down to an acceptable level.

Some of the most potent, well known antihypertensive drugs lower blood pressure by inhibiting the activities of an enzyme known fondly as ACE. ACE is an acronym that stands for **a**ngiotensin **c**onverting **e**nzyme. This enzyme plays a major role in regulation of blood pressure. Drugs that inhibit ACE have been clearly shown to not only lower blood pressure, but also to reduce the size of enlarged (overworked) hearts and reduce mortality.

Recently, fermented milk products have been noticed to lower blood pressure in both hypertensive rats (Yamamoto et al., 1994) and humans (Hata et al., 1996). Interestingly, some strains of probiotics produce their own ACE-inhibiting substances during the fermentation process.

Although most bacteria that produce lactic acid produce ACE inhibitors during milk fermentation, out of 26 different strains that were tested, *Lactobacillus helveticus* was identified as the most effective. However, it is important to note, compared to the blood pressure lowering effects of prescription ACE inhibitors, the magnitude of ACE inhibition with probiotics is really quite low. Perhaps for some individuals with mild hypertension who are intolerant of side effects associated with prescription drugs, fermented milk products may be an acceptable form of antihypertensive therapy (Fuglsang et al., 2003).

Dental Caries (Cavities)

Lactobacilli suppress growth of many bacteria in the mouth including mutans streptococci, a species known to contribute to dental cavities. A study was carried out in 594 children attending daycare to determine whether supplementing milk with *Lactobacillus rhamnosus* GG would affect the number of dental caries these children experienced during a 7 month period compared to children who drank normal milk. During the study, neither the children nor the dentists knew which group of children was drinking the probiotic-supplemented milk. At the end of the study, there were significantly fewer dental caries in the probiotic-treatment group, as well as significantly less mutans streptococci. Thus, *Lactobacillus rhamnosus* GG reduced the risk of dental caries, presumably by suppressing the growth of this particular streptococcal species. Beneficial effects were particularly dramatic for three and four year old children (Nase et al., 2001).

Chronic Kidney Failure

Chronic kidney failure is often accompanied by bacterial overgrowth in the small intestine known as small bowel bacterial overgrowth (SBBO). SBBO causes high concentrations of toxic compounds (including dimethylamine and nitrosodimethylamine) to accumulate in the blood stream. This condition begins when kidney function falls below 20% and worsens as kidney function declines. By the time kidney function reaches 5%, patients are forced to begin dialysis to remove toxins and fluids that accumulate. At this point, SBBO is well-established and not reversible by dialysis alone. Although the direct cause of SBBO is unknown, results from human studies have found various strains of

Lactobacillus acidophilus sufficiently restore gut normal flora, reduce concentrations of toxins in the blood stream, and greatly improve the quality of life for patients with kidney disease (Dunn et al., 1998).

Hepatic Encephalopathy

Hepatic encephalopathy is a term that describes the detrimental effects that liver failure has on the brain and the entire central nervous system. Symptoms of hepatic encephalopathy can range from mild confusion to complete unresponsiveness or coma. This condition occurs when there are high levels of ammonia in the blood, a complication that develops as a consequence of liver failure.

Ammonia is produced in the gastrointestinal tract by intestinal bacteria. Usually, it is the liver's job to detoxify ammonia from the blood stream. However, in folks with liver failure, toxic levels of ammonia build up in the blood. Some researchers have found *Lactobacillus acidophilus* and *Enterococcus* decrease activities of the bacteria that produce ammonia in the gut. These bacteria do this, possibly, by producing short chain fatty acids. Acidic intestinal conditions are beneficial not only because growth of harmful bacteria is suppressed, but also because acids tend to draw ammonia out of the bloodstream and into the colon, where ammonia is then converted into a more readily excretable form. Probiotics lower ammonia levels in the blood and improve mental status of patients suffering from liver failure (Loguercio et al., 1987; Rolfe, 2000).

Autism

Another area where probiotics may exert a positive influence over a central nervous system disorder is the treatment of autism. Autism is a devastating and largely untreatable disorder. It is usually diagnosed in children prior to the age of 2 1/2 years. Children with autism have severe difficulties in communication, forming relationships with people, developing language, and understanding abstract concepts. Repetitive and limited patterns of behavior, marked by obsessive resistance to miniscule changes in familiar surroundings, are also features of this disorder. The obvious question probably going through your head right now is "How in the world could this psychiatric disorder possibly be related to abnormal bacteria in the gut?"

After several parents reported to researchers that their children were normal and met typical developmental milestones until given a prolonged course of antibiotics near the age of 18 months, a theory was born. Some have surmised that prolonged or repeated use of antibiotics could disrupt the normal gastrointestinal microorganisms, allowing colonization by a bacterial strain that secretes neurotoxins. No specific bacteria have been implicated, although *Clostridium tetani* (tetanus), *Clostridium botulinum* (botulism poisoning) and *Clostridium difficile* have all been suggested as possibilities. According to Dr. Thomas Borody at the Probiotic Therapy Research Centre in Sydney, Australia, "Autism becomes apparent in children around the ages of 18-24 months after they have used antibiotics." Borody and others believe autistic symptoms occur when a neurotoxin, the toxin produced by *Clostridium tetani* (this is the microorganism that causes tetanus), is produced by bacteria in the gut and travels up the vagal nerve to the temporal lobe of the brain. The temporal lobe is a "speech" center in the brain. According to Borody, "Imaging studies show less blood flow to the temporal lobe in autism."

If it is true that bacterial toxins cause autism, then perhaps appropriate antimicrobial therapy could reduce autistic symptoms. Indeed, at least one group of researchers have identified gut bacterial imbalances in children with autism (Sandler et al., 2000). Additionally, appropriate antibiotic therapy (directed towards difficult-to-eradicate clostridial species) improved autistic behaviors in several children *while taking antibiotics*, only to regress within two weeks of stopping antimicrobial therapy (Sandler et al., 2000). This is consistent with spore-forming bacteria that survive during antibiotic therapy, only to germinate and begin growing again once antibiotics have been stopped.

Further studies also confirm the clostridium-autism association. When fecal flora of children with autism was compared with that of normal children, clostridial counts were higher in the autistic children. In fact, children with autism had 9 species of *Clostridium* in their intestines that aren't even found in healthy children. Additionally, fecal flora from autistic children contained substantial numbers of spore-forming anaerobes and microaerophilic bacteria, whereas there was a complete absence of these bacterial types in healthy children (Finegold et al., 2002). This is where appropriate selection of probiotics might be useful. At least in theory, some probiotic regimens may be able to correct underlying bacterial imbalances and improve outcomes for autistic children.

In a few instances, Dr. Borody's method of human probiotic infusions has been helpful for some autistic children. Borody kindly shared some of the details with me. One child, supplemented with 18 different laboratory-grown bacteria and oral probiotics went from speaking only 20 words to speaking over 800 words in a matter of weeks. Another 7 year old autistic child had major behavioral issues; he used to scream and shriek and was completely out of control. His mother has been giving him fecal enemas periodically —probably 17 or 18 so far — and his behavior has completely resolved. According to Dr. Borody, "This child has completely normal behavior now, but missed a lot during the past 6 years. He still has a lot to learn."

Immune Enhancement

Immunizations

Since, as we know, probiotics modify immune responses, it has been suggested that a dose of oral probiotics taken simultaneously with vaccinations would enhance the immune system's response to vaccinations. Initial experiments in human infants seem to support this notion. *Lactobacillus* GG did, in fact, increase the immune system's antibody response to oral vaccination with a rotavirus vaccine. These results suggest that *Lactobacillus* GG might also have the potential to increase immune responses to other oral vaccinations, such as the poliovirus vaccine (Isolauri et al., 1995).

Respiratory tract infection prevention

The bulk of investigation regarding probiotic benefits in preventing respiratory infections has focused on experimental animal models. For obvious ethical reasons, it isn't acceptable to intentionally cause a respiratory infection in humans. Researchers have found that orally administered *Lactobacillus casei* in mice prevents respiratory infections caused by a bacterium known as *Pseudomonas aeruginosa*. This bacterium is especially problematic for children with cystic fibrosis. Lactobacilli protect against pseudomonal infections by nonspecifically stimulating activities of the immune system (Alvarez et al., 2001).

In a human study, 571 children aged one to six years who attended daycare participated in a clinical trial to determine whether lactobacilli supplements reduced the frequency of respiratory infections. For these children, milk was supplemented with either placebo or *Lactobacillus* GG. Over a period of seven months, children who consumed the probiotic experienced significantly fewer respiratory infections (Hatakka et al., 2001) and the infections that they did get were less severe compared to children who did not receive probiotic supplementation.

Ecoimmunonutrition

Recently, a group of Swedish scientists developed an **enteral** nutrition formula obtained by fermentation of *Lactobacillus plantarum*. Scientists are referring to this as a product that provides ecoimmunonutrition. The goal of such a product is to non-specifically stimulate the immune system, while simultaneously providing balanced nutrition. Potential reasons to use such a product are: major surgery, trauma, liver or pancreatic disease, multiple organ failure, prematurity in infants, radiation therapy, antibiotic therapy, cancer, HIV, inflammatory bowel disease, old age, etc. (See Bengmark 1998, for a complete list). So far, data suggest that this formula stimulates gut immunity and prevents infections (Bengmark, 1998).

Rheumatoid arthritis

Rheumatoid arthritis is another area currently being explored to determine whether or not probiotic microorganisms may have positive effects. As you may be aware, rheumatoid arthritis is an autoimmune disease, meaning the immune system actually starts making antibodies that attack "self" rather than targeting foreign invaders. In rheumatoid arthritis, the normal and necessary proteins of the body's joints are suddenly recognized as "foreign invaders" and are attacked!

The immune system's inflammatory pathways are critical for initiation and development of rheumatoid arthritis. As long ago as 1968, researchers in Sweden noted two-thirds of patients with rheumatoid arthritis had abnormal gut flora, some of them having large numbers of disease-causing *Clostridium perfringes* in their intestines. In fact, these researchers mentioned that, even back then, it was known that up to 20% of people with intestinal inflammation or colitis, also suffer from arthritis. These ideas led to the drastic, but sometimes successful, practice of curing rheumatoid arthritis by *removing the colon.* (Olhagen and Mansson, 1968).

If you think surgical removal of your large intestines seems like a bit of overkill for treating rheumatoid arthritis, perhaps probiotics are more your style. Recently, in experimental mice with arthritis, oral administration of *Lactobacillus casei* strain Shirota reduced the incidence and progression of arthritis. The probiotic was successful, presumably by altering secretion of key pro-inflammatory cytokines — specifically suppressing IFN-γ secretion (Kato et al., 1998).

In humans, enzyme markers for various patterns of bacterial colonization within the gut were compared between 26 individuals with juvenile chronic arthritis and other healthy adults (Malin et al., 1996). It turns out that patients with arthritis have elevated levels of urease in their fecal matter. Urease is an enzyme produced largely by anaerobic bacteria. Urease enables disease-causing bacteria to survive in the gastrointestinal tract and damages the intestinal wall. Importantly, treatment with *Lactobacillus* GG corrects high urease levels (Malin et al., 1996) and returns fecal urease levels to normal. These results suggest there is a relationship between gastrointestinal bacteria and joint diseases (Malin et al., 1996). Additionally, in some patients with juvenile arthritic disease, probiotics have caused symptoms to go completely into remission (personal communication, D. Shellenberger). Certainly, further study is needed before any recommendation can be made to the millions of people that suffer from painful, debilitating arthritis.

Diabetes mellitus

Like rheumatoid arthritis, insulin-dependent diabetes mellitus is also an autoimmune disease. In this case, antibodies inappropriately attack the pancreas, the organ required for manufacturing insulin. Following pancreatic destruction, patients require daily insulin injections in order to control blood sugar.

Using a mouse strain that develops diabetes — a situation that mimics the onset of human insulin-dependent diabetes mellitus — researchers recently investigated whether or not administration of the immunomodulatory probiotic strain, *Lactobacillus casei,* would prevent these mice from developing diabetes.

Oral administration of heat-killed *Lactobacillus casei* did, indeed, reduce development of diabetes in these mice. Furthermore, unlike the mice that developed diabetes, the probiotic-treated mice gained weight normally, the probiotic-treated mice did not have evidence of pancreatic destruction, and the probiotic-treated mice exhibited different patterns of cytokine release. Specifically, probiotic-treated mice produced more IL-4, IL-5, IL-6, IL-10, and less IFN-γ (Matsuzaki et al., 1997). These results suggest that under this experimental condition, *Lactobacillus casei* prevented diabetes by regulating immune responses. The exact mechanisms by which these immunomodulatory actions prevent diabetes remain to be understood.

Serious Staph infection prevention

Staphylococcus aureus causes a variety of human infections. Staph infections range from minor skin abrasions to serious, life-threatening infections of bone and soft tissues (especially after surgery), infections of the blood, and infections of the heart and its surrounding tissues. Unfortunately, *Staphylococcus aureus* infections are becoming increasingly difficult to treat because the bacteria have acquired resistance to most antibiotics. As a result, new antistaphylococcal agents are desperately needed.

In a recent experimental study in mice, the probiotic *Lactobacillus fermentum* RC-14 and its secreted surfactant successfully inhibited infections caused by *Staphylococcus aureus* following a surgical implant. In these experiments, it appears that a surfactant secreted by the probiotic inhibited disease-causing Staph microorganisms from adhering to surgically-implanted surfaces in the body (Gan et al., 2002). It is possible that this surfactant may eventually serve as the prototype for a new class of antibiotic drugs, or that surgically implanted devices could be coated with this lactobacilli-secreted biosurfactant to prevent post-surgical infections caused by *Staphylococcus aureus.*

Future Directions

For all the disease states mentioned in this chapter, there is a small amount of evidence supporting the use of probiotics. However, more carefully controlled human studies are needed before a recommendation can be made to use a specific probiotic for any of these conditions.

There are some other wonderful new avenues of research currently ongoing with probiotics. Some investigators have genetically engineered the bacterium *Lactococcus lactis* to produce the anti-inflammatory cytokine IL-10, for its actions locally on intestinal epithelial cells (Steidler et al., 2000). Using two different mouse models of intestinal inflammation, this genetically engineered probiotic has reduced and prevented intestinal inflammation. So far, this approach has only been evaluated in experimental mice, but implications for humans are huge, especially for individuals suffering from inflammatory bowel disease! Along the same lines, it may also be possible to genetically modify probiotic bacteria to secrete digestive enzymes like lactose or lipase to aid in digestion of sugars and fats (Drouault et al., 2001).

As mentioned in a previous chapter, immunocompromised individuals may have a greater tendency to experience unwanted adverse effects when using probiotics. For this reason, some investigators have begun to evaluate the effects of inactivated — or heat killed — probiotics. Inactivated microorganisms have merits in terms of safety and a longer shelf-life. While inactivated probiotics have successfully shortened the duration of viral or bacterial diarrhea, these products are expected to stimulate the immune system less effectively than viable probiotics (Isolauri et al., 2002). However, in some diseases that involve bacterial toxins, inactivated probiotics may be even more effective than live microorganisms (el-Nezami et al., 1998). So, for immunocompromised individuals, heat-killed probiotics may be a safer choice.

On the other hand, there may be other reasons why inactivated microorganisms are not a good choice. A recent study comparing the effects of heat-inactivated and viable *Lactobacillus* GG in infants with eczema found that both live and inactivated microorganisms decreased the severity of eczema similarly. However, the heat-inactivated microorganisms caused severe gastrointestinal symptoms; so severe, in fact, that the clinical trial had to be stopped early. While it is not entirely clear why this occurred, it has been suggested that high numbers of *Bacteroides* or clostridia in the guts of these infants may have responded antagonistically to the inactivated *Lactobacillus* — and secreted toxins against it. Those children who received viable microorganisms did not experience gastrointestinal disturbances because live *Lactobacillus* GG responded and counter-acted by secreting its own bacteriocins against the antagonistic bacteria (Kirjavaninen et al., 2003). These explanations, while plausible, are purely speculative at this time. Clearly, more studies are needed in this area. It will be exciting to watch new developments unfold in the probiotic arena — an area of medicine that is truly an ancient medical practice revisited!

Notes

Notes

References

Aiba Y, Suzuki N, Kabir AM. Lactic acid-mediated suppression of *Helicobacter pylori* by the oral administration of *Lactobacillus salivarious* as a probiotic in a gnotobiotic murine model. Am J Gastroenterol. 1998;93:2097-2101.

Alvarez S, Herrero C, Bru E, et al. Effect of *Lactobacilus casei* and yogurt administration on prevention of *Pseudomonas aeruginosa* infection in young mice. J Food Prot. 2001;64:1768-1774.

Andrews PJ, Barnes P, Borody TJ. Chronic constipation reversed by restoration of bowel flora. A case and a hypothesis. Eur J Gastroenterol Hepatol. 1992;4:245-247.

Andrews PJ, Borody TJ. "Putting back the bugs": Bacterial treatment relieves chronic constipation and symptoms of irritable bowel syndrome. Med J Austral. 1993;159:633-634.

Armuzzi A, Cremonini F, Bactolozzi F, et al. The effect of oral administration of *Lactobacillus* GG on antibiotic-associated gastrointestinal side-effects during *Helicobacter pylori* eradication therapy. Aliment Pharmacol Ther. 2001a;15:163-169.

Armuzzi A, Cremonini F, Ojetti V, et al. Effect of *Lactobacilllus* GG supplementation on antibiotic-associated gastrointestinal side effects during *Helicobacter pylori* eradication therapy: A pilot study. Digestion. 2001b;63:1-7.

Aso Y, Akaza H, Kotake T, et al. Preventative effect of a *Lactobacillus casei* preparation on the recurrence of superficial bladder cancer in a double-blind trial. Eur Urol. 1995;27:104-109.

Bengmark S. Immunonutrition: Role of biosurfactants, fiber, and probiotic bacteria. Nutrition. 1998;14:585-594.

Benno Y, Mitsuolka T. Impact of *Bifidobacterium longum* on human fecal microflora. Microbiol Immunol. 1992;36:683-694.

Bodana AR, Rao DR. Antimutagenic activity of milk fermented *by Streptococcus thermophilus* and *Lactobacillus bulgaricus*. J Dairy Sci. 1990;73:3379-3384.

Borody T, Noonan S, Cole P, et al. Oral vancomycin can reverse idiopathic constipation. Gastroenterol. 1989;96:A52.

Bouchnik Y, Flourie B, Andrieux C, et al. Effects of *Bifidobacterium* sp fermented milk ingested with or without inulin on colonic bifidobacteria and enzymatic activities in healthy humans. Eur J Clin Nutr. 1996;50:269-273.

Bukowska H, Pieczul-Mroz J, Jastrzebsk K, et al. Significant decrease in fibrinogen and LDL cholesterol levels upon supplementation of the diet with *Lactobacillus plantarum* (Pro Viva) in subjects with moderately elevated cholesterol concentrations. Atherosclerosis. 1998;137:437-438.

Canducci F, Armuzzi A, Cremonini F. A lyophilized and inactivated culture of *Lactobacillus acidophilus* increases *Helicobacter pylori* eradication rates. Aliment Pharmacol Ther. 2000;14:1625-1629.

Celik AF, Tomlin J, Read NW. The effect of oral vanomycin on chronic idiopathic constipation. Aliment Pharmacol Ther. 1995;9:63-68.

Challa A, Rao DR, Chawan CB, et al. *Bifidobacterium longum* and lactulose suppress azoxymethane-induced colonic aberrant crypt foci in rats. Carcinogenesis. 1997;18:517-521.

Cremonini F, DiCaro S, Covino M, et al. Effect of different probiotic preparations on anti-*Helicobacter pylori* therapy-related side effects: A parallel group, triple blind, placebo-controlled study. Am J Gastroenterol. 2002;97:2744-2749.

De Simone C, Bianchi Salvadori B, Negri R, et al. The adjuvant effect of yogurt on production of gamma-interferon by Con A-stimulated human peripheral blood lymphocytes. Nutr Rep Int. 1986;33:419-433.

de Vrese M, Stegelmann A, Richter B, et al. Probiotics-compensation for lactase insufficiency. Am J Clin Nutr 2001;73:421S-429S.

Drouault S, Juste C, Marteau P, et al. Oral treatment with *Lactococcus lactis* expressing *Staphylococcus hyicus* lipase enhances lipid digestion in pigs with induced pancreatic insufficiency. Appl Environ Microbiol 2002;68:3166-168

Dunn SR, Simenhoff SL, Ahmed KE, et al. Effect of oral administration of freeze-dried *Lactobacillus acidophilus* on small bowel bacterial overgrowth in patients with end-stage kidney disease: Reducing uremic toxins and improving nutrition. Int Dairy J. 1998;8:545-53.

Eizaguirre I, Urkia NG, Asensio AB, et al. Probiotic supplementation reduces the risk of bacterial translocation in experimental short bowel syndrome. J Ped Surg. 2002;37:699-702.

el-Nezami H, Kankaanpaa P, Slaminen S, et al. Physiochemical alterations enhance the ability of dairy strains of lactic acid bacteria to remove aflatoxin from contaminated media. J Food Prot. 1998; 61:466-468.

Finegold SM, Molitoris D, Liu SY, et al. Gastrointestinal microflora studies in late-onset autism. Clin Infect Dis. 2002;35:S6-S16.

Fuglsang A, Rattray FP, Nilsson D, et al. Lactic acid bacteria: Inhibition of angiotensin converting enzyme *in vitro* and *in vivo*. Antonie van Leeuwenhoek. 2003;83:27-34.

Gan BS, Kim J, Reid G, et al. *Lactobacillus fermentum* RC-14 inhibits *Staphylococcus aureus* infection of surgical implants in rats. J Infect Dis. 2002;185:1369-1372.

Giaccari S, Tronci S, Falconieri M, et al. Long-term treatment with rifaximin and lactobacilli in post-diverticulitic stenoses of the colon. Riv Eur Sci Med Farmacol. 1993;15:29-34.

Goldin BR, Gualtieri LJ, Moore RP. The effect of *Lactobacillus* GG on the initiation and promotion of DMH-induced intestinal tumors in the rat. Nutr Cancer. 1996;25:197-204.

Goldin BR, Gorbach SL. Effect of *Lactobacillus acidophilus* dietary supplements on 1,2-dimethylhydrazine dihydrochloride-induced intestinal cancer in rats. J Natl Cancer Inst. 1980;64:263-265.

Goldin B, Gorbah SL. The effect of milk and *Lactobacillus* feeding on human intestinal bacterial enzyme activity. Am J Clin Nutr. 1984;39:756-761.

Goldin BR, Gorbach SL. Saxelin M, et al. Survival of *Lactobacillus* species (strain GG) in human gastrointestinal tract. Dig Dis Sci. 1992; 37:121-128.

Halpern GM, Prindiville T, Blackenburg M, et al. Treatment of irritable bowel syndrome with Lacterol fort: A randomized, double-blind, cross-over trial. Am J Gastroenterol. 1996;91:1579-1585.

Harms HK, Bertele-Harms RM, Bruer-Kleis D. Enzyme-substituted therapy with the yeast *Saccharomyces cerevisiae* in congenital sucrase-isomaltase deficiency. NEJM. 1987;316;1306-1309.

Hata Y, Yamamoto M, Ohni M, et al. A placebo-controlled study of the effect of sour milk on blood pressure in hypertensive subjects. Am J Clin Nutr. 1996;64:767-771.

Hatakka K, Savilahti E, Ponka A, et al. Effect of long term consumption of probiotic milk on infections in children attending day care centers: Double blind, randomised trial. BMJ. 2001;322:1327-1331.

Hosoda M, Hashimoto H, Morita H, et al. Studies on antimutagenic effect of milk cultured with lactic acid bacteria on the Trp-P2-induced mutagenicity to TA98 strain of *Salmonella typhimurium.* J Dairy Res. 1992;59:543-549.

Isolauri E, Joensuu J, Suomalainen H, et al. Improved immunogenicity of oral D x RRV reassortant rotavirus vaccine by *Lactobacillus casei* GG. Vaccine. 1995;13:310-312.

Isolauri E, Kirjanaiene PV, and Salminen S. Probiotics: A role in the treatment of intestinal infection and inflammation. Gut. 2002;50:iii54-iii59.

Johansson M-L, Molin G, Jeppsson B, et al. Administration of different Lactobacillus strains in fermented oatmeal soup; *in vivo* colonization of human intestinal mucosa and effect on the indigenous flora. Appl Environ Microbiol. 1993;59:15-20.

Kasper H. Protection against gastrointestinal diseases—Present facts and future developments. Int J Food Microbiol. 1998;41:127-131.

Kato I, Endo K, and Yokokura T. Effects of oral administration of *Lactobacillus casei* on antitumor responses induced by tumor resection in mice. Int J Immunopharacol. 1994;16:29-36.

Kato I, Endo-Tanaka K, and Yokokara T. Suppressive effects of the oral administration of *Lactobacillus casei* on type II collagen-induced arthritis in DBA/1 mice. Life Sciences. 1998;63:635-644.

Kato I, Kobayashi S, Yokokura T, et al. Antitumor activity of *Lactobacillus casei* in mice. Gann. 1981;72:517-523.

Kirjavainen PV, Salminen SJ, Isolauri E, et al. Probiotic bacteria in the management of atopic disease: Underscoring the importance of viability. J Ped Gastrenterol Nutr. 2003;36:223-227.

Longuercio C, Blanco DV, Coltorti M. Enterococus lactic acid bacteria strain SF68 and lactulose in hepatic encephalopathy: A controlled study. J Int Med Res. 1987;15:335-343.

Lorca GL, Wadstrom T, Valdez GF. *Lactobacillus acidophilus* autolysins inhibit *Helicobacter pylori in vitro.* Curr Microbiol 2001;42:39-44.

Malin M, Vernnonen P, Mykkanen H, et al. Increased bacterial urease activity in faeces in juvenile chronic arthritis: Evidence of altered intestinal microflora? Br J Rheumatol. 1996;35:689-694.

Mombelli B and Gismondo MR. The use of probiotics in medical practice. Int J Antimicrobial Agents. 2000;16:531-536.

Marteau PR, deVrese M, Celier J, et al. Protection from gastrointestinal diseases with the use of probiotics. Am J Clin Nutr. 2001;73:430S-436S.

Matsuzaki T, Nagata Y, Kado S, et al. Prevention of onset in an insulin-dependent diabetes mellitus model, NOD mice, by oral feeding of *Lactobacillus casei*. APMIS. 1997;105:643-649.

Matsuzaki T, Yokokura T. Inhibition of tumor metastasis of Lewis lung carcinoma in C57BL/6 mice by intrapleural administration of *Lactobacillus casei*. Cancer Immuno Immunother. 1987;25:100-104.

Matsuzaki T, Yokokura T, and Mutai M. Antitumor effect of intrapleural administration of *Lactobacillus casei* in mice. Cancer Immunol Immunother. 1988;26:209-214.

Mollenbrink M, Bruckschen E. Treatment of chronic constipation with physiologic *Escherichia coli* bacteria. Results of a clinical study of the effectiveness and tolerance of microbiological therapy with the *E. coli* Nissle 1917 strain (Mutaflor®). Med Klin. 1994;89:587-53.

Morotomi M, Mutai M. *In vitro* binding of potent mutagenic pyrolysates. J Natl Cancer Inst. 1986;77:195-201.

Mrda Z, Zivanovic, Rasic J, et al. Therapy of *Helicobacter pylori* infection by *Lactobacillus acidophilus*. Med Pregl. 1998;51:343-345.

Mukai T, Asasaka T, Sato E, et al. Inhibition of binding of *Helicobacter pylori* to the glycolipid receptors by probiotic *Lactobacillus reuteri*. FEMS Immunol Med Microbiol 2002;32:105-110.

Nase L, Hatakka K, Savilahti E, et al. Effect of long-term consumption of a probiotic bacterium, *Lactobacillus rhamnosus* GG in milk on dental caries and caries risk in children. Caries Res. 2001;35:412-420.

Niedzielin K, Kordecki H, Birkenfeld B. A controlled, double-blind, randomized study on the efficacy of *Lactobacillus plantarum* 299V in patients with irritable bowel syndrome. Eur J Gastreoenterol Hepatol. 2001;13:1143-1147.

Nobaek S, Johansson M-L, Molin G, et al. Alteration of intestinal microflora is associated with reduction in abdominal bloating and pain in patients with irritable bowel syndrome. Am J Gastroenterol. 2000;95:1231-1238.

Okawa T, Niibe H, Arai T, et al. Effect of LC9018 combined with radiation therapy on carcinoma of the uterine cervix: A phase III, multicenter, randomized, controlled study. Cancer. 1993;72:1949-1954.

Olhagen B, Mansson I. Intestinal *Clostridium perfringes* in rheumatoid arthritis and other collagen diseases. Acta Med Scand. 1968;184:395-402.

Orrhage K, Sillerstrom E, Gustafsson JA, et al. Binding of mutagenic heterocyclic amines by intestinal and lactic acid bacteria. Mutat Res. 1994;311:239-248.

O'Sullivan MA and O'Morain CA. Bacterial supplementation in the irritable bowel syndrome. A randomised double-blind placebo-controlled crossover study. Dig Liver Dis. 2000;32:294-301.

Pimentel M, Chow EJ, Lin HC. Eradication of small intestinal bacteria overgrowth reduces symptoms of irritable bowel syndrome. Am J Gastroenterol. 2000;95:3503-3506.

Pool-Zobel BL, Bertram B, Knoll M, et al. Antigenotoxic properties of lactic acid bacteria *in vivo* in the gastrointestinal tract of rats. Nutr Cancer. 1993;20:271-282.

Pool-Zobel BL, Neudecker C, Domizlaff I, et al. *Lactobacillus* and *Bifidobacterium* mediated antigenotoxicity in the colon of rats. Nutr Cancer. 1996;26:365-380.

Probiotic Therapy Research Centre. http://www.probiotictherapy.com.au/physicians/diseases_2.html

Rasic J, Klem I, Jovanovic D, et al. Antimicrobial effect of *Lactobacillus acidophilus* and *Lactobacillus delbrueckii* subsp. *bulgaricum* protiv *Helicobater pylori in vitro*. Arch Gastroenterohepatol. 1995;14:158-160.

Renner HW, Munzer R. The possible role of probiotics as dietary mutagens. Mutat Res. 1991;262:239-245.

Rolfe RD. The role of probiotic cultures in the control of gastrointestinal health. J Nutrition. 2000;130:396S-402S.

Sakamoto I, Igarashi M, Kimura K, et al. Suppressive effect of *Lactobacillus gasseri* OLL 2716 (LG21) on *Helicobacter pylori* infection in humans. Antimicrob Chemother. 2001;47:709-710.

SandlerRH, Finegold SM, Bolte ER, et al. Short-term benefit from oral vancomycin treatment of regressive-onset autism. J Child Neurol. 2000:15;429-435.

Steidler L, Hans W, Schotte L, et al. Treatment of murine colitis by *Lactococcus lactis* secreting interleukin-10. Science. 2000;289:1352-1355.

Stein J, Schroder O, Bonk M, et al. Induction of glutathione-*S*-transferase-pi by short chain fatty acids in the intestinal cell line caco-2. Eur J Clin Invest. 1996;26:84-87.

Takahashi T, Kushiro A, Nomoto K, et al. Antitumor effects of the intravesical instillation of heat killed cells of the *Lactobacillus casei* strain Shirota on the murine orthotopic bladder tumor MBT-2. J Urol. 2001;166:2506-2511.

Teitelbaum JE and Walker WA. Nutritional impact of pre-and probiotics as protective gastrointestinal organisms. Annu Rev Nutr. 2002;22:107-138.

Uejima M, Kinouchi T, Kataoka K. Role of intestinal bacteria in ileal ulcer formation in rats treated with a nonsteroidal antiinflammatory drug. Microbiol Immunol. 1996;40:553-560.

Vanderhoof JA, Young RJ, Murray N, et al. Treatment strategies for small bowel bacterial overgrowth in short bowel syndrome. J Pediatr Gastroenterol Nutr. 1998;27;155-160.

Williams AB, Yu C, Tashima K, et al. Evaluation of two self-care treatments for prevention of vaginal candidisis in women with HIV. J Assoc Nurses AIDs Care. 2001;12:51-57.

Wollowski I, Rechkemmer G, Pool-Zobel BL. Protective role of probiotics and prebiotics in colon cancer. Am J Clin Nutr. 2001;73:451S-455S.

Yamamoto N, Akino A, and Takano T. Antihypertensive effect of the peptides derived from casein by an extracellular proteinase from *Lactobacillus helveticus* CP790. J Diary Sci. 1994;77:917-922.

Zhang XB, Ohta Y. *In vivo* binding of mutagenic pyrolyzates to lactic acid bacterial cells in human gastric juice. J Dairy Sci. 1991;74:752-757.

Summary

Probiotics have been remarkably beneficial for many folks; they have saved lives of people who had no hope. As you embark on probiotic therapy keep in mind that each one of us has different normal flora (or abnormal, as the case may be). We do not all respond the same way to prescription drugs, nor will we all respond alike to the same probiotic. You may have to search for the right probiotic, the appropriate number of microorganisms, or the necessary combination of probiotics until you find the right mix to successfully fill the bacterial niche missing in your gastrointestinal tract.

Remember, too, probiotics are not created equally. Some microorganisms are more beneficial for treating one disease than another. When selecting a probiotic, be certain to choose a strain with documented efficacy in treating the condition for which you intend to use it.

Remarkably, most practicing physicians pay little or no attention to probiotics. To be fair, the word "probiotic" is not even mentioned in most medical textbooks. On the other hand, the term is well known among those in the agricultural industry. It was the dairy industry that coined the term "probiotic" in the 1950s. Farmers and veterinarians know that it is more cost-effective to keep animals well by using probiotic supplements than to treat an entire herd of animals after a disease has set in.

Hopefully, prescribing practices among physicians will soon change now that some prominent doctors are beginning to take notice of the very effective "natural" therapy that has been used safely for thousands of years. You can take a pro-active role in your health by sharing this book with your physician and asking if probiotics may be right for you.

Appendix A

Inflammatory Bowel Disease

Additional Case Scenario

A.P. was a 72 year old man who developed symptoms of bloody diarrhea rather late in life at age 67. He was diagnosed with ulcerative colitis. Although he was treated with typical prescription drugs, he never had a complete remission of symptoms. He decided to enter a study in which his intestinal flora was "wiped" out by several antibiotics and antifungals and subsequently recolonized with probiotics, including 2 strains of non-disease-causing *Escherichia coli, Lactobacillus acidophilus* strain DDS-1, *Lactobacillus bulgaricus*, and *Bifidobacterium bifidum.*

After initiating probiotics, over the next 2 months, A.P.'s symptoms recovered. Annual endoscopies and biopsies over the next 7 years showed no evidence of disease.

However, despite giving his doctor a note from his previous physicians indicating that he *could not tolerate antibiotics* because they would disrupt his gut flora, an orthopedist prescribed an antibiotic *prophylactically* during A.P.'s hospitalization for hip replacement surgery. After being discharged from the hospital, sure enough, symptoms of ulcerative colitis gradually returned over the next 3 months.

A.P. was again treated with the same regimen of probiotics and he recovered completely. As of June 2003, A.P. is a healthy and well 85 year old gentleman who continues to take *Lactobacillus acidophilus* only.

Glossary

Achlorhydria Absence of stomach acid (hydrochloric acid)

Aerobe Any organism that requires oxygen for growth

Amino acids Fundamental components of proteins

Amylase An enzyme found in saliva and pancreatic secretions that breaks down sugars

Anaerobe An organism that is able to live and grow in the absence of oxygen. An *obligate anaerobe* can grow *only* in the absence of oxygen. A *faculatative anaerobe* grows best in the presence of oxygen, but can grow without it.

Anaphylaxis An abnormally extreme allergic reaction in which swelling, constriction of the bronchioles, heart failure, and sometimes death occurs

Antibiotic A substance that destroys or inhibits the growth of microorganisms

Antibody A special type of protein made in lymph tissues in response to the presence of a particular antigen. The purpose of antibodies is to attack foreign antigens and render them harmless.

Antigen Any substance that the body regards as foreign and potentially dangerous. Most often, antigens are proteins, but any substance may become antigenic.

Apoptosis A genetically-determined, orderly, programmed cell death

Bacillus A term used to describe the rod-like shape of some bacteria

Bacteria A group of microorganisms that lack a membrane-bound nucleus and are considered more primitive than animal and plant cells. Bacteria may be characterized by their shape as either *cocci* or *bacilli*.

Bile A thick alkaline fluid, secreted by the liver and stored in the gallbladder. It is ejected periodically into the duodenum where it helps emulsify fats and stimulate peristalsis.

Bolus A soft mass of chewed food

Carbohydrate Any one of a group of compounds, including sugars and starches. They are important sources of energy. All carbohydrates are eventually broken down into the simple sugar, glucose, which takes part in energy-producing metabolic processes.

Carcinogen Any substance that can cause cancer

Cardiovascular The heart and its network of blood vessels

Chymotrypsin An enzyme secreted by the pancreas that digests proteins

Cocci A term used to describe the round or spherical shape of some bacteria

Colitis Inflammation of the colon. Usual symptoms include diarrhea, blood, mucus, and lower abdominal pain.

Colon The main part of the large intestine which consists of four main sections: ascending, transverse, descending, and sigmoid. The colon has no digestive functions but absorbs large amounts of water and electrolytes.

Colonoscopy A procedure for examining the inside of the colon using a flexible, illuminated fiberoptic instrument (colonoscope) that is introduced by the anus

Crossover In this type of clinical trial, participants receive active drug treatment for a finite period of time and then also receive placebo for another similar period of time. Typically, study participants are not aware of which treatment they are receiving at any given time. This type of clinical trial design allows study participants to serve as both the "treatment group" and the "control group". In this way, each study participant serves as his/her own control.

Cytokines Pharmacologically-active, small proteins that are secreted by one cell for the purpose of altering the function of the cell itself or an adjacent cell

Cytoskeleton A network of proteins inside cells that help maintain cell shape and provide support to cells

Differentiation The process by which unspecialized cells become specialized for specific functions. With regard to cancer development, it is the degree of similarity of tumor cells to the organ from which the tumor arose.

Diverticulitis Inflammation of the diverticula in the colon. Diverticula are sacs or pouches that form at weak points in walls of the digestive tract.

Double-blind In this type of clinical trial, neither doctors conducting the study nor patients know who is receiving the trial drug or the inactive placebo until after study completion.

Duodenum The first of the three parts of the small intestine. It extends from the stomach to the jejunum.

Dysbiosis An abnormal population of gut bacteria

Dysphagia A situation where swallowing is difficult or painful, or food is hindered from passing through the throat to the stomach.

Emulsify To disperse fine droplets of one liquid (such as fats) throughout another liquid (such as water)

Endogenous Already existing within the body

Endoscopy A procedure used to view, examine, or treat the interior of the body (via an endoscope)

Enteral Pertaining to the digestive tract

Enzyme A protein that speeds up the rate of a biological reaction, but does not participate actively in the reaction. To function, enzymes require certain conditions for optimal activity — like correct temperatures, for example. Enzymes are easily inactivated by heat or by certain chemicals.

Epithelial Cells Cells that line the hollow structures of the body (like the digestive tract). The cells rest on a basement membrane, which separates the cells from underlying connective tissues.

Erosion The process of wearing away by abrasion

Facultative A term that describes an organism that is not restricted in one way or another. A *facultative* parasite can live as either a parasite or a non-parasite, surviving without a host. A *facultative* anaerobe can live in the presence or absence of oxygen.

Fermentation The biochemical process by which substances, especially carbohydrates, are decomposed by enzymes to provide chemical energy

Gall bladder	A pear-shaped organ that lies underneath the liver and stores bile
Gene	The basic unit of genetic material found at special locations on chromosomes
Genus *pl.* **genera**	A category used to classify living things such as plants, animals, bacteria, and viruses. A genus consists of several closely related, similar species.
Gram stain	A method of staining bacterial cells, primarily for the purpose of identification. **Gram-positive** bacteria retain the initial stain and appear violet in color under a microscope. **Gram-negative** bacteria lose the initial stain, but take up a counterstain so that they appear red.
Gut-Associated Lymph Tissues	Peripheral lymph organs comprised of lymph tissues associated with Peyer's Patches, tonsils, lymph nodes, and the appendix of the gut. It is especially rich in antibody-secreting cells and is responsible for localized immunity to bacteria, viruses, and parasites. Often abbreviated **GALT**.
Homeostasis	The physiologic process by which the body maintains equilibrium, despite variations in surroundings
Ileocecal valve	The muscular valve that separates the small and large intestines
Ileostomy	A surgical operation that bypasses the colon. The ileum is brought through the abdominal wall to create an artifical opening through which intestinal contents are eliminated. A bag is worn to collect wastes.
Ileum	The lowest portion of the small intestines. It runs from the jejunum to the ileocecal valve.
Immunoglobulin (Ig)	Any one of a group of proteins that acts as an antibody
Immunology	The study of immunity and defense mechanisms of the body
Interleukin (IL)	A family of proteins that control aspects of immune responses
Interferon (IFN)	A group of proteins produced by cells exposed to the activities of bacteria or viruses

Jejunum	The middle portion of the small intestines that connects the duodenum to the ileum
Lamina propria	The layer of connective tissue that lies under the epithelial cells of the gut
Lipase	An enzyme that breaks down fats
Liver	The largest gland of the body. It synthesizes bile, regulates blood sugar, and detoxifies chemicals and unwanted substances.
Lumen	The inner, open space within a tube. For example, it is the open space inside the intestines.
Lymph	The fluid within the vessels of the lymphatic system that bathes tissues and transports water, electrolytes, and proteins from tissues back into the blood stream. It is similar to plasma but contains less protein and more white blood cells.
Lymphocyte	A variety of white blood cells present in the lymph nodes, spleen, thymus gland, gut wall and bone marrow. They are involved in immunity and are subdivided into B-lymphocytes which produce antibodies and T-lymphocytes which are responsible for cell-mediated immunity. T-lymphocytes can differentiate into helper, killer, and suppressor cells.
Lysozyme	A enzyme that catalyzes destruction of bacterial cell walls
Macrophage	A scavenger cell found in connective tissue and many body organs that removes bacteria and other foreign bodies from blood and other tissues
Microorganism	Any organism too small to be seen with the naked eye. Examples include bacteria, fungi, viruses, etc.
Motility	The action of moving spontaneously. The gastrointestinal tract constantly propels and moves food downward, through the digestive tract.
Mucosa	The mucus tissue lining the digestive tract
Mucosal barrier	Epithelial cells, antibodies, mucus, immune cells, cytokines and other chemicals that form a critical barrier between the host and potentially injurious contents of the gut lumen

Mutagen Any external agent that increases the rate of mutations

Mutation A change in genetic material (DNA) not caused by normal genetic processes

Normal Flora The mixture of microorganisms regularly found at any anatomical location

Obligate A term that refers to organisms that are restricted to one particular way of life. For example, an obligate anaerobe cannot survive in the presence of oxygen.

Open-label In this type of clinical trial, doctors and patients know who is receiving the active drug and who is getting placebo. In other words, this type of trial is not "blinded."

Oral tolerance A term that describes the situation in which mature white blood cells recognize, permit, and are rendered ineffective against antigens

Organelle A structure within a cell that is specialized for a particular function

Pancreas A gland that secretes various digestive juices, enzymes that aid in digestion, and the hormones insulin and glucagon

Pathogen A microorganism that produces disease

Peptidase A group of digestive enzymes that splits proteins in the stomach and the intestines into individual amino acids

Peyer's patches Oval masses of lymph tissues on the mucous membrane lining the small intestines

Phagocytosis The process of engulfment and digestion of bacteria and other foreign particles by a cell

Placebo A substance or medication that does not contain active ingredients. Often, a placebo is referred to as a "sugar pill". Placebos look, taste, smell, and feel just like active drugs so patients and physicians don't know which treatment is being given. New drugs or therapies are often compared to placebos. Sometimes, a beneficial response is seen when a placebo is used — simply because people have faith in its ability to heal.

Placebo-controlled A type of clinical trial design in which new drugs are compared to inactive sugar pills in order to assess true benefits of the drug that is being studied

Pouchitis An inflammatory condition of the intestines that occurs after a portion of the intestines has been surgically removed, and a pouch has been created for storage of stools

Prebiotic A nondigestible food ingredient that stimulates growth of beneficial bacteria in the digestive tract

Probiotic Live microorganisms, that when ingested, produce therapeutic or preventative health benefits

Procarcinogen A chemical substance that becomes a carcinogen after it is altered by metabolic processes

Pseudo-membranous colitis Bacterial-toxin-induced inflammation, nodules, or loose plaques lining the interior of the intestines. It is evident during colonoscopic examination. This condition is associated with severe, sometimes life-threatening diarrhea. The cause is attributed to the presence of toxin-producing *Clostridium difficile*.

Receptor A structural protein on or inside cells that binds to specific factors like drugs, hormones, or antigens

Retrospective Looking backwards in time

Ribosome A particle consisting of RNA and proteins that is involved with cellular protein synthesis

Secretion The process of releasing a substance, especially one that is not a waste product, from cells

Sepsis Tissue death caused by disease-causing bacteria or their toxins

Species The smallest unit in the classification of living things

Spore A dormant or resting state of microorganisms

Sprue disease A disease of the small intestines in which there is insufficient digestion and absorption of food. Symptoms include stunted growth, distended abdomen, and pale, foul-smelling stools.

Substrate A specific substance upon which enzymes act

Symbiotic An intimate association between two different species resulting in mutual aid and benefit

Synbiotic The combination of a prebiotic and a probiotic

Synthesis The process of combining individual pieces to make a coherent whole

Tight junctions Cell-to-cell junctions that seal adjacent epithelial cells together, preventing passage of most molecules from one side of epithelial cells to the other

Trypsin An enzyme secreted by the pancreas that digests proteins, breaking them down into smaller peptide chains

Urinary tract infection An infection within any of the ducts or channels that conduct urine from the kidneys to the outside of the body, including the ureters, bladder, and urethra

Urogenital The organs or tissues involved with excretion and reproduction, which are anatomically close together, including the bladder, kidneys, urethra, periurethra, vagina, and cervix

Vaginitis Inflammation of the vagina, often caused by an infection

Vaginosis Infection of the vagina, most often caused when there are too few lactobacilli and too many other anaerobic bacteria overgrow. There may be itching, pain, or vaginal discharge.

Vulva External female genitalia including the two pairs of fleshy folds that surround the openings of the vagina and urethra

Printed in the United States
113649LV00003B/175/P

9 781412 009256